Nutrition Therapy

by

Kathy King Helm, RD, LD
Private Practitioner, Author, Speaker, Publisher
Lake Dallas, TX

Bridget Klawitter, MS, RD, FADA
Manager, Department of Clinical Dietetics
All Saints Healthcare System, Racine, WI

Helm Seminars
Lake Dallas, TX

To my parents Iris and Lee, my daughters Savannah and Cherokee, and my husband Carter, the flowers in my garden. **KKH**

One's future is built upon those who color the rainbow around us and give meaning to all our endeavors. Without the strength and determination I have learned from my husband, Kurt, and the support and encouragement of my parents Joe and Patracia Swik, this project would have seemed overwhelming. It is with much love and gratitude I dedicate this work to them and God, for the inspirations, faith, hope and love that have made my rainbow shine through the most difficult times. **BK**

Nutrition Therapy

Cover design: Mark Wyatt
Major content editor: Gill Robertson, MS, RD
Copyediting: Paul Kamps
Interior book design and typesetting: Darcy Kamps

For information or to order books or study guide, call or write:
Helm Seminars
P.O. Box 1295
Lake Dallas, TX 75065
phone & fax 817-497-3558

ISBN 0-9631033-1-8

TABLE OF CONTENTS

TABLE OF CONTENTS

Preface

Our Professional Imperative As Nutrition Experts
Sue Rodwell Williams, PhD, MPH, RD

When I was asked to contribute my views on how we can best collectively and individually advance our profession, I happily accepted, using the above title as a starting point. During my career in nutrition, covering over four decades of experience as a clinical nutritionist, teacher, and writer, I have had the pleasure of witnessing and participating in the wonderful and dramatic growth of our profession.

In the 1940s, when I began my career, our field was little more than hospital meal service for patients and various "home economics" studies in some colleges. Both the field itself and those of us working in it had no real clinical acceptance and stature, other than in a purely auxiliary role, in the arena of patient care. But compare that picture with today. Today, nutrition is increasingly able to be a full-fledged "profession." In many places it is a recognized clinical and therapeutic specialty in its own right, most clinical nutrition practitioners have advanced degrees or specialized training, and the variety of roles that nutritionists fill continues to expand.

But what now? Two key questions immediately confront us: Collectively, where does our profession need to be in these challenging times? Individually, as nutrition experts, how must we conduct our practice?

For answers to these questions, I look to my own career experiences.

Through my years of practice as a clinical nutrition specialist—I have learned a great deal about my chosen profession. I learned about people with varied cultural backgrounds and needs from my clients and patients. I learned about team care from the group of medical specialists with whom I worked as the nutrition authority. In California, I had the good fortune to come in on the pioneer beginnings of what was to become one of the largest Health Maintenance Organizations (HMO) in the United States, with a growing group practice of medical specialists who viewed me as a peer specialist. With them I was able to build and head a clinical nutrition division, establish clinical training for dietetic interns and Public Health field work, and participate in research. But mostly I learned more about myself, my love for my work and my thirst to know more, not just through two earned graduate degrees but daily on the job. All of my experiences have taught me that with the rapid advance of scientific knowledge, the true professional never stops learning. The excitement is to always be on the "cutting edge."

My first purpose here is to encourage you, whatever your working situation, to be proactive, ahead of the trend.

Return to our title and consider the meanings of three key words:

Profession. This word comes from the Latin verb "profiteri" which means—to declare or avow publicly—A true profession is a vocation based on knowledge of a specific area of learning or science that requires advanced education and training and involves intellectual skills. As nutrition professionals, we must not only possess this high standard of knowledge and skills, but also be committed personally to the profession's ideals and values. Public professional registration and state laws of certification or license govern and protect our practice. We, through our professional organization, control our own practice and conduct.

Imperative. This word, from the Latin verb "imperare" meaning to command, conveys two meanings: (1) authority or power and (2) urgency, absolute necessity. Thus, as professional nutrition authorities, we are compelled and entitled to maintain our high standards of practice in our own right, and to carry individual responsibility for these high standards.

Expert. Two interesting Latin roots form this key word: (1) the prefix "ex," meaning from, and (2) "periri", meaning peril, danger, harm, or injury. Thus, as the nutrition expert, we use our professional knowledge, skills, and commitment to promote the health of our clients and patients and help protect them from harm or illness.

My second purpose here is to inspire you.

In my own clinical experience, three professional basic actions in some form have become imperative:

Search for all possible information and clues to help identify individual needs. Develop communication skills, especially learn to listen, not only for what is said but also for what is often unsaid. Try to see the situation through the client's personal and social lens. This is the person-centered base of our work.

Research the problems presented through every available resource. Check the person's clinical chart. Communicate with other medical team members. Use any medical and university sources at hand for current scientific and practice information about the medical problem. Here in my office, for example, my computers can access the statewide University of California library system, through my personal account, to review any journal source and receive any desired printouts. Beyond that, the worldwide databases and professional forums of the Internet are available. This is the growing knowledge base of our work.

Develop a working plan based on your initial search and research. Then constantly update the plan with client feedback, new knowledge, and ongoing medical team communications. This is the action base of our work.

Some personal experiences in my own clinical work may serve as illustrations of this type of nutritional practice:

Nutritional care plan. In my years of clinical work at the large HMO, our health plan physicians simply referred their patients to me with their clinical data records. It was my responsibility to establish the nutritional care plan, based on these data and my own interview and history, to monitor the person's progress, and to adjust the care plan as needed. For example, in our Northern California regional metabolic newborn screening program, as soon as initial testing and medical examination identified the genetic disease, the parents were immediately referred to me for ongoing nutritional care, since that constituted the basic treatment. Following our team protocol, I was then responsible for selecting and calculating the initial special formula, for immediately giving phone instructions to the parents in various areas of Northern California, for monitoring blood levels of the involved nutrient or metabolite, for recalculating formula needs according to the infant's growth rate, and for calling parents with the adjusted formula. I also made home visits and held periodic outreach nutrition clinics with our team nurse coordinator. Quarterly metabolic clinics at our central medical center, and morning clinic visits involved all members of the regional metabolic disease team: pediatrician specialists in genetics and endocrinology, clinical nutritionist, nurse coordinator, and pediatric social worker.

In my private practice, I continued this special metabolic work under a personal consultant contract. Other clients have come to me by referral or on their own. In either case, I follow the same procedure, sending a copy of my findings, nutritional care plan, and periodic progress notes to the physicians involved, who often respond with additional referrals.

Charting. Nutrition charting has also come a long way. In the beginning, the usual practice in our hospital was to place nutritionist chart entries in the section of the patient chart reserved for miscellaneous nursing comments. But that changed after one dramatic high-risk patient incident. In that case, our specialist team had carefully managed the high-risk pregnancy of one of our clients with insulin-dependent diabetes mellitus (IDDM) that she had developed in early childhood. She had suffered two prior stillbirths in the efforts she and her husband were making to have a child. In this pregnancy, she was hospitalized early to prepare for the obstetrician's carefully planned delivery. But one day, I discovered to my astonishment that the patient's blood sugar control had been dangerously compromised and mishandled. My previous nutrition charting had been ignored, staff resident physicians had given wrong routine diet orders, and my specifically ordered interval foods had not only not been served to the patient, but had actually been eaten by night staff who thought it was just leftovers to be discarded! I immediately comprehensively charted my findings, this time in the physician notes section of her medical record, outlining and documenting in full my nutritional care plan to meet her diabetes and pregnancy needs. During her remaining hospital days, all medical and nursing staff followed my nutrition care plan notes to the letter, and our patient was able for the first time to deliver a healthy baby.

After that incident, I always placed my charting notes and instructions in the same section of the chart as that used by the attending physician, and made sure that my instructions, as the clinical nutrition specialist, were known and followed.

Laboratory tests. As part of my clinical nutrition work at a large HMO health care center, I always ensured that appropriate laboratory tests were specifically written into the protocol for each nutrition-related program. In some instances I helped to write the initial protocol itself. Periodically, as part of team management, each program physician and I reviewed the protocols and added or revised appropriate tests for nutrition assessment. In private practice, this same function of ordering lab tests requires that the practitioner must be recognized as a clinical nutrition specialist by the medical community, with similar protocols written jointly by the clinical nutritionist and a physician and filed with a nearby reputable clinical laboratory.

So what is our answer to the initial question of nutrition imperatives? Where must our profession be focused? Essentially, in our changing world we must stretch our boundaries. We must continue to shed any lingering subservient attitudes and roles. We must work with physicians as nutrition specialists in our own right, viewing them as team peers, not patrons—but we must earn that right individually. It is past time that we accept full ethical, moral, and legal responsibility for our own practice as full professionals. We must collaborate with all other health professionals, physicians and nonphysicians, as team partners with common goals of patient/client care, provide expert nutritional care, and demonstrate a high level of skill and competence.

Our professional imperative flows from the inner drive and dedication of each of us. Our profession can advance in responsibility and stature and value only as far as we advance as individual nutrition experts.

Sue Rodwell Williams, Ph.D., M.P.H., R.D.

President, SRW Productions, Inc., and Clinical Nutrition Consultant, Davis California; Formerly Chief, Clinical Nutrition Division, Kaiser-Permanente Medical Center, Oakland, California and Metabolic Nutritionist, Kaiser-Permanente Northern California Regional Newborn Screening and Metabolic Porgram, and Field Faculty, M.P.H.—Dietetic Internship Program and Coordinated Undergraduate Program in Dietetics, University fo California, Berkeley, California

Introduction

As Nutrition Therapists, we make our living because what to eat and how much to eat are not simple choices for many people. Factors such as taste preferences, family and cultural habits, psychological relationships to food, disease processes, the affordability and availability of food, and a person's ability to chew, digest and absorb food affect what he or she eats.

Today's marketplace and competitive health care environment demand that our counseling skills evolve at a fast pace. The days of the "one session miracle" should be a thing of the past except when the client only needs basic nutrition survival skills or until the client can return for a more extensive consultation. Basic nutrition information and lists of foods are readily available to both the public and other health professionals. As clinical dietitians our job is not just the dissemination of information. If that's all we do, we will be easily replaced by a floppy disk, on-line service, preprinted food list, or health educator. We must advance our clinical practice through becoming highly qualified and effective nutrition therapists in counseling. We must seriously consider creating clinical NutritionD doctoral programs whose graduates can diagnose nutritional deficiencies and toxicities, and interpret biochemical and genetic nutrition assessments of the human body.

We must help produce successful outcomes in a larger proportion of our client populations, and we must market our successes! No one else will do this for us; it is our responsibility.

Origin of this Book

When co-author Bridget Klawitter and I acted as content experts for The American Dietetic Association's "Counseling" self-assessment module, developed by Pennsylvania State University, we were awed by the enormity of the project. What counseling theories? What counseling skills? What body of knowledge or book would most practitioners agree is the state-of-the-art in nutrition counseling? What questions could we ask that would "stretch" but not fail the majority of practitioners? Our committee had to write four "typical" counseling scenarios with subtle counseling "mistakes" interspersed in conversation with over 400 rationales on why each answer was best or incorrect. It took two and a half years, extensive input from Penn State's staff and consultants, review by over 100 registered dietitians, and untold hours to produce the final product.

This book is an outgrowth of the above process. While we worked on the module, I telephoned across the country talking to and interviewing dietitians on what they were doing with their patients or clients. I also conducted surveys at state dietetic meetings and at other group meetings of dietitians on how often they saw patients, on their counseling skills, and on perceived barriers to success. I wanted to know what a "typical" interview entailed. Many shared their counseling resources, their strategies, and their client protocols.

I found highly successful practitioners in acute care settings as well as outpatient clinics, and of course, private practice. Most had evolved to more comprehensive skills by observing what worked in their practice or through training in advanced degrees in counseling. Some had been practicing that way for over 20 years. Many of these people are now authors of chapters, case studies, or side bars in this book.

My questionnaire and informal surveys found that too many dietitians spent too little time actually working with clients to help them achieve the necessary benefits. For example, the majority of hospital-based practitioners usually only saw their patients once and often for less than 30 minutes. They reported they seldom referred patients to an outpatient department unless the hospital had an on-going diabetes group or in-house cardiac rehabilitation program. They also rarely referred patients to a private practice or managed care dietitian for follow-up at home.

Nutrition Therapy

Thirty-six highly qualified practitioners share their practical skills and years of knowledge in the pages of this book. We do not presume to have all of the answers, we struggle at times like everyone else but we have learned through trial and error what works most of the time with our client populations. Contributing authors give many examples of counseling strategies and business skills they learned from their own efforts, and from books, published research, and other professionals.

This book is meant to challenge readers to try new "helping" and counseling skills, as well as give role models for nutrition "therapy." What do you talk about after you review the food record and patient's weight? How often should you see a patient? How do you help a patient sliding into relapse? How can you attract patients back for revisits? When should a patient be referred for psychotherapy? How do you work with other counselors for the benefit of the client?

Since obesity is the number one malnutrition problem in the U.S., we have added many examples of the different approaches used to manage this problem. As you will see, not all of them agree in approach or philosophy, but there are many common threads. This book also includes many examples from the prevention, chronic care, and outpatient settings since we believe that the market is moving in those directions. For that reason and the fact that in outpatient settings a nutritionist usually will see far more overweight women as clients, a chapter has been included on women and weight issues.

It is hoped that as you read the pages, they will validate what you presently do while stretching you to conquer new or traditional areas of practice with renewed excitement.

This book is intended to help readers reduce the time spent developing the necessary skills to become an effective nutrition therapist in any setting. However, each counselor must generate his or her own philosophy and style in the nutrition therapy process.

It is understood that even with the best of knowledge and skills, some work situations are not easily changed to the ideal. Our contributing authors started in similar situations, but they did what was necessary to make their counseling more conducive to "positive patient outcomes." That also will be your strongest argument as you negotiate for better counseling space, more time to conduct counseling sessions, and sufficient, well-trained staff. Positive patient outcomes should be the motivating factor for your professional efforts in counseling.

Kathy King Helm, Publisher

Kathy King Helm, RD

To order "Counseling" self-assessment module: call ADA Sales 1-800-877-1600

We want to thank all of the people, especially the contributing authors, who helped bring this project to fruition and provided input into its content and philosophies.

Part I
The People Involved

1
The Nutrition Therapist
Kathy King Helm, RD, LD

After reading this chapter, the reader will be able to:
- ☐ identify the helping skills and their role in nutrition therapy
- ☐ define transference and list two examples in the nutrition counseling setting
- ☐ list five ethical guidelines for the counseling of clients on nutrition
- ☐ identify three core conditions for building counseling relationships
- ☐ identify the basic themes underlying five common counseling theories

---

THE EVOLUTION OF COUNSELING IN DIETETICS

Nutrition counseling skills began evolving for the profession as a whole more than 20 years ago when the growth of the wellness philosophy empowered people to take responsibility for their own health and to seek nutrition care outside the acute care hospital setting. These clients had to make the effort to walk into the outpatient or private practice dietitian's office and pay for the visit themselves with little hope of being reimbursed by insurance or government funding.

The clients' high expectations for change and their willingness to return and pay for revisits quickly changed the expectations of the providers of care–the consulting dietitians. This was a new revelation. However, it soon became apparent to nutrition counselors that what they had been trained to do in counseling only took one or two visits to cover at most. What appeared to work in the hospital setting only scratched the surface in outpatient counseling.

To help improve their skills, these budding nutrition therapists started reading about counseling in other fields, attending conferences, and joining individual and group therapy sessions for their own personal growth or problems. They hired psychologists and exercise specialists to speak at their group weight loss programs. They also listened to their clients. As is often the case, these early therapists were taught how to address clients' needs and work with them personally based on simple comments like, "You know what you said that really worked for me?" or "You are trying to push me too fast; I'm not ready for that yet."

Trial and error taught clients and therapists what worked and what didn't work for that client. Soon the therapist started seeing commonalties between certain types of problems and therapies that were tried by many clients. This body of experience helped the therapist become more effective in working with each new challenging person who walked through the door for help. The client played a very active role in the entire process. Therapists and clients found that often psychological needs exerted more influence on food habits than logic. (1) It also became clear that the interaction, mutual respect, and genuine caring shared between the client and the counselor were as therapeutic as the printed diet information.

Research Supports Evolution

In the 1970's the first significant body of research and published books on the "helping" skills (new, more successful strategies for counseling), emerged. (2,3,4,5,6) They were in response to conclusions from the 1960's that later became disputed, that traditional psychotherapy and counseling skills only produced favorable outcomes in a small percentage of clients. Researchers concluded that "helping" is simply a learning or relearning process leading to change or gain in the behavior of the helpee. (2)

Leaders in the helping skills concept also supported the philosophy that many professionals (police, teachers, dietitians, nurses, and so on) in the course of their normal jobs are in the position to psychologically interact with people and enter into caring relationships with them for the benefit of that person. To facilitate the helping process, communication and interactive skills were identified so the process was not left to random whims that might do more harm than good. In fact, active, caring listening skills form the basis for "helping." Often just talking about a problem to another person will help someone find solutions to their problems. This new philosophy supported the nutrition therapist as he or she stretched formerly accepted practice boundaries.

BALLARD STREET
By Jerry Van Amerongen

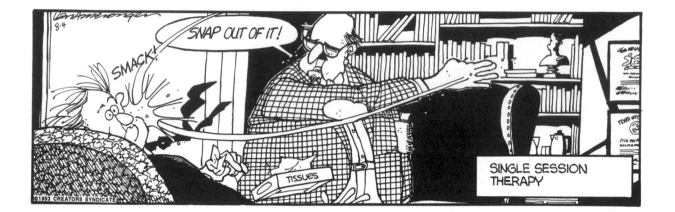

Used with permission Jerry Van Amerongen and Creators Syndicate.

In the 1980's nutrition research and literature broadened the generally accepted scope of nutrition counseling practice even more to include a strong emphasis on behavior modification. (7,8,9,10) However after a time, it was agreed that dietitians should not only ask about someone's eating behaviors and other lifestyle habits, but they should also encourage their clients to come to new awareness about their food habits. This included when they were growing up, their recent normal and not so normal eating habits, their inability to handle stress and interpersonal relationships without misusing food, and a myriad of other food-related issues. Dietitians began helping clients find coping strategies, new behaviors, and new ways of thinking. This then caught up to the level of counseling practiced by many of dietetics' pioneers.

Advancing beyond the understanding of nutrition science to understanding human nature brings new growth and stature to dietetic practice. In fact Curry reports, "Some health professionals call dietitians semi-professional technicians when we carry out orders and provide only advice (education) instead of confronting emotional connections with food and function as a counselor." (1)

Dietetics in the 1990's is now in a transition where many of these new helping and psychotherapy skills are being integrated into all counseling settings. Coupled with this, health care is changing at an alarming pace and more patient education is being transferred to outpatient clinics, private practices, Health Maintenance Organizations (HMOs), physicians' offices, long-term care settings and patients' homes. Disordered eating, a new term covering a variety of weight related eating habits, is growing in interest and concern among nutrition professionals.

> **Definition: Disordered Eating is characterized by eating without regard to internal hunger and satiety cues or physical needs and may involve counter-compensatory behaviors to manipulate weight. Restrained eating, repeated dieting, diet-induced obesity, compulsive eating, bulimia nervosa and anorexia are included in this category.**
>
> *Karin Kratina, MS, RD 1995*

Holding Nutrition Counselors to the Light

According to Donna Israel, licensed counselor and registered dietitian with a Ph.D. in nutrition, "There is another developmental stage that our dietetic profession needs to embrace along with more training in counseling—professional supervision of our skills. Just like any other counseling profession, we need to 'hold ourselves up to the light.' In other words, we must begin to feel comfortable with having other mental health professionals or nutrition therapists with more skill and practical experience than ourselves, look over our shoulders and evaluate how we work with our clients."

Not only do our skills need to be evaluated, but also our "baggage"—the biases, "blind spots" and underdeveloped emotional growth of our own (called *countertransference* issues). *Transference* refers to feelings and thoughts the client has toward the counselor. (11) Sometimes without realizing it, either the client or the counselor sabotages the effectiveness of the counseling efforts. For example, either one may have negative ideas about the other brought on by how he or she is dressed, or the client may whine too much and upset the counselor's unwritten code of acceptable behavior thus changing how the client is treated. As a counselor, you have the responsibility to identify and control your countertransference issues and try to keep them out of your clients' therapy sessions. You can also help clients identify and work through their issues, so that together you can establish better rapport and facilitate collaboration. Your supervision could be carried out by a mental health professional, i.e., psychiatrist, psychologist, psychiatric social worker, or licensed counselor or a dietitian skilled in the psychotherapeutic model. (See FYI on page16.)

NUTRITION THERAPY

Experience has shown us that handing out lists of foods and meticulously calculated diets will not guarantee compliance or motivate clients to change their behaviors. It is not that simple. At best it will produce "first order change," which means removal of the symptoms. (14) People are intertwined with their food and eating habits. Human nature, a person's will, and mental health can play major roles in the change process. The goal is to produce "second order change," which means to address and change the causes of the problem. (14) (See side bar on the responsibilities of the nutrition therapist.)

Clients are often "stuck" in ways of thinking and acting around food. A counselor can help them "explore" new ways of thinking, which in turn can help them try new actions, respond to stimuli differently, choose foods based on new criteria, handle stress without turning to food, and take more responsibility for their lifestyle choices.

Curry states, "Nutrition counseling involves a process, a sequence of events, and the elements of the interpersonal relationship between the counselor and client. The most important aspect of counseling is the interpersonal relationship between the counselor and client. It is also the most difficult to understand and master." (1)

The traditional medical model is fast, short-term intervention primarily of a content-oriented educational nature with minimal relationship development or input by the client, little or no follow-up, and everyone with the same diagnosis gets the same plan of action. We know what's best for them and it's their problem or lack of motivation if they don't follow it! *This approach works when the client makes the effort to read, learn and apply the content. (1)* Dietitians can't take much of the credit except for teaching the content. Advanced counseling skills and the psychodynamic model of therapy empower the dietitian to become an active facilitator in the therapy process enabling a larger percentage of clients to successfully make and sustain lifestyle choices that will improve their health, and possibly, longevity and quality of life. (See Table 1-1 comparing nutrition education to a psychotherapeutic style of counseling.)

Advanced counseling skills include:

- relationship building skills: empathy, warmth and genuineness
- helping skills: attending, helping a client explore, active listening responses
- ability to gain collaboration and empower the client
- sensitivity to multicultural and other client-specific uniqueness
- ability to sustain a long-term counseling relationship
- ability to assess and teach developmental skills

Table 1-1   Comparison of Nutrition Education and Psychotherapeutic Counseling

Nutrition Education	*Psychotherapeutic Counseling*
1. Short-term	Open-ended
2. Content-based	Process (continuous series of interdependent events)
3. Goal-oriented	Relationship-oriented
4. Improve knowledge & skills	Resolution of issues & barriers that inhibit a person from making healthy choices
5. Work on behaviors	Work on thoughts, feelings, behaviors
6. Address cognitive deficits	Addresses motivation, denial, resistance
7. Success measured objectively (e.g. knowledge, behavior change, or health parameters)	Success measured subjectively (e.g., happiness, mood shift, movement, relationships)

Adapted from © 1993, Johanna H. Roth, RD, LD, CHES, CAS, Bethesda, MD. Used with permission.

Responsibilities of the Nutrition Therapist

1. Assessment, diagnosis and supportive feedback
    a. level of malnutrition (ICD-9 codes or human condition nutrition codes—see Chapter 9)
    b. dietary adequacy
    c. caloric requirement (including growth and exercise)
    d. physical and psychological symptoms of starvation
    e. healthy weight range/ set-point range
    f. perceptions of hunger and satiety
    g. belief system and cognitive distortions (food, body image, physiology, etc.)
    h. family interactions
2. Education about recovery endpoint, for example, metabolism, food acceptance, weight, menstruation, gastrointestinal function, reduction of hunger and obsessive thinking, normal exercise, and resumption of social eating
3. Non-coercive guidance in making incremental changes in weight and behaviors, as the need for the behaviors diminishes
4. Acknowledgment of and compassionate support for anxiety over anticipating and making behavioral changes
5. Assistance with learning the difference between thoughts and feelings, identifying feelings, and understanding the connection between feelings and behaviors.
6. Communication with physician and interpretation of medical information for the psychotherapy treatment team.

Used with permission. Copyright 1993, Johanna H. Roth, RD, LD, CHES, CAS, Bethesda, MD. Adapted from: Reiff D, Reiff KL. *Eating Disorders: Nutrition in the Recovery Process.* Gaithersburg, MD: Aspen Pub, Inc.; 1992. (11)

All of these skills can be taught to counselors. However, a therapist's own personality and ability to work with clients determines his or her effectiveness as a counselor more than years of dietetic experience.

The client has the right and responsibility to make choices about his or her own health care. The nutrition therapist's role is to *facilitate* the process by which patients or clients more clearly identify where they are, where they want to be, what they need to learn to get there, help identify the pros and cons of the various options, and step-by-step guidance on how to get to where they want to be.

To accomplish the "facilitator" role, the therapist must become a trainer (one who facilitates growth and change in the patient or client through guidance and practice) instead of a teacher who only discusses content (diet lists, exchange system, etc.).

See how to become a National Certified Counselor and Licensed Psychotherapist in Appendix 1-A and Appendix 1-B.

Ethics and Responsibility

The core of ethical responsibility is to *do nothing that will harm the client or society. (6)* As the counselor, you carry the responsibility to be professional, knowledgeable, and skilled. The client is more vulnerable and is coming to you for help and assistance. Following are some ethical guidelines: (6,8,11)

1. *Maintain confidentiality.* The client trusts that what he or she tells you will be held in confidence. You have the responsibility to not disclose information shared by the client or about the client's therapy without the client's permission. If you are a student, you do not have legal confidentiality, and your clients should be made aware of this. (6)
2. *Recognize your limitations.* It is important that you talk to your clients about the process you want to use to help them improve their nutritional intake and give them the option of stopping at any time. Know your limitations, as described in this book, in the areas of counseling and exercise recommendations. Nutrition therapy deals with what a person eats or doesn't eat, weight and body image issues, the availability of adequate wholesome, safe food and the behaviors, thoughts, and feelings that affect a client's decisions in these areas. With training it can include other health related lifestyle choices, such as adding physical activity, stress management, and smoking cessation. It is about helping others, not examining and delving into their lives. (6)
3. *Seek consultation.* Counseling is very private. As mentioned earlier, hold yourself to the light in order to grow personally and improve your skills. Review ethical standards frequently.
4. *Treat the client as you would like to be treated.* Every person deserves to be treated with respect, dignity, kindness, and honesty. (6)
5. *Be aware of individual and cultural differences.* One diet does not fit all just because the diagnosis is the same!

The Goals of Counseling

Many sources identify what they believe are the goals of nutrition counseling or therapy. These goals help the client or patient to: (15,16)

*   increase self-awareness and decrease denial that problems exist, which effect the person's nutrition or weight, and that these problems can be resolved.
*   become aware of inner strengths so the person can function independently and challenge old beliefs about how to eat or change weight.
*   increase feeling responsible for his or her own feelings, thoughts, behaviors, and relationships instead of staying in the "victim" role.
*   learn to take risks like being more flexible and tolerating more incongruities.
*   learn to trust more and give new behaviors and thoughts a chance before discounting them.
*   become more conscious of alternative choices when responding to stress and other stimuli, or choosing foods based on new criteria.

- "have a functional lifestyle where his values (what he believes to be true) and his behaviors (what he does) are consistent; there is a good level of self-acceptance. He is doing what he believes he should be doing, and feels good about it," states Beckley. (16) (See Table 1-2)

Table 1-2 Functional vs. Dysfunctional Lifestyles (16)

Functional: (Self-acceptance)	*Dysfunctional: (Denial, low self-esteem, depression, anger)*
Values are consistent with behavior	Values conflict with behaviors
Values are semi-flexible	Values are rigid
Behaviors are moderate	Behaviors are extreme

Used with permission. Copyright 1992, Lisa Beckley, RD and Nutrition Dimensions, in *Diet, Addiction and Recovery* (2nd ed.) 1993.

Core Conditions and Skills for Building Relationships

In the context of therapy, client growth is associated with high levels of three core or facilitative, relationship conditions: empathy (accurate understanding), respect or warmth (positive regard), and genuineness (congruence). (6,17,18) When these conditions exist in a counseling relationship positive change often takes place irrespective of the philosophical orientation of the counselor. Successful clients in behavior therapy, psychotherapy and most others rate their personal interaction with the therapist as the single most important part of treatment. (6) If these conditions are absent, clients may not only fail to grow, they may deteriorate. (2,19) In recent years, researchers like Carkhuff, Egan, Gazda and Ivey have developed concrete, teachable skills that have made it possible for people to learn how to communicate these core conditions to clients. (2,5,19,4,20)

Empathy means the counselor truly tries to understand what the patient feels from their frame of reference, and responds accurately to that person's concerns and problems. For example, if a client says, "I have really tried to eat differently when I'm at school, but by the time I get home I'm too starved and I overeat," an empathetic response would be something like, "You feel if you cut calories at noon time at school you don't have control that afternoon." In contrast, if you say something like, "You ought to try harder," you are responding from your frame of reference, not the client's.

Empathy serves the following purposes: it builds rapport, elicits information by showing understanding, and fosters client self-exploration through conveying that the environment is safe and confidential. You can convey empathy to clients through certain verbal and nonverbal messages.

Verbally, you can show a desire to comprehend by asking for clarification about the client's experiences and feelings. You can discuss what is important to the client and respond with statements that show you understand the client's concerns. Refer to the client's feelings or add on to implicit client messages. (6,17) For example, you might say, "Food seems to mean love and anger to you. Love because it reminds you of the special foods your grandmother baked for you, and anger because at times when you binge, you are angry at the food and your attraction to it. Is that right?"

Attentive nonverbal behavior also conveys empathy. Such things as direct eye contact (but not staring), a forward-leaning body position (at times), facing the client, and an open-arm position all show interest in the other person. (6,17,8) See Table 1-3 on nonverbal cues of warmth and coldness.

Genuineness means being yourself without being phony or playing a role. The counselor is honest and straightforward with the client. You act human and collaborate with the client, which reduces the emotional distance between you and the client. There are at least five components of genuineness: (6,17)

- nonverbal behaviors (mentioned in Table 1-3),
- honest interest in helping people (not just a role to play for the moment),
- congruence (your words, actions, and feelings match and are consistent), for example, if you become uncomfortable about something that is being said or how the client handles a situation in a violent manner, you tactfully address it instead of feigning comfort,
- spontaneity
- openness and self-disclosure (the ability to be open, to share yourself, and to disclose certain information about yourself when its appropriate). See side bar on self-disclosure.

Respect or warmth or positive regard means the ability to prize or value the client as a person with worth and dignity. (21) The four components of positive regard are: (6)

- commitment (you are interested in working with the client and show up on time, reserve private quiet time for the appointment),

Table 1-3 Nonverbal Cues of Warmth and Coldness (U.S. Anglo)

Nonverbal cue	Warmth	Coldness
Tone of voice	Soft, soothing	Callous, reserved, abrupt
Facial expression	Smiling, interested	Poker-faced, frowning, disinterested
Posture	Relaxed, leaning toward the other person	Tense, leaning away from the other person
Eye contact	Looking into the other person's eyes (intermittently)	Avoiding eye contact
Touching	Touching the other softly and discreetly	Avoiding all touching
Gestures	Open, welcoming	Closed, guarded
Physical proximity	Close (arm's length)	Distant

Adapted from *Reaching Out: Interpersonal Effectiveness and Self-Actualization* (3rd ed.), by D.W. Johnson. Copyright 1986 by Printice-Hall. Reprinted with permission.

- understanding (you act interested by using techniques mentioned earlier, and by using specific listening responses such as paraphrasing and reflecting client messages), (see Chapter 7).
- nonjudgmental attitude (you suspend judgment of the client's motives and actions to avoid condemning or condoning the client's thoughts, feelings, or actions. You are able to remain objective and not become involved in the client's personal affairs. If a female client discloses that she hates her husband when he makes derogatory comments about her weight, you might answer something like, "You feel hurt when your husband isn't sensitive about your weight.")
- warmth (most clients, even hostile ones, usually respond with warmth if you offer it first. Without verbal and nonverbal warmth many helping strategies are therapeutically impotent.) (22)

COUNSELING THEORIES

It is estimated there are over 40 different therapy models or theories with seven or so being the most commonly used: (6,8,17)

Psychodynamic theory is primarily associated with its founder, Sigmund Freud. This long-term therapy works by getting to the unconscious roots of present behavior. Today, derivatives of this theory such as attachment theory (how securely an infant or child was attached to his or her mother), object relations theory (our relationships with key people in our lives), and ego psychology (helping people balance between their id—unconscious rebellion--and their superego--conscious rules–giving the person more power to control his or her own life), have the most immediate impact on practice. Free association of words or ideas (say whatever comes to mind), regression (clients return to past traumatic experiences) and dream analysis are commonly used strategies. (23) A major drawback to this type of therapy is that the client is not typically oriented to transfer learning from the interview to daily life and present day problems. That may happen as a result of therapy but it often takes extended periods of time to make breakthroughs.

Existential-humanistic best known through Carl Rogers' and Viktor Frankl's work (also includes Gestalt). Frankl holds that the critical issue for humankind is not what happens, but how one views or thinks about what happens (cognitive change), but he also believes in taking action. From his concentration camp experience during World War II, he learned to help people who are faced with problems that cannot be solved, like rape or AIDS, and to find love and meaning in their lives.

Rogers is the listening or attending therapist. He is the founder of person-centered therapy that focuses on each person's worth and dignity, and accepts that the person's perceptions are reality. The emphasis is on the ability to direct one's own life and move toward self-actualization, growth and health. (24)

Gestalt—was developed by Frederick (Fritz) Perls. Counselors want to operate in the "here and now" instead of retelling stories from the past. The client may be asked to close his or her eyes and describe a typical incident that needs work. The client may retell a recent conversation and then be asked to create a more suitable ending to the problem. The client may be asked to rehearse messages to an empty chair so that it will be easier to say them to others. The goal is for clients to take responsibility for change. (25)

Cognitive-behavioral (includes psychoeducational and rational-emotive therapy)—with the evolution of cognitive (what a person thinks) along with behavioral (what a person does) therapy, therapy became "brief" in comparison to the long-term commitment of psychoanalysis. Once problem behaviors or irrational beliefs are identified, strategies for change can be made more quickly. It helps clients define their problems and promote cognitive, emotional and behavioral changes, and prevent relapse. (See Chapter 8)

Psychoeducational therapy—"implies a process of learning about oneself, self understanding (one's physical and mental impulses, instincts, and/or patterns of behavior), and gaining new knowledge (i.e. the number of grams of fat in a teaspoon of butter), and learning to regulate one's behavior in accordance with some standard" (definition by Kiy, MS, RD see Chapter 8 for more detail). Guerney, Stollak, and Guerney (26) developed this technique as a method, not focused on "curing," but rather, on "managing" physical and mental impulses appropriately. Nutrition therapists help clients integrate individualized nutrition knowledge through cognitive and behavioral change.

Rational-Emotive Therapy (RET), developed by Albert Ellis, believes irrational ideas and negative self-talk are a major cause of emotion-related difficulties. Emotion must be present along with logic and rational thought in order for change to likely occur. In other words, you may know that your serum cholesterol is too high and that you prefer foods high in fat but unless you feel emotion (fear, frustration, etc.), change may never occur. (27)

Multicultural therapy (MCT) recognizes that traditional theories of helping, developed in a predominantly white male Northern European and North American context, have gender and cultural limitations when working with clients from other cultures, women, and minorities in the US, and they give little consideration to family issues. MCT draws upon the above therapies but tries to respect multiple perspectives and give culturally appropriate treatment. (17)

Feminist Therapy— is eclectic, endorsing theoretical positions which encourage empowerment and self-growth, but also recognizing woman's more interdependent way of living and relating to others. (See Chapter 4)

Family counseling recognizes that the family of origin is where the client's culture manifests most clearly. For clients with problems related to their relationship or function in the family, working within the family context helps clients have fewer relapses and quicker improvement than when treated individually. (17) This type of therapy has proven to be the only consistently successful mode of therapy in adolescent obesity.

Today, psychoeducational, multi-cultural and family counseling counseling are growing in popularity as more therapists become aware of and trained in these methods. Empowerment and self-growth are being integrated in many other therapy styles.

NUTRITION COUNSELING APPROACHES

As you can see by the overlap in theories, and from your experience with clients and their problems, no one therapy or model holds all the answers for each client. The counselor's personal and professional judgment is crucial to the outcome of the therapy. (1) For more consistent success in counseling, Gilliland et.al. (28) suggest a flexible, client-centered problem-solving approach that merges the best ideas from the most popular models (see Chapters 2, 7 and 8). The assumptions of this eclectic approach to counseling include: (28)

- no two clients or client situations are alike;
- each client and counselor is in a constant state of change and flux—no person or situation in counseling is or can ever be static;
- the effective counselor exhibits a flexible repertoire of activity on a continuum from directive (telling the client what to do) to nondirective;
- the client is the world's greatest expert on his or her problems;
- the counselor uses all the available personal and professional resources in the helping situation, but is fully human in the relationship and cannot ultimately be responsible for the client;
- counselors and the counseling process are fallible and cannot expect to observe overt or immediate success in every counseling or client situation;
- competent counselors are aware of their own personal professional qualifications and deficits and take responsibility for ensuring that the counseling process is handled ethically and in the best interest of the client and public;
- client safety takes precedence over need fulfillment of the counselor;
- probably there is no one best approach or strategy in dealing with each problem;

Self-disclosure

Self-disclosure is any information you share about yourself with the client. The information may be general in nature like the fact that you also have children or what college you went to, or it can be personal in nature and either positive or negative. For example, a positive self-disclosure is "I used to eat whether I was hungry or not, so I can relate to what you are saying. Now I eat according to my appetite and you can too." Negative self-disclosure provides information about personal limitations, unsuccessful or inappropriate behaviors and situations, and experiences dissimilar to the client's. (6) An example of negative self-disclosure is "I, too, have a hard time telling people 'no' and taking time for myself."

Self-disclosure can increase the client's level of disclosure, close the distance between you and the client, and bring about changes in the client's perception of their behavior. On the negative side, too much can take too much time away from working with the client's needs, it may appear the counselor is lacking in discretion, or needing therapy as much as the client. (6)

The best rule of thumb until you have more experience in this area is to make your self-disclosure at the same depth and intensity as the information shared with you by your client. (6,17) Clients who are white professionals in America usually are very open about sharing intimate facts, but other cultures take more time to get to know someone. Self-disclosure too early in the counseling relationship will be a problem with more private individuals.

- many problems in the human dilemma appear insolvable, but there is always a variety of alternatives, and some alternatives are better for the client than others;
- generally, effective counseling is a process that is done *with* the client rather than *to* or *for* the client;
- for most people requiring changes that are basic to their lifestyle, three months is probably a minimum and six months should not be considered too long a time for counseling. Weight control can often take years to accomplish, and it is time that the need for long-term attention to this problem is recognized. (1)
- when the client and therapist believe it is time to stop therapy, the client should identify his or her "red flags" that will signal a need to return to therapy, and the door should be left open for future informal contact by either party.

The Helping Model

One of the first and best known researchers in the helping-type therapy movement was Robert R. Carkhuff. Many have adopted his model to explain the process. There are four phases in Carkhuff's Helping Model that identify the interpersonal stages of a counseling relationship: (29)

Pre-Helping Attending: The counselor "attends" to the needs of the client or patient by giving undivided attention, listening, observing, and physically showing interest through positive body language. This helps the client become interested and involved in the process.

Responding: The client's apparent interest triggers the counselor to respond with empathy, respect, and sometimes concreteness (specificity as opposed to vagueness) in focusing the client's attention on experiences. As the client becomes comfortable, the counselor can help him or her *explore* their experiences and develop insight. Exploring is a pre-condition of understanding, giving both counselor and client an opportunity to get to know where the client is in the world. Exploration is a self-diagnostic process for the client. Exploration is an art under the control of the counselor and in part under the control of the client. High-level functioning clients explore themselves independent of the level of interpersonal skills offered by the counselor while moderate to low-level functioning clients are dependent upon the counselor's skills for their level of exploration.

Personalizing: These skills involve filtering the client's experiences through the counselor's experiences, which serves to facilitate client understanding. Clients go from *exploring* where they are in relation to their experience to *understanding* where they are in relation to where they want or need to be. The basic foundation for understanding rests with insights, which reveal the client's own deficits and role in the situation. This may increase the probability that related behaviors will occur. Unfortunately, action does not always follow insight.

Initiating: This phase involves developing a course of action to resolve the client's problems. It emphasizes the action-oriented counseling dimensions of honest assessments, self-disclosure (the counselor sharing personal revelations), specific problem solving and program development and, under some conditions, confrontation of discrepancies in client's behaviors.

It must be said here that not all client or patient situations call for extensive interaction and problem solving, especially when the person is motivated and is already somewhat knowledgeable about the content. When the person is not ready or willing to hear the content or to become more involved, that is his or her right, and does not reflect poorly on the therapist if concerted effort is made to give the person or the family as much information and support as desired.

Using Psychology

Nutrition therapy should contribute to a client's good mental health, not sacrifice it. Psychiatrist Scott Peck, author of *The Road Less Travelled,* writes, "Mental health is an ongoing process of dedication to reality at all costs. Giving up is the most painful of human experiences. . .giving up personality traits, well-established patterns of behavior, ideologies, and even whole lifestyles." (30) Think how often in the past we nutritionists asked clients to change all of those factors at once!

Peck goes on to explain that it is easier to work with patients who have neurotic tendencies (they take too much responsibility for what happens) than patients with character disorders (they take no responsibility for what happens and blame it on someone or something else). (30) That is one explanation why some clients are so much more difficult to work with than others.

In their article on "Incorporating Psychological Principles into Nutrition Counseling," Stuart and Simko clearly outline how psychology can be used in nutrition counseling: (31)

> It is very important to encourage self-help and self-responsibility, thereby putting the client or patient in control. Having a sense of control is an essential component of self-esteem. Clients will exhibit less self-destructive behavior and think about themselves as responsible and able to care for themselves (and follow dietary guidelines better).

The nutrition counselor briefly helps the client define problems, accepts the client's feelings, gives permission for normal responses, expects the client to handle the problems, and suggests specific follow-up assignments and tasks. By giving permission and information that normalizes the client's reactions, providing specific suggestions, and making a contract to continue to work on the problem, the counselor is creating highly therapeutic conditions. Providing supportive psychotherapy in this manner can only benefit a client.

BOUNDARIES BETWEEN NUTRITION TREATMENT AND PSYCHOTHERAPY

Saloff-Coste, Hamburg and Herzog give examples of practice boundaries in their article, "Nutrition and psychotherapy: Collaborative treatment of patients with eating disorders." (32)

In general, the dietitian's territory properly includes almost any issue related to food, weight, eating patterns, and body image. So, for example, if a patient with anorexia nervosa who has achieved a safe, stable weight laments that she will never be happy because she is not tall and beautiful like her sister, it is well within the nutritionist's domain to challenge the patient's underlying notion that happiness depends on physical appearance. The nutritionist may also remind the patient that she possesses other qualities that impart value to her life.

It may also be appropriate for the dietitian to challenge a patient's view of herself and the world when it specifically perpetuates inappropriate eating patterns. In this instance, the nutritionist's nonnutrition interventions serve to provide necessary room for discussions concerning improved eating behavior.

When to Make Referrals to Other Mental Health Professionals

Referral to other mental health professionals is indicated when the patient or client discloses information such as suicidal tendencies, physical abuse, severe marital difficulties, feelings of depression, past unresolved sexual abuse, recurring self-destructive behaviors, eating disorders, and other severe problems that are beyond the scope of nutrition practice.

The patient or client may or may not choose to see a mental health professional. If they go to see another therapist, you may continue to see them concurrently or you may wait until the other issues are resolved. If they choose *not* to seek other help, your options are to continue seeing the person for his or her nutrition-related problems that you can work with (in hopes that you will be able to influence the person to seek help at some future date), or to explain that you must terminate your nutrition therapy until the larger issues are handled (and risk alienating the patient). If the situation is very severe and urgent (like for threatened suicide), you may have to be more forceful and seek help for patients or clients *with their permission* as they sit in your office. Either call their physician or therapist or refer the patient to an emergency psychiatric service. (32) See side bar on how to work with a psychotherapist or treatment team.

THE COUNSELOR OR THERAPIST

The terms nutrition counselor and therapist are used interchangeably in this book just as they are by members in the counseling field. The term *therapist* is also consistent with other allied health professionals, such as physical therapist and occupational therapist.

The nutrition counselor or therapist takes on a large responsibility when he or she decides to help other people with their problems and needs. The directive managerial skills that make a dietitian good at running and managing a food service are not usually the skills that make a dietitian good at counseling patients. Collaboration and patience are necessary to be a counselor. Also, some people like working with other people and their problems while others find it depressing and tedious. Not every dietitian that likes nutrition education will be good at or interested in patient counseling. Our profession and institutions need to do a better job of identifying and training dietitians who show interest and skill in counseling.

Whether we intend it or not, patients and clients look to therapists as role models. It is therefore important that the nutrition counselor be mature and emotionally stable, and obviously, eat healthy. Each therapist should look at his or her own abilities to appropriately cope with stress, to successfully handle interpersonal relationships, and to relate with others to see if areas need improving.

Many counselors have found invaluable assistance with personal problems, which may impact their ability to counsel others by seeking help from a psychiatric social worker, psychologist, or psychiatrist.

HERMAN

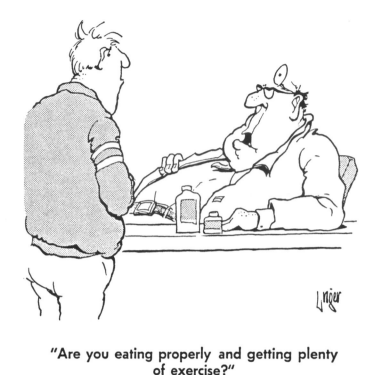

**"Are you eating properly and getting plenty
of exercise?"**

This author went to see a psychiatric social worker 15 years ago upon referral of a social worker colleague. I found my personal and professional lives were too intertwined. The skills that made me a good counselor—empathy, caring, and personal strength—also made me attract people in my personal and professional life who needed to be taken care of (a problem I have been told is common among caretaking-type people). Also, because of my childhood experiences, which were nothing out of the ordinary, I had a need to be loved and needed. All of this is pretty common human nature. My patient load confirmed that I was needed, but I was being drained emotionally. I allowed many people to make demands of me and I tried to be understanding when they did not pull through on what they had committed to do. My problem was that I had never learned how to set boundaries in this area of my life. I soon realized that no one benefited from my present way of thinking.

In just a couple of counseling sessions, I became aware of the problem, I tested new behaviors that I still use today, and I had new counseling strategies to use in helping my patients with similar problems. From that time on, I was an advocate of having someone in turmoil seek the therapy of a good, empathetic counselor.

Just as it is not necessary to have been a pregnant female to be a good obstetrician, it is not necessary to have been overweight or anorexic to be a good counselor for people with those problems. However, it is imperative that each counselor become familiar with his or her patient populations, their common needs and nutrition-related problems, their usual food supplies, and customs. It is the counselor's responsibility to adapt educational materials and nutrition counseling to the patient, not the patient's responsibility to interpret what the counselor probably meant.

A good counselor uses power appropriately and does not dominate patients or clients, is able to give and receive love, is willing to admit mistakes, uses humor, and is not afraid to seek counsel and supervision from other qualified professionals.

Reiff and Reiff summarized what qualities people with eating disorders want in a nutrition therapist; the list is adapted for nutrition problems in general: (11)

- patient, caring and nonjudgmental
- flexible, not perfectionistic
- makes sensitive comments
- does not have unrealistic expectations

- will work at a pace the client can handle
- experienced with the problems the clients face
- understands fears about food and weight
- optimistic and hopeful
- works in a collaborative manner

The next time you go to a lecture on a topic of interest to you, think about how many details you remember the next day, or the next week. Compare that to how much more you have retained from a session where the other person talks about you, and you not only freely interact but also summarize the key points and identify what you will work on for the next visit. That is what a good counseling session can do for a client.

The need for nutrition counseling skills in dietetic practice is being widely recognized. Two different groups have formed recently in The American Dietetic Association to promote and support practitioners with the desire for increased expertise in counseling. They are the Nutrition Therapists subgroup of the Nutrition Entrepreneurs Dietetic Practice Group and the Disordered Eating Networking Group within the Sports and Cardiovascular Nutritionists (SCAN) Practice Group. Their purposes are to lead, support, and train practitioners to be high-level therapists. You can find out more information or join the DPG groups by calling ADA at 1-800-877-1600.

Learning New Counseling Skills

Danish suggests from his experience teaching dietitians new counseling skills that the best way to learn skills is in a situation like a two-day seminar or a course where skills can be taught, modeled, practiced, evaluated, and refined. Afterward, the practitioners must use them upon returning to work and incorporate them into daily counseling sessions. He gives four steps that must occur to learn a new counseling skill: (33)

1. Name and describe the skill
2. Understand the rationale for the skill
3. Demonstrate the skill—what it should be and what it should not be
4. Practice extensively under supervision

To further improve your counseling style, read books on assertiveness, boundaries, and getting in touch with feelings. Take a psychology class that is beyond the basics to learn about personality disorders, cognitive-behavioral interventions, family systems theory, and different counseling styles. Attend conferences that can expand your skills. Conferences on disordered eating usually explore counseling and psychological issues extensively. (12)

Five Significant Barriers to Becoming an Effective Counselor

Dietitians have identified their biggest barriers to becoming effective counselors in questionnaires passed out at dietetic meetings. (34) Those barriers have included:

- patients don't keep initial appointments
- patients don't return for follow-up appointments
- physician conveys to patient that "diet probably won't help"
- patients not motivated
- patients do not receive insurance reimbursement

Each one of these barriers will be discussed in detail in the pages of this book through case studies and chapters.

Although these barriers seem universal to counseling, many therapists' counseling strategies and business skills are so effective *they do not have these problems.* For example, Philomena Koulbanis, RD, was in private practice in Mystic, CT for seven years before she retired, and in those years, she reports only having four "no-shows" for appointments. In a busy clinic it's not unusual to have that many people who do not show for appointments before noon some days.

Just Starting to Counsel?

Kim Reiff, psychologist, gives very good suggestions on what to do if you are just starting to counsel: (15)

- understand that it's normal to have anxiety—confidence builds with experience;

Establishing a relationship with a psychotherapist or treatment team

Karin Kratina, MA, RD

Continuing collaboration with therapists and/or becoming part of a treatment team will increase your effectiveness with clients. Legal and ethical standards require a signed release from your patient in order to communicate with others about his or her case in a private practice setting.

To begin a collaboration, make contact with the patient's therapist to schedule an appointment in person or on the telephone. Discuss philosophy of treatment, length of time expected to work with clients, expectations of treatment, and assessment tools used such as body fat analysis and computer diet analysis. Determine the therapist's expectations of nutrition counseling: A one time visit and meal plan? On-going nutrition counseling? Exploration of feelings behind the food and weight related behavior by the dietitian? (12)

Establish boundaries with the therapist. Determine mutual responsibilities of treatment. Who will weigh the client? What happens when the client asks the therapist a nutrition related question? When working as a treatment team there is potential for "splitting," a situation in which the client pits one member of the team against another. Effective communication helps avert this. If a client tells you that she doesn't like the therapist or she feels the therapist is not listening well, encourage the client to bring up her feelings at the next visit with her therapist. Don't take sides. Listen but let the client take action. Let a problem between the therapist and client remain a problem between just the two of them. It is ethical, however, to encourage the client to seek help from another therapist if he or she is unhappy.

While you are seeing a client who also sees a therapist on issues that may relate to nutrition, maintain contact with the therapist, in person or by phone, with brief progress notes, or by leaving a message on the therapist's voice mail (make sure it is a confidential line). If you are seeing several of a therapist's clients, you may want to set up a standing lunch meeting. (12)

- no one expects you to be perfect;
- set limits on your time and accessibility, and maintain a good quality of life for yourself;
- one therapist may not cultivate a patient's whole healing process—the person may need to see several different therapists;
- it is a mistake to think that advice (telling the person what to do) is counseling;
- results may come slowly—don't get frustrated;
- accept that you won't succeed with every patient;
- it is painful for every therapist when patients don't return.

CONCLUSION

For the dietetic profession and for practitioners looking for new career avenues, nutrition counseling or therapy is potentially an enormous area of growth. With the current emphasis on prevention, health promotion, genetic testing for disease markers, and nutritional assessment of the whole human body, nutrition counseling will only grow in importance to the health care system and to the public.

With organized, supervised training and experience, we can elevate the clinical counseling practice of dietetics and bring more practitioners to the therapist level. It is not too soon for practitioners to think about supporting the move to create a Clinical Nutrition Doctorate with a clinical residency and strong counseling component or a certification as a Nutrition Therapist.

LEARNING ACTIVITIES

1. With a colleague, discuss your personal limits and boundaries in regards to nutrition therapy, using the sample questions/ issues listed in FYI on page 16.
2. In a nutrition counseling session in which you function as an observer, identify at least six nonverbal and verbal cues that convey empathy.
3. Demonstrate the effective use of nonverbal behavior in a role-play nutrition counseling session.
4. Identify attitudes or behaviors about yourself that may facilitate or interfere with establishing a successful counseling relationship (hold yourself "to the light").
5. Which would you choose as the most effective method of teaching counseling skills to students?
   a. Abbreviated classroom lecture with observation of working practitioners
   b. All classroom study with modeling by video and instructor, practice in the classroom, and evaluation
   Read the answer to this question in How Students Learn Counseling Skills Best in FYI on pages 16-17.

REFERENCES

1. Curry KR. *Dietetic Practitioner Skills: Education, Counseling, Business Management*. New York: Macmillan; 1987.
2. Carkhuff RR. *Helping and Human Relations*. Vol. 1. New York: Holt, Rinehart & Winston; 1969a.
3. Danish S, Hauer A. *Helping Skills: A Basic Training Program*. New York: Behavioral Publications; 1973a.
4. Egan G. *The Skilled Helper*. Monterey, CA: Brooks/Cole; 1975.
5. Ivey A, Authier J. *Microcounseling*. (2nd ed.). Springfield, IL: Charles C. Thomas; 1971, 1978.
6. Cormier WH, Cormier LS. *Interviewing Strategies for Helpers*, (3rd ed.) Pacific Grove, CA: Brooks/Cole; 1979, 1985, 1991.
7. D'Augelli A, D'Augelli J, Danish S. *Helping Others*. Pacific Grove, CA: Brooks-Cole; 1981.
8. Snetselaar L. *Nutrition Counseling Skills: Assessment, Treatment, and Evaluation*, (2nd ed.) Gaithersburg, MD: Aspen Pub; 1989.
9. Pace PW, Russell ML, Probstfield JL, Insull W. *Intervention specialist: New role for dietitians' counseling skills*. J Am Diet Assoc. 1984; 84: 1357.
10. Brammer LM. *The Helping Relationship: Process and Skills*. Englewood Cliffs, NJ: Prentice-Hall; 1985.
11. Reiff D, Reiff K. *Eating Disorders: Nutrition Therapy in the Recovery Process*. Gaithersburg, MD: Aspen Pub.; 1992.
12. Kratina K, Albers M, Meyer R. *Treatment of Eating Disorders*. Chapter in The Florida Dietetic Association Diet Manual: Manual of Clinical Dietetics. Tallahassee, FL: FDA; 1995.
13. King N, Kratina K. *Student Fact Sheet Series: The Disordered Eating Fact Sheet*. Chicago, IL: Amer. Dietetic Assn.; Sports, Cardiovascular and Wellness Nutritionists, In Press.
14. Carl Greenberg, MS, Behavior Science Faculty, Family Medicine, University of Washington, Seattle, Phone interview January 1995.
15. Reiff K, Reiff D. *Advanced Counseling* Workshop, Pre-Amer.Dietetic Assn., Orlando, FL, October 17, 1994.
16. Beckley L. *Diet, Addition and Recovery*, (2nd ed.) San Marcos, CA: Nutrition Dimension; 1993.
17. Ivey AE, Ivey MB, Simek-Morgan L. *Counseling and Psychotherapy: A Multicultural Perspective*. (3rd ed.) Boston: Allyn and Bacon; 1993.
18. Truax CB, Carkhuff RR. *Toward Effective Counseling and Psychotherapy*. Chicago, IL: Aldine; 1967.
19. Carkhuff, RR. *Helping and Human Relations*. Vol. 2. New York: Holt, Rinehart and Winston; 1969b.
20. Gazda GM, Asbury FS, Balzer FJ, Childers WC, Walters RP. *Human Relations Development*. (2nd ed.). Boston: Allyn & Bacon; 1977.
21. Ivey AE, Ivey MB, Simek-Downing L. *Counseling and Psychotherapy: Integrating Skills, Theory and Practice*, (2nd ed.). Englewood Cliffs, NJ: Prentice-Hall; 1987.
22. Goldstein AP. Relationship-Enhancement Methods. In Kanfer FH, Goldstein AP (Eds.), *Helping People Change* (3rd ed.). New York: Pergamon Press; 1986.

23. Freud S. *A General Introduction to Psychoanalysis*. New York: Washington Square Press; 1952. (original work published in 1900.)

24. Rogers C. *Client-centered Therapy*. Boston: Houghton-Mifflin; 1951.

25. Perls FS. *The Gestalt Approach and Eyewitness to Therapy*. Palo Alto, CA: Science and Behavior Books; 1973.

26. Guerney B, Stollak L, Guerney L. The practicing psychologist as educator: An alternative to the medical practitioner model. *Professional Psychologist*. 1971; 2: 276-282.

27. Ellis A. *Reason and Emotion in Psychotherapy*. New York: Lyle Stuart; 1962.

28. Gilliland BE, James RK, Roberts GR, Bowman JT. *Theories and Strategies in Counseling and Psychotherapy*. Englewood Cliffs, NJ: Prentice-Hall; 1984.

29. Carkhuff R. *The Art of Helping VII*, (7th ed.). Amherst, MA: Human Resource Development Press; 1993.

30. Peck MS. *The Road Less Travelled*. Great Britain: Hutchinson & Co; 1983.

31. Stuart M, Simko M. A technique for incorporating psychological principles into the nutrition counseling of clients. *Topics in Clinical Nutrition*. 1991; vol. 6: 4; 32-39.

32. Saloff-Coste C, Hamburg P, Herzog D. Nutritionnn and psychotherapy: Collaborative treatment of patients with eating disorders. *Bulletin of the Menninger Clinic*. Fall 1993; 57: 4: 504-516.

33. Danish S. Advanced Counseling Skills. Presentations at American Dietetic Assn. Convention, Orlando, FL, October, 1994.

34. Unpublished surveys of *Counseling Habits and Barriers* taken at various state and regional dietetic meetings in 1993-94 by Kathy King Helm, RD.

FOR YOUR INFORMATION

Developing a Psychotherapeutic Style of Counseling

Karin Kratina, MA, RD

To develop the psychotherapeutic style of counseling, dietitians need to receive some form of supervision to discuss specific cases. This provides feedback around treatment interventions, and an opportunity to discuss limits and boundaries. It will help you understand and deal with the denial, manipulative behavior, power struggles, transference, countertransference and other issues that may arise. In long-term work with clients, dietitians are more likely to come across negative emotions. The client may also be overly compliant or defensive. Dealing with these emotions effectively has not been part of our training. Rather than dealing with these feelings, we try to change them, avoid them, or re-direct them.

Examples of issues that can be explored around personal limits and boundaries are:

- How do you decide if a client is too difficult or complex to work with?
- What kind of contracts, if any, do you set with your clients?
- What are consequences for broken contracts? How do you enforce them?
- How do you identify the limits of your competency?
- How comfortable are you saying no?
- How aware are you of your own comfort level with personal limits and boundaries?
- How much of yourself do you share in session?
- What are your personal limits regarding physical contact, extra sessions, contact with client's family members, fees, grounds for termination, etc.?

Supervision can be accomplished one-on-one or in groups. One-on-one supervision allows more time to explore individual cases, and more opportunity to explore personal issues. Group supervision can be when several dietitians meet together to discuss cases, facilitated by a skilled therapist occasionally or on an on-going basis. Another format that dietitians may find helpful is to meet with their therapists at work. The dietitian can explore their own cases, as well as observe and learn from therapists discussing cases. The fee a therapist or dietitian will charge for supervision is usually similar to the fee they charge clients.

Many dietitians feel it is invaluable to experience the counselor/client relationship first hand. Locate a respected therapist; and commit to a specific time period of therapy; assess your own relationship with food, weight, exercise, body image, and size acceptance. Discover what techniques, approaches, and counseling styles you prefer.

FOR YOUR INFORMATION

How Students Learn Counseling Skills Best

Nancy Cotugna, D.r. Ph., RD and Connie Vickery, PhD, RD,
Department of Nutrition and Dietetics, University of Delaware

Classroom Practice Versus Modeling Practitioners

Nutrition counseling is an integral part of a clinical dietitian's responsibility. The techniques of interviewing and counseling are both knowledge and performance requirements of dietetic education programs. (1) The typical training for dietetic counseling skills includes modeling where students observe practitioners in action and imitate their behaviors. *This is an acceptable method of training if the student is observing a role model with adequate counseling skills*. However, observations of practicing dietitians counseling surrogate patients (2,3) and of those in actual clinical practice (4,5) have underscored the poor instructional quality used by many of these health professionals. This may, in part, explain poor dietary compliance rates among patients.

Counseling skill techniques have improved dramatically in the last years. However, research has suggested that practicing dietitians need supplemental training to learn the new skills and improve the quality of their patient education. (5) Many dietitians do not routinely use the techniques known to help patients learn and use information better. With this in mind, we designed a project to evaluate the effectiveness of a counseling course versus role-modeling with practicing dietitians. We compared the counseling skills of students who had only classroom lecture and simulation experiences with those in a coordinated program who had little classroom training but actual practice of skills learned primarily through modeling practitioners in healthcare settings.

Methods of Comparison

To briefly review the methods, a one-semester counseling course was presented in lecture format with the integration of a number of video-based nutrition counseling programs and tapes (see references 6,7,8,9) and demonstration by a skilled instructor. Mock counseling sessions were conducted and evaluated. At the end of the course, sessions were videotaped.

In the other group, coordinated students were presented basic lecture information on counseling during a one-week orientation program with limited role-play. From there, they were placed in supervised practice experiences with the opportunity to observe dietitians counseling patients and to practice these skills.

Results

The data collected were evaluated using a counseling skills rating checklist adapted from Pichert. (10) A more complete description of the project is detailed elsewhere. (11) Results showed that students who completed the nutrition counseling course that included technique modeling and skills identification presented via videotapes or live demonstration by a skilled instructor, practice and evaluation, performed significantly better than coordinated students in all counseling skills evaluated. This included areas of establishing relationships with clients, needs assessment, communication techniques, and behavior change strategies.

Students in both groups demonstrated respect for their clients which is in agreement with research noting that dietitians do have effective interpersonal skills. (4,5) However, our study detected significant differences in the use of behavior change strategies between the groups. Students who had taken the course demonstrated effective use of contracting, cue elimination, reflective listening, relanguaging, and visualization. The students who modeled their behavior on practitioner observations were more likely to develop instructional plans with little input from their clients. Students who completed the course were more likely to encourage client participation and assess commitment to change, while coordinated students typically queried, "Do you think you will be able to do this?" or "Do you have any questions?", failing to recognize or acknowledge signs of doubt or concern expressed by the client.

Problem With Today's System

Do we have a case of "the blind leading the blind?" Many dietitians completed their academic and professional experience before counseling skills received the attention they do in current curricula. (4,13) Thus, the professionals serving as counseling preceptors may not have been adequately prepared themselves. It cannot be assumed that because they are employed, they have up-to-date counseling skills. We agree with others who recommend that a course in nutrition counseling is a necessary addition to dietetics curriculum and should be recommended for practicing dietitians along with supervision. (14,15) Many universities are starting to offer courses on helping skills and effective patient education.

Components of an Effective Course

In our nutrition counseling course, we find it most effective to combine lecture and discussion with modeling, role-playing, and evaluation. As part of the introduction to basic components of a nutrition assessment, the instructor models the skill of conducting a dietary history as the counselor with a willing student serving as the client. Roles are then reversed. As students become comfortable, they are invited to assume these roles with the remainder of the class evaluating their performance by reinforcing positive attributes and identifying negative practices.

Videotapes of counseling sessions are useful in helping the class analyze the needs of the client and identify potential obstacles to making necessary lifestyle changes. In class scenarios, the "counselor" must interview the "client"; using appropriate strategies. Then the "counselor" identifys whether the problem is related to a knowledge or skill deficit, lack of social support, competing activities, treatment costs, or stress.

Communication techniques are demonstrated throughout the course. Such behavioral strategies as relanguaging, reflective listening, reinforcement, and self-esteem building are practiced. Students learn to conduct a cost-benefit ratio and to develop a contract. Negotiation strategies, also an essential component of the nutrition counseling course, are illustrated using videotaped counseling sessions with appropriate and inappropriate scenarios. Throughout the course we stress there is not one correct way to counsel per se. Repeated videotaping allows students to see themselves as others see them and to become comfortable with evaluation. Near the end of the course, each student is videotaped conducting a session from start to finish. *The student's grade is based on a self-evaluation of the counseling scenario rather than on the actual performance.*

Resources for Advanced Training

Three-day course on Effective Patient Teaching through Diabetes Research and Training Center, Vanderbilt University. Call (615) 936-1149 for more information.

Check with the meetings department and NE or SCAN groups of American Dietetic Association, state and local dietetic association conventions, your local universities, and programming produced by experienced nutrition therapists, eating disorder and weight control experts.

REFERENCES

1. *Accreditation/Approval Manual for Dietetic Education Programs.* (2nd ed.). Chicago, IL: The American Dietetic Association; 1991.
2. Danish SJ, Ginsberg MR, Terrell A, Hammond MI, Adams SO. The anatomy of a dietetic counseling interview. *J Am Diet Assoc.* 1979; 75: 626-630.
3. Snetselaar LG, Schrott HG, Albanese M, IasielloVailas L, Smith K, Anthony SL. Model workshop on nutrition counseling for dietitians. *J Am Diet Assoc.*18 1981; 79: 678-682.
4. Roach RR, Pichert JW, Stetson BA, Lorenz RA, Boswell EJ, Schlundt DG. Improving dietitians' teaching skills. *J Am Diet Assoc.* 1992; 92:1466-1473.
5. *Stetson* BA, Pichert JW, Roach RR, Lorenz RA, Boswell EJ, Schlundt DG. Registered dietitians' teaching and adherence promotion skills during routine patient education. Patient Educ Couns. 1992; 19: 273-280.
6. *Nutrition Counselor: Strategies for Results* (videotape). Philadelphia, PA: ARA Services, Inc., 1991.
7. *Nutrition Counseling* (videotape). Boston, MA: Joslin Diabetes Center, Inc., 1982.
8. Dow RMc. Simulations teach management and nutrition counseling skills. J Am Diet Assoc. 1981; 79:453-455. 9. *Gaining Collaboration in Nutrition Counseling* (videotape). Flushing, MI: DGH Productions, 1992.
10. Pichert JW. Teaching strategies for effective nutrition instruction. In: Powers MA, ed. *Handbook of Diabetes Nutritional Management.* Rockville, MD: Aspen Pub.; 1987.
11. Vickery CE, Cotugna N, Hodges PAM. Comparing counseling skills of dietetic students: A model for skill enhancement. *J Am Diet Assoc.* (in press)
12. Danish SJ, Lang D, Smiciklas-Wright H, Laquatra I. Nutrition counseling skills: Continuing education for the dietitian. *Top Clin Nutr.* 1986; 1: 25-32.
13. Lorenz RA, Pichert JW, Boswell EJ, Jamison RN, Schlundt DG. Training health professions students to be effective patient teachers. *Med Teach.* 1987; 4: 403-408.
14. Isselmann MC, Deubner LS, Hartman M. A nutrition counseling workshop: Integrating counseling psychology into nutrition practice. *J Am Diet Assoc.* 1993; 93: 324-326.
15. Lewis NM, Hay AL, Fox HM. Evaluation of a workshop model for teaching counseling skills to nutrition students. *J Am Diet Assoc.* 1987; 87: 1554-1557.

APPENDIX 1-A

The National Certified Counselor (NCC) Credential

Alison Murray Kiy, Ed.M., NCC, RD, Counselor, Deaconess Hospital, Boston, MA
and Adjunct Instructor, Behavioral Sciences, Quincy College, Quincy, MA

The National Board for Certified Counselors (NBCC), a nonprofit organization formed in 1982 and accredited in 1985, functions with three purposes. The NBCC monitors national certification procedures, and represents and maintains a current register of counselors to both the public and professionals. NBCC administers the National Counselor Exam (NCE) which is used by licensing boards in approximately thirty states.

National Certified Counselor (NCC) certification may be achieved by successfully completing graduate-level course work, a counseling practicum, the NCE, and 2,000 hours of postgraduate counseling, supervised experience. Prior to sitting for the exam, one must complete a minimum of 32 hours of graduate-level course work in eight of ten subject areas, two of which are required.

The counseling practicum, a component of required course work must be completed during the graduate degree program. Students gain up to 500 hours of practical counseling experience in a variety of settings. All counseling is performed under the supervision of a licensed professional from a related mental health discipline.

The National Counselor Exam is a two hundred item, multiple choice test offered in the spring and fall of each year. The exam assesses one's *knowledge* of counseling theory and practice, and covers the course work areas described above. Thus, the test assesses the degree to which a counselor possesses information, which should be known by all counselors, regardless of specialty. Many state level licensing boards use the NCE as a regulatory requirement.

The final component of the NCC package is completing an approved and supervised counseling work experience. The minimum required hours is 2,000. The supervisor, as described above, notifies the board in writing that the counseling experience was completed. This requirement must be met no later that two years after completing the NCE.

After certification is obtained, it is maintained by completing 100 hours of continuing education every five years. The NBCC publishes a list of approved providers of continuing education. Continuing education records are maintained by each counselor, and are subject to auditing every five years. The cost of certification is currently $25 annually. The NCC certification is useful in that it provides the dietitian an opportunity to perform advanced level counseling. The NCC is also a basic requirement for licensure as a counselor in approximately 30 states. Licensure may require additional education and training in one of four specialty areas including National Certified Career Counselor (NCCC), National Certified Guidance Counselor (NCGC), National Certified School Counselor (NCSC), and/or Certified Clinical Mental Health Counselor (CCMHC).

For more information contact:
National Board for Certified Counselors
3-D Terrace Way
Greensboro, NC 27403
(910) 547-0607

Appendix 1-B

How to Become a Licensed Psychotherapist

Lisa Dorfman, MS, RD, LMHC, Athlete, Lecturer, Media Spokesperson, and Licensed Mental Health Counselor/Licensed Nutritionist, Food Fitness International, Inc.

Although practicing "Nutrition Therapy" appears a great deal more glamorous than "doing a diet consult," it takes several years of education and training to be qualified to be a Licensed Mental Health Counselor (LMHC) and provide psychotherapy. I became interested in this area of expertise in 1983, when I graduated from Florida International University with a B.S. in Dietetics and Nutrition and a minor in Psychology. Since I loved to work with people diagnosed with eating disorders and mental health issues, I began to pursue the licensure requirements for mental health counseling. I chose these credentials because it was broad enough to allow me to work with many populations.

Being a Licensed Mental Health Counselor means incorporating the use of scientific and behavioral science theories, methods and techniques for the purpose of describing, preventing and treating undesired behavior and enhancing mental health and human development. Mental Health Counseling includes but is not limited to counseling, psychotherapy, behavior modification, hypnotherapy, sex therapy, consultation, client advocacy, crisis intervention and/or providing needed information and education to clients. The counseling can be given to groups, families, individuals, couples, organizations and/or communities.

Although the terminology for the title may vary between states, the license requirements are similar. In the state of Florida, "Psychotherapist" can also be used in place of Licensed Mental Health Counselor, Clinical Social Worker or Marriage and Family Therapist. Check with your state Mental Health Licensing organization for requirements in your state.

The preparation for the licensing credential, L.M.H.C., includes a Master's Degree from a fully accredited university; 32 hours of graduate course work in counseling theories and practice, human development theories, personality theory, psychopathology, human sexuality, group theories and practice, ethics and individual evaluation and assessment; 3 years clinical experience in mental health counseling, (2 years at the postmasters level under the supervision of a LMHC or the equivalent) and a passing grade on the state examination. After the completion of these requirements and a successful examination grade, a LMHC must take a 3 hour state approved HIV course, and maintain 30 CEU hours every 2 years.

In addition to being a member of the national and local Mental Health Counselors Association, I belong to the American Psychological Association and North American Association of Master's in Psychology. I've been a Licensed Mental Health Counselor for 5 years now and I am very satisfied with my credentials because it allows me to practice both diet and mental health counseling, charge higher fees for my expanded expertise, secure third party reimbursement for mental health issues which affect eating and maintain a practice which never has a dull moment.

2

Counseling and Learning: Child, Adolescent, Adult, Elderly and Family

Bridget Klawitter, MS, RD, FADA

After reading this chapter, the reader will be able to:
☐ identify basic differences in principles of learning for children versus adults
☐ list at least six developmental skills that should be considered when counseling adolescents
☐ identify the role of family in the nutrition counseling process
☐ apply learning principles in various counseling environments across the lifespan
☐ identify four evaluation methods and their application in nutrition counseling

Our challenge as nutrition therapists is to adapt our counseling style, language, and nutrition information to different individuals of various ages. Children learn differently from adolescents, who learn differently from adults at different ages. If we, as nutrition therapists, understand how people learn, we may be better able to predict when and how learning is facilitated and arrange for its occurrence. The initial formal education of children is referred to as pedagogy, and androgogy is defined as the art and science of helping adults learn. (1)

CONSIDERATIONS SPECIFIC TO CHILDREN
Children learn a new skill or body of knowledge when they are physically and mentally mature enough to do so. That is why it can be frustrating for a parent to watch while a small child learns to run without falling or to catch a ball. Throughout childhood, academic learning is traditionally organized around certain fundamental subjects (i.e., math, reading, writing). The child accumulates facts and has a subject-centered focus on learning, quite different than the problem-focused learning of the adult.

Children in different development age groups and different cultures perceive the world in different ways.(2) The major task to be accomplished is full mastery of whatever a child is doing, whether it's making a mud pie or memorizing a song on the piano. The child can experience mastery through personal accomplishments and interaction with peers. They also need love, guidance and emotional support to develop a sense of worth and of understanding him or herself.

Parents and Family
Parents and family should serve many functions in the life of a child: as sources of unconditional love and acceptance, morale boosters, and role models. They should teach and mold the child with such important lessons as delayed gratification, discipline, problem-solving techniques, and traditional values. They should provide a safe environment with adequate food, shelter, and clothing.

Unfortunately, these positive things do not always happen. Although children are not always aware that their home environments are less than ideal, they often carry "baggage" from those formative years for the rest of their lives. Specific to food and lifestyle choices, the child may learn by example to console himself with food when he is sad or frustrated; he may learn to "pig out" on the holidays and at other family gatherings; he may crave or avoid certain foods which remind him of home. Many children are greatly influenced by how they see their parents reacting to life's problems and stresses. Others see, recognize, and vow never to repeat inappropriate behavior they see in their parents.

Family counselors today report an increase in the number of children growing up without good role models and adequate, balanced guidance due to the increase in single parent households, or overly tired, or guilty, working parents. In these circumstances the parent(s) abdicates the parent role to become a peer to the child providing little or no guidance or rules. On the other end of the spectrum are the inflexible families (that have been around for a long time) with rigid rules and roles that often produce children who are not ready for responsibility and/or decision making. (3)

The Foundation of Good Mental Health

As Peck states in his book, *The Road Less Travelled*, (4)

"Life is a series of problems. Do we want to moan about them or solve them? Discipline is the basic set of tools we require (beginning in childhood) to solve life's problems. What makes life difficult is that the process of confronting and solving problems is a painful one. Problems, depending upon their nature, evoke in us frustration or grief or sadness or loneliness or guilt or regret or anger or fear or anxiety or anguish or despair. Yet it is in this whole process of meeting and solving problems that life has its meaning. Problems call forth our courage and our wisdom; indeed they create our courage and our wisdom. It is only because of problems that we grow mentally and spiritually.

Fearing the pain involved, almost all of us, to a greater or lesser degree, attempt to avoid problems. We procrastinate, hoping that they will go away. We ignore them, forget them, pretend they do not exist. We attempt to get out of them rather than suffer through them. This tendency to avoid problems and the emotional suffering inherent in them is the primary basis of all human mental illness. Since most of us have this tendency to a greater or lesser degree, most of us are mentally ill to a greater or lesser degree, lacking complete mental health. Some of us will go to quite extraordinary lengths to avoid our problems and the suffering they cause, proceeding far afield from all that is clearly good and sensible in order to try to find an easy way out, building the most elaborate fantasies in which to live, sometimes to the total exclusion of reality."

The use of defense mechanisms like denial (deny the reality) or distortion (reject or change the perceived reality) often occurs when a person has difficulty dealing with the reality of an experience. Often these responses are at an unconscious level and they help the person feel better by avoiding reality. Dietitians may see these kinds of responses in people with new diagnoses of diabetes, cancer, or eating disorders. Other commonly seen defense mechanisms are fixation and regression where the person stays at the present stage of development or returns to an earlier stage, respectively, that seemed safer. Some young women will choose to be very thin and young looking, or very overweight in order to avoid facing growing up and being sexually attractive. Rationalization is where the person makes excuses instead of facing reality. For example, a male client may blame his increased blood lipid levels and weight gain on his wife's cooking or dislike for cooking instead of on his hearty appetite.

The way out of this fog is to face reality and work through the problems. If the layers of self-deception are severe, the person may need psychotherapy in order to identify and "unpeel" the layers and face the reality and possible suffering. The nutrition therapist can help other more typical clients by helping them learn lifeskills like assertiveness and setting boundaries that were never fully developed while growing up (perhaps due to lack of good role models), but which affect how they take care of their health. The nutritionist can help the person confront irrational dieting and self-perceptions like, "It's not fair that I can't eat as much as my sister, the marathon runner. I walk," or "I can only lose on 500 calories per day, that's the way I lost the other three times." As therapist, you will see many clients who want the results that a food or lifestyle change will give them, but since childhood they have never been able to delay gratification. They want it NOW!

Nutrition therapy can serve as a reality check for clients and their lifelong beliefs and habits. That is why cognitive (thoughts), behavioral (habits) and psychoeducational therapies (applying psychological or helping skills to learning a body of knowledge) are so important to nutrition counseling. Albert Ellis teaches through his Rational-Emotive Therapy that, it is too bad if something awful happened to you as a child, but it is worse if as an adult, you do nothing about it. (5) A mentally well person works through, confronts, forgives, forgets, or reinterprets things that bother him or her instead of letting them fester and become wounds.

When a Child Needs Nutrition Counseling

Clients of all ages have difficulty in accepting and adjusting to changes in health or lifestyle habits. Children, because of a limited reasoning ability, may have an even harder time. Children do not always understand the reasons why they must change habits or perform certain tasks. Allowing children to have some part in the planning of their care may assist them in feeling they have control over the situation.

Previous hospital experiences can also modify a client's behavior. Children are especially influenced by how they were cared for during prior hospitalizations. Children particularly remember the attitudes of those who took care of them in great detail, especially related to truthfulness. (6) A child's sense of trust is largely influenced by any past relationships with adults. Any previous experiences with a nutrition counselor can influence the child's expectations. A child, just like an adult, fears the unknown and the experienced pediatric nutrition counselor can alleviate these fears in a manner the child can understand through telling a little about yourself or your own children, by asking about the child and his or her family and establishing rapport first.

Children, like many adults, are quick to express their feelings. It becomes very important to listen to these feelings and discern their meanings in the situation at hand. All behaviors have meaning, but the meanings to a child may be more of a challenge to decipher, like when a child speaks very little. Is the child shy, totally satisfied, angry, or ready to go?

Many strategies for teaching young children center on play, the primary way in which children learn. A child may be motivated to learn by playing games, reading books, or using dolls and puppets. When a child, even as young as five years old, understands and "buys-into" solving a nutritional problem, he or she may actually prove to be more disciplined than the parents. Some children take "rules" very seriously, so be sure to assess the child and choose your words carefully so that "guidelines" don't become "rigid rules" unless that are meant to be.

Also, one parent, sometimes unknowingly, will sabotage the efforts of a child and the other parent through offering trips to the ice cream store as reward for good grades or for other reasons. The counselor must then work to help that parent (who often will not come in) to find other ways to show love and share special times with the child without turning to high calorie foods.

In some instances the counselor may be placed in the position of role model or surrogate parent by a child or adolescent (or an adult) client. Coaches of youngsters on athletic teams often serve the same function. It is important that the counselor recognize the potential influence he or she may have in the child's life and do no harm, while modeling mature, rational, caring behavior. (See Appendix 2-A Counseling the pediatric patient.)

Parent/Child Considerations

It is important to take into consideration the relationship between a child and his or her parents as well as the parental expectations of the counseling experience. The nutrition counselor should also learn as much as possible about a child from the parents, especially facts about his or her feeding and toilet habits and social environment.

Throughout the counseling experience, the nutrition counselor should seize opportunities to observe the child-parent interaction and gather information relative to the child's learning needs, any cultural factors that may impact interventions, interaction patterns within the family, the child's level of development, and the parents' level of understanding and coping capabilities. (7) Counseling in the pediatric setting also entails an understanding of adult learning principles to work with the parents and to solidify the entire family-counselor relationship.

The major goal in counseling parents is to help them increase their competence and confidence in meeting the needs of their child. Consequently, the nutrition counselor must establish rapport and trust in the relationship with the parents. Hornby (8) proposes a three stage counseling model based on a general approach which can be used with children and adults in a wide variety of settings. The three stages are: listening, understanding and action planning. The rationale for using the model is based on the premise that any problem or concern parents bring to counseling can be dealt with by going through the three stages and determining the solution that best suits the family unit.

Ivey and Matthews (9) describe a five-stage decisional framework to facilitate counseling. They argue that effective counseling and therapy tend to cover these five points over the time span of the counseling experience. Table 2-1 lists the general guidelines for counseling children using the five-stage model.

Lipkin and Cohen outline potential approaches and helpful tips for working with pediatric clients in the health care setting: (6)

- Establish a friendly relationship with the child. Take time to talk to the child without the parents present. Respect the child's unique feelings and needs and show an interest in his or her interests. Be open to the child's way of doing things if it does not interfere with the goals of therapy.

- Help the child deal with problems as they arise. Provide information in simple terms and honestly.
- Do not overwhelm the child with facts and explanations. Encourage discussion using drawings, pictures or food models to help the child understand basic concepts. Answer questions as they are asked, simply and concisely.
- Recognize that children may view any limitation (such as food or fluids) as punishment. Limitations may be met with anger or resentment. Continue to approach the child with gentle kindness and genuine concern.
- Provide outlets for a child's anger or hostile feelings. Encourage the child to draw pictures or act out feelings with dolls or puppets.
- Give a child choices, but only if you can respect their decisions as part of the counseling experience. Build trust by acting on the child's decisions and providing for some control over the situation.
- Encourage the parents to ask questions. Provide factual explanations that assist parents in support of the counseling experience.
- Be flexible. Flexibility is particularly important when working with children. Short-term goals that can be accomplished easily are vital as the counseling relationship develops.

Table 2-1 Interviewing Children Using the Five Stage Model

Stage 1   Establish rapport
Establish rapport in your own way: Use facial expressions (i.e. smile, laugh), play activities or drawing

Stage 2   Data gathering emphasizing strengths
Paraphrase, reflect child's feelings, summarize frequently. Keep questions and concepts concrete, avoid abstract talk. Identify positive aspects.

Stage 3   Determine goals
Ask what the child wants to happen. Accept a child's goals but focus on concrete short-term goals. Allow a child to explore the ideal world and discover fantasies and desires.

Stage 4   Generate alternative solutions and actions
Utilize creative brainstorming techniques. Try small groups with children having similar problems. Imagine the future and explore various alternatives.

Stage 5   Generalize
Maintain concrete goals day to day. Homework assignments are useful. Observe behavior and interactions with others.

Adapted from Ivey AE, Ivey MB, Simek-Morgan L. *Counseling and Psychotherapy: A Multicultural Perspective*, 3rd ed. Boston: Allyn and Bacon; 1993. Used with permission.

CONSIDERATIONS SPECIFIC TO ADOLESCENTS
Developmental Skills
The extent to which developmental tasks (2) are completed or resolved successfully influence the adolescent's success in finding an identity. Developmental skills that should be learned are:
- Identifying needs (what makes him or her feel stable, happy, secure, loved)
- Active listening (focused, involved listening that enhances communication and relationship building)
- Assertiveness (the ability to stand up and be proactive; it means you believe your opinions have merit)
- Separation (seeing yourself as an individual with needs and wants that are valid but possibly different from parents, siblings and peers, and the ability to function alone)
- Limit setting (the ability to set boundaries to your actions and those you allow in others that involves you)
- Decision making (the ability to look at the facts and draw your own conclusions and commit yourself to timelines, appointments and other responsibilities)
- Organization (the ability to prioritize and structure random information and commitments in order to manage time or complete tasks better)

- Appropriate pacing (this involves the management of time and physical and mental capabilities to promote good health and productive work output)
- Support systems (this acknowledges that other people are very important to each of us, and our happiness and productivity are often highly influenced by the people we choose to be around and whether they positively support us)
- Delegation (the ability to manage your time and energy better by asking or allowing other people to share some of the responsibility by doing tasks they do best)

Adolescents can be most challenging as they struggle to emerge from the role of dependent child to that of independent adult. Through their peers, adolescents learn about life beyond the family unit. Peer groups offer the adolescent the opportunity to try new roles, different identities, and behaviors not experienced at home. Children progress from a strong conformity to what parents mandate, to an equally strong conformity to their peers, and eventually move to their own identity with the maturity and independence of adulthood.

The central task of adolescence is the establishment of identity, with the primary risk being identity confusion, which means the adolescent wants to be like someone else (a movie star, favorite friend, or popular kid in school). (2) Adolescents feel the need to establish their personal identity and with this desire comes increased assertiveness. The adolescent increasingly sees him or herself as able to make decisions regarding his or her well-being including the choice of food, activity, clothes and friends. Psychological influences on health decisions are ultimately related to developmental processes.

Adolescents often understand the whole notion of health differently than adults do. Health compromising behavior decisions like riding a motorcycle or drinking alcohol can represent a way of controlling the environment or testing one's independence from family or peers. Advice about reducing health compromising behavior, like cutting down on candy bars and high fat snacks, may be viewed as adult methods to limit the adolescent's independence and freedom of choice.

Adolescents establish autonomy when they search for avenues to express their free will. The adolescent needs to feel autonomous and have a true sense of commitment to any proposed lifestyle changes. Adolescents tend to be concerned about their physical development, appearance, and emotions. In terms of cognitive development, early adolescents think in the concrete here and now. Abstract or long-range consequences of health behaviors are difficult for adolescents to comprehend. Emphasis for nutrition counseling must be on the immediate, concrete, personal impact of health-compromising behaviors. An emphasis on restrictions and negatives are counterproductive; effective health promotion messages emphasize personal power and control by the adolescent.

Potential approaches to the adolescent client in the health care setting have been outlined by Lipkin and Cohen. (6) Several can be adapted and applied directly to nutrition counseling practice:

- Understand the adolescent's need to mature. It is important to include an adolescent in decisions and goal setting as well as keeping him or her informed about progress during therapy.
- Do not impose your value and belief system (counter-transference issue on your part). Allow the adolescent to verbalize his or her opinions and feelings and agree or disagree without becoming judgemental.
- Recognize that adolescent problems usually involve family interaction issues. Assist the adolescent in evaluating his surroundings and praise and encourage them when they make independent decisions.
- Treat the adolescent with dignity and respect. Stress positive aspects and allow adolescents to express their ideas and concerns openly without criticism.
- Set limits that are fair and enforce them consistently. Recognize the adolescent's individual needs and set goals realistically.
- Do not work with adolescents unless you genuinely like and care about them. Adolescents are going through many conflicts, physically, emotionally and psychologically, and need assistance in guiding them through this difficult period. Adolescents need to feel secure in any relationship and guided by individuals they can trust.

CONSIDERATIONS SPECIFIC TO FAMILIES AND NETWORKS

Traditional counseling in North America has centered on the individual and too little on his or her family and network of friends or significant others like a work group. Many times a spouse, friend, or peers at work play a significant role in whether a client is able to make and sustain eating behavior changes. In some cultures it is most appropriate to work through the family to facilitate changes. In some types of cases such as adolescent obesity counseling, if the family dynamics, rigid rules, or alcoholic parent are the major problem creating stress for the child, working with just the child will not necessarily make the child's life more comfortable. In such cases, nutrition counseling is often not the type of counseling that needs to be instituted first!

The family unit is both affected by an ill member and it has an impact on that family member. (10) For example, having a child with diabetes or PKU usually affects parents' entire lives, and how the parents respond to the child and his or her needs will have an important bearing on the child's behavior and coping skills. Another example might be having an older parent with several diet limitations come to live with a family, requiring more time being spent on meal planning and preparation, and more money being spent on special foods. In these instances, nutrition counseling for parents or other family members is intended to help normally functioning individuals better cope with the additional demands of living with a family member struggling with a health alteration. If the nutritionist perceives that family members are not coping, it is appropriate and ethically responsible to suggest a referral to a family counselor skilled in this area.

It is important to consider the effects of an alteration in health status or behavior changes on the family unit as a whole. The social as well as potential economic impact must be recognized and dealt with. An understanding of the process by which family members adapt to change is essential. It is also important to understand the ways in which the family unit typically functions.

A client's readiness to learn can be enhanced by identifying and utilizing the client's support system to assist the individual in coping with change. Family counseling has been shown to be the most effective therapy for treating adolescent obesity. (11) (See "Family counseling: The ShapeDown approach to adolescent weight loss" in Appendix 2-A.) The nutrition counselor can encourage family and friends to create a supportive environment in which the client works to make lifestyle changes. If they will not agree to that, try to have them agree that they will not sabotage the client's efforts. Studies indicate that an individual's support system is helpful in long-term adherence to diet regimens. (12,13)

In practice you may work in a clinic or on a team with a family counselor, or you may refer clients and their families to a private practicing family counselor. Trained family counselors come from many disciplines, i.e. psychiatry, psychology, psychotherapy, psychiatric social worker. They all must have a minimum of a master's in counseling with special emphasis and supervision in family dynamics and counseling. (3) It is not an easy job to step into the emotional dynamics of a family that has been functioning only marginally for many years. Without proper training, a nutrition therapist should not attempt it. It is appropriate, however, to work with a client and his or her supportive family members on nutrition-related issues if the client wants the help.

OVERVIEW OF ADULT LEARNING CONCEPTS

The field of adult learning has grown and expanded as the need for lifelong learning became more widely recognized. It wasn't until the late 1960's and early 1970's that attitudes about teaching adults began to change. Those involved in education began to see an important difference between the initial formal education of children and how adults learn. The commonly recognized principles of adult learning are:

1. Adults like to determine their own learning experiences.
2. Adults want to have efficient use of their time.
3. Adults are more motivated to learn if they see a purpose or need.
4. Adults can learn from the experiences of others as well as their own.
5. Adults desire practical solutions to problems they encounter.
6. Adults like physical surroundings conducive to their comfort.
7. Adults operate from a problem-solving mode.
8. Adults want to be active participants in their learning experiences.
9. Adults draw on their own experiences when evaluating a learning environment.
10. Adults do not like to be treated like children.
11. Adult learning is an active and continuous process.
12. Adults learn at different rates and in different ways.
13. Adults like to know whether progress is being made.

These assumptions have many implications for the planning, implementation and evaluation of nutrition counseling interventions. See Table 2-2 on Adult Learning Concepts and Nutrition Counseling.

Self Concept and Learning

As individuals mature, independence develops as adults take control of their lives. Adults in our society develop a deep psychological need to be perceived by others as being self-directing. Therefore, in situations that do not allow them to be self-directing, adults experience tension between the situation and their self-concept. The typical reaction is bound to be tainted by resentment and resistance to change. Adults "tend to avoid, resist and resent being placed in situations in which they feel they are treated like children—told what to do and what not to do, talked down to, embarrassed, punished and judged." (14)

Table 2-2 Adult Learning Concepts and Nutrition Counseling

Concept	*Counseling Strategy*
Clients want to be treated as adults	Do not reprimand or talk down to clients
Every client is an individual	Individualize teaching plan for each client's situation
	Avoid "standardized" materials unless they can be individualized
Most adults prefer objectivity and a business-like approach	The use of titles or surnames is appropriate unless the client mentions otherwise
	Treat the client with respect
Clients have difficulty with change	Explain that change will minimize threat rather than insist on change
Some clients lack confidence	Lack of education, fear of failure, distrust of the medical community may be barriers
	Patience, answering questions, and realistic goals may help promote a sense of confidence
Some clients are overconfident	Important to set realistic goals
Adults need positive reinforcement and feedback	Assists in overcoming fear and anxiety
	May improve compliance

Used by permission. Dietitians in General Clinical Practice, 1992. In: Klawitter B. The Dietetic Practitioner as Adult Educator: An Overview. *DGCP Newsletter.* 1992; 9; 4: 4-9.

Clients who discover nutrition "truths" on their own are more likely to accept, integrate, and apply these concepts. (15) The level of learning may also be related to the level of trust and rapport that exists between the counselor and the client. This process includes collaboration with the counselor in decision-making in regards to the client's nutritional needs. Nutrition therapists must involve the client in selecting what to learn, how to present the information, and what evaluative tools to utilize to determine the achievement of learning goals.

Evaluation can evoke anxiety in many adult clients. In adult learning, the best evaluative methods are those that are not intimidating, allow for determination of what is learned (such as having the client verbally list basic concepts) and elicit how newly learned information will be incorporated into daily activities (for example, selecting foods from a sample restaurant menu). Individuals need to participate in choosing the methods used to assess their learning and see their own progress towards established goals and objectives.

Life Experience
The effect of the environment is to arouse behaviors already learned and to teach new behaviors. Behavior changes reflect learning in specific situations; for example, strategies for incorporating increased physical activity into daily routines. The past experiences of adults have a tremendous impact, positively and negatively, on learning. In androgogy, there is less emphasis on the transmittal techniques found in traditional educational settings like lectures, canned audiovisual presentations and extensive reading, and an increased emphasis on experiential techniques to tap the experience of adult learners and involve them in analyzing their experiences. Due to the fact that individuals learn in different ways, it is important that content be presented in a variety of formats. Table 2-3 lists some general points to consider when selecting printed or audiovisual materials for adult learners. Table 2-4 gives teaching strategies for individuals with limited literacy skills.

Table 2-3 Media Considerations for the Adult Learner

Printed Materials	*Nonprint Materials*
Is content written at an appropriate level for clientele?	Are they appropriate for the topic?
Is content clear and concise?	Are they accurate yet appealing?
Is material organized in a logical sequence?	Are important points easy to identify?
Is important information highlighted?	Can opportunities for cognitive practice be provided?
Are visuals attractive and do they contribute to understanding?	Are the sound and /or color acceptable?
Is the print easy to read and the type large enough?	
Is the content accurate?	
Does the material allow for patient participation/ interaction?	

Used by permission. Dietitians in General Clinical Practice, 1992. In: Klawitter B. The Dietetic Practitioner as Adult Educator: An Overview. *DGCP Newsletter.* 1992; 9; 4: 4-9.

In their initial assessments, nutrition counselors need to determine the clients' feelings and experiences related to the counseling process they are about to be involved in. For example you might ask, "Have you attempted to make any of these changes before?" The counseling plan must incorporate this knowledge and be built on positive experiences in order to overcome any negatives that may block learning or change.

Table 2-4 Teaching Strategies

Needs Of Individuals With Limited Literacy Skills	How To Meet Those Needs
Use of relevant material	Base materials on learner needs and interests
	Link information to learner's experience
Flexible learning pace	Allow individuals the time they need
	Keep sessions short, amounts of information small
	Avoid sudden surprises or changes
Involvement in learning process	Encourage clients to set goals and discover resources
	Promote client's responsibility for learning
	Use discovery techniques (hand-on experience)
Organized, useful materials	Encourage group problem-solving, simulation
	Use information and materials with practical meaning
Evaluate efforts	Recognize achievements, Minimize chances of failure
	Provide regular feedback

Used by permission. Copyright 1994, James A. Fain, RN. In: Fain JA. Assessing nutrition education in clients with weak literacy skills. Nurse Practitioner Forum. 1994; 5: 1: 52-55.

Some literature indicates adults prefer one-on-one interventions which allow for individualized counseling strategies and content based on the individual's limitations and barriers. If a counseling strategy is unfamiliar to a client, like the exchange system or keeping extensive behavioral records, evaluate whether the client has difficulty using it, since trying to master content and learn a new skill at the same time might inhibit learning and change.

Readiness to Learn

Androgogy assumes learners are ready to learn those things that they *need* to learn because of developmental phases they are approaching in their roles as workers, spouses, parents and the like. Before pursuing a counseling relationship, the counselor should determine if the client is prepared to make changes in his or her health behavior. A candid discussion with the client about his or her readiness may prevent frustration and misunderstandings down the road.

Stages of Change: Model for Nutrition Counseling Clients arrive at our doors with varying levels of interest in making lifestyle changes. The stages of change model (See Figure 2-1) has been utilized to describe the processes of health behavior change. Prochaska and DiClemente and others (16,17,18) have studied groups of people trying to change risky lifestyle behaviors such as smoking, consuming alcohol, adopting more exercise, and weight loss. They found that participants were more successful making changes if the strategies more closely matched each person's stage of change.

You can identify which stage a client is in by asking very simple questions like, "Are you concerned about your cholesterol level being high?" (A negative answer here would show that the client is in the *Precontemplation Stage* and had not accepted or personalized the risk involved.) Clients in the *Contemplation Stage* believe they have a problem but aren't sure where to begin, and they need lots of help identifying what needs to be done. The *Preparation Stage* is where clients are ready to make a change but haven't yet taken any action, and they need encouragement to make small steps and draw from their past successes. In the *Action Stage*, clients have taken the first steps to change and now need help reinforcing the decision. The *Maintenance Stage* is typified by increasing the coping skills and self-rewards to support sustained change. In the *Relapse Stage*, clients return to old ways and need renewed commitment and motivation. Table 2-5 shows this model adapted to nutrition counseling. (14)

Research has shown that major events (such as illness) stimulate adult learning; however, more research is needed on when is the best time to counsel individuals following an illness. Certainly, we believe in providing the most crucial "survival" information close to the time it is needed in the acute care setting. However, counseling the client more completely when he or she is physiologically and psychologically stable and free from discomfort is much more logical.

A number of factors affect an individual's readiness to learn (see Table 2-6) and some may be more appropriately addressed in an outpatient setting. Readiness to learn is greatly influenced by clients' interpretations of their health problems and treatments. It may be necessary for you to talk with the client regarding these concerns before further counseling can take place. Learning readiness can be influenced by many factors such as pain or anything else that affects the client's physical or psychological comfort level. Attempting to proceed with counseling efforts without understanding these circumstances is usually futile.

Figure 2-1 Stages of Change Model Emphasizing Points of Entry, Relapse, and Reentry.

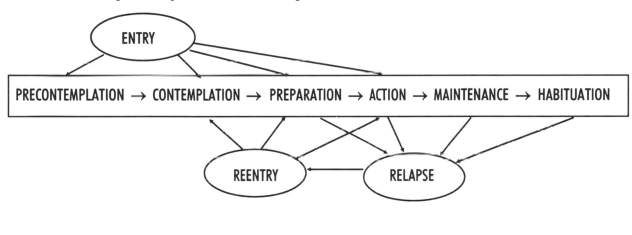

Used with permission. Copyright 1994, Aspen Publishers, Inc. Sandoval W, Heller K, Wiese W, Childs D. Stages of Change: A Model for Nutrition Counseling. *Topics in Clinical Nutrition.* June 1994, vol 9:3; 64-69.

Acute Care Setting. When attempting to counsel the critically ill patient in the acute care setting, there are two counseling issues that should be addressed: (16) the nutrition counselor must develop an awareness of what the client is feeling and the counselor must understand her or his own emotional responses to critical illness.

If you are unsure how rigid to make diet limitations for a 78-year-old woman with multiple chronic illnesses, ask her! Say, "How aggressive do you want to be with your food intake now that you understand how it can effect your different medical problems? What are you willing and able to do at home?" You may be surprised! Too often medicine writes off people over a certain age and does not expect patients will want to make changes that won't increase their life expectancies. But many simple food and lifestyle changes will improve the quality of their lives. It is our responsibility to make patients aware of their nutrition-related options so they can make informed decisions.

It is extremely important that a counselor remain flexible in the acute care setting and return at another time if the patient is vomiting, arguing with a family member, or sleeping during the day when the chart states that the patient has been unable to sleep at night. It is equally important for the intern or dietitian to check the patient's chart and talk to the charge nurse, if possible, about whether the patient knows his or her new diagnosis before entering the room to give a discharge diet instruction.

Many patients and their families are devastated when they find out the patient has diabetes, heart disease, or other life-threatening diseases, and they may not want to talk. The opposite also may be true; they may want and need to talk to someone about what to do. If that is the case, it is a good time to establish rapport by showing concern and empathy, and set their minds at ease by answering their most pressing questions. Of all times this is a time when the you must avoid overwhelming or confusing the patient with too much information given too fast. If time permits, schedule a second more comprehensive consultation the next day, or if they are leaving that day, let the patient choose which two or three changes he or she will agree to make and schedule an outpatient consult. See Table 2-7 Communication Techniques for Counseling the Critically Ill.

Orientation to Learning

Maslow's hierarchy of needs describes physiological needs as being the most basic.(20) Safety, belongingness and love, esteem and self-actualization are needs on the progressive steps of the hierarchy. Esteem needs and the motivation to learn are closely related. Consequently, the motivation to learn or change behavior may increase as the clients' self-esteem increases. That is why most counselors try to reinforce or build a client's self-esteem during therapy.

Table 2-5 Application of the Stage of Change Model With Goals and Strategies

Stage	Goal	Strategies
Precontemplation	Personalize risk	1. Create supporting climate for change 2. Discuss personal aspects for poor-eating behavior 3. Assess nutrition knowledge and beliefs in myths 4. Build on prior nutrition knowledge
Contemplation	Increase self-efficacy	1. Identify problematic behaviors 2. Priotritize behaviors to change 3. Discuss coping strategies 4. Discuss motivations 5. Identify barriers to change and possible solutions 6. Elicit support from family and friends
Preparation	Initiate Chnage	1. Encourage initial small steps to change 2. Discuss earlier attempts to change and ways to succeed
Action	Commitment to change	1. Reinforce decision 2. Encourage self-rewarding behavior 3. Discuss relapse and coping strategies 4. Reinforce self-confidence
Maintenance/habituation	Continued commitment	1. Plan follow-up to support changes 2. reinforce self-rewarding behaviors 3. Increase coping skills 4. Discuss relapse and techniques
Relapse	Reinforce commitment	1. Reassess motivation and barriers 2. Discuss importance of maintaining change 3. Explore new coping strategies

Used with permission. From Sandoval W, Heller K, Wiese W, Childs D. Stages of Change: A Model for Nutrition Counseling. *Topics in Clinical Nutrition.* June 1994, vol 9:3; 64-69

Nutrition counseling does not guarantee learning and learning can occur without counseling. The "teachable moment" for the adult occurs when he or she recognizes that a problem needs to be solved. However, a client may be motivated to learn by a creative and dynamic counselor. It is important for you to approach adult clients with a positive attitude and believe that they can learn and that learning will have a positive impact on improving their function and well-being. Clients' receptiveness to the counseling experience is influenced by their personalities, attitudes, educational backgrounds, physical characteristics and even economic situations. (21) See FYI at the end of this chapter on Personal Styles and Relationship Strategies pages 38-44.

CONSIDERATIONS SPECIFIC TO THE OLDER ADULT

The issue of counseling the older adult presents the potential for ageism. Ageism can be defined as imposing one's own beliefs and values about what an individual can or should be able to do at various ages. A good nutrition counselor must realize there are wide varieties and differences in individual development and that restricting strategies by age may not be valid. Peterson and Eden (22) report that numerous studies have conclusively shown that intelligence does not decline substantially over the lifespan and that healthy older individuals arc typically capable of continuing to learn and change behavior into their 60's, 70's and 80's.

Table 2-6 Factors Which Can Affect Readiness to Learn

Physical	***Pain, fatigue, disability, sensory deprivation***
Psychological	Health and illness beliefs, attitude, values, acceptance of illness, motivation to change
Cognitive	Educatioanl level, reading ability, ability to comprehend
Cultural/ environmental	Ethnic background, religion, health values, social roles, support system, financial standing, home environment

Used by permission. Dietitians in General Clinical Practice, 1992. In: Klawitter B. The Dietetic Practitioner as Adult Educator: An Overview. *DGCP Newsletter.* 1992; 9; 4: 4-9.

Table 2-7 Communication Techniques for Counseling the Critically Ill

Communication Technique	***Suggested Rationale***
1. Learn to listen to the patient	Ask patients directly what problems exist
	Determine problems then find solutions
2. Repeat information at least once	The more times a patient hears information, the more it is remembered
	When first diagnosed, many people can only remember the most basic information
3. Provide all pertinent information in written form	Write down pertinent brand names to aid retention
	Provide dietitian's phone number for future questions
4. Urge patients to write down questions	Anxiety of a hospital visit often blocks the memory
5. Include family members as care providers	This emphasizes importance of recommendations
	Provides additional support for patient
	Often therapeutic for family to be involved
6. Always be direct and keep it simple	Avoid medical or nutrition jargon
	Do not expect patient to remember names or details
	Explain physiology in simple manner to justify changes
	Pictures may often be appropriate
7. Compensate for shorter attention span	Medications may make patient unable to concentrate
	Make important points first
	Reduce length of visit and return more often
8. Know when enough has been said	Do not pursue counseling when patient is angry or indifferent
	Revisit patient on another day

Used with permission. Copyright 1986 Aspen Publishers, Inc. Adapted from Luann Bell Gilmore LR. Nutrition Counseling: The Critically and Terminally Ill Patient. *Topics in Clinical Nutrition.* 1986; 1:1: 1-6.

Eldergogy (23) or gerogogy (24) refer to an evolving specialized approach to learning in older adults that utilizes strategies or techniques best suited for the aged. This field of study takes into account the distinct concerns and traits of old age that need to be incorporated into nutrition counseling for the older adult population. Some older adults may appear to have decreased learning abilities because they are physically slower. Speed of perceptions, initiating a response, and of movement are all affected by the neural changes due to aging. (25) In older adults, a brief functional assessment of psychomotor skills (ability to cook food, shop, add more physical activity, and so on) should be carefully done by the nutrition therapist before goals are set and counseling initiated, especially if behavior change necessitates any of these skills.

Research has found inconclusively that the aging adult has increasing difficulty with transfer of information from primary to secondary memory, and particularly in search land retrieval cf information from long-term memory. (26)

Particular teaching strategies have been identified to assist the older adult to adapt to age-associated memory decline and they are very similar to the guidelines for communicating with a critically ill patient: keep in information clear and simple, speak slowly and repeat your major points, support major points with easy-to-understand printed materials, eliminate environmental distractions, and correct wrong answers immediately to maintain clarity of your message.

Counseling the older adult includes attention to the sensory changes of aging. The changes that have the most significant impact on the teaching-learning process are the declines in vision and hearing. These changes are common physiological deficits in the older age group but may not always correlate with the client's chronological age. Particular strategies to overcome these sensory deficits are listed in Table 2-8.

Table 2-8 Visual and Auditory Barriers to Learning

Changes Of Aging	Teaching Strategies
Decreased visual acuity	Use high-density lighting
	Use sharp, contrasting colors
	Use large print and low vision aids
	Encourage use of glasses
	Use taped cassettes as aids
Distorted color perception	Avoid using the colors blue, green and violet in teaching aids
Increased glare	Avoid using shiny surfaces or plastic in teaching aids
Inability to hear high-pitched sounds	Speak slower with greater separation of words
	Speak in low-pitched tones
	Use nonverbal communication techniques
	Use audiovisuals for content communication
	Avoid background noise

Used by permission. Dietitians in General Clinical Practice, 1992. In: Klawitter B. The Dietetic Practitioner as Adult Educator: An Overview. *DGCP Newsletter.* 1992; 9; 4: 4-9.

Research suggests that, with increasing age, the majority of individuals do become more rigid or set in their ways as one way of coping with stress. (28) Consequently, an older adult client may be hesitant to learn something new or make changes because they are afraid of failure. Counseling strategies should focus on assessing the client's abilities and pacing the amount and type of information so that success is almost guaranteed. Several studies have identified areas of concern for older adults that can be assessed in the counseling session (29) and may assist the nutrition counselor in the initial assessment process such as age related physiologic changes (i.e. decreased response time, decreased visual acuity) as well as psychosocial changes (i.e. depression, retirement).

THE LEARNING PROCESS
The focus and purposes of health and wellness counseling are to define the problems, suggest coping behaviors, and facilitate client mastery and control. A counseling process based on a client-centered problem-solving model uses three steps: establish rapport with the client, assess the problem(s), then plan strategies, to include: goals and objectives, content, counseling strategies, implementation and evaluation.

Rapport
As mentioned in Chapter 1, possibly the most important single factor that influences the outcome of a consultation is the relationship between the client and the therapist. You can establish rapport with clients by actively listening to what they have to say, by being genuinely interested in the clients as people not just their health or nutritional problems, by showing an interest and concerted effort in their nutritional well-being, and by being honest, reasonable, and supportive.

Assessment
Assessments serve many functions such as identifying a client's problems or strengths, physical or biochemical abnormalities, abilities or limitations, health risks and so on. As a therapist you choose how much time and how much value you place on the assessment phase. Some good therapists spend only a few minutes on formally assessing a client at the beginning of the initial consult and instead casually assess the client through one or more sessions. Others using the more

medical model, choose to define the situation at that point in time and design future therapy. Whichever style you use is not so important as making sure the results of the assessment actually affect therapy (one diet should not fit all), and that the client is reassessed at each visit to finely tune the therapy to his or her needs.

Assessment is a two-step process: first, information gathering and second, data interpretation by both the therapist and the client. A *learning need* is defined as the difference between the information the client already knows and the information necessary to perform a task or care for oneself. An assessment to determine the client's learning needs is essential so the counseling plan can address the client's deficit in skill or knowledge.

In order to plan and evaluate nutrition counseling, therapists need to assess diet intake with a reasonable degree of accuracy. An evaluation of intake before intervention may help identify problems and target specific areas for modification. Repeating the assessment periodically after intervention will indicate any behavior changes and will provide information to evaluate the effectiveness of counseling.

Assessment should also consider the individual's cognitive function, attitudes, and physical abilities. In certain locales, cultural assessment may also be indicated to elicit detailed cultural factors that may influence intervention strategies.

Not all clients may be ready to learn or change behavior and dietetic practitioners do not always have the time to counsel individuals who are not ready either physically or emotionally. With decreasing lengths of stay in the acute care setting, the most that may be accomplished is to assess the level of readiness, document what has been assessed, and communicate this to the appropriate referral source after discharge.

Behavioral diagnosis (30) is the systematic identification of health practices that appear to be causally linked to health problems identified in the medical diagnosis. The behavioral diagnosis makes possible the identification of factors that have an influence on health behavior and can aid in selecting appropriate strategies to aid the client in changing or improving health status. Specific steps in conducting behavioral diagnosis include:

1. distinguishing between behavioral and nonbehavioral causes of the problem,
2. defining those behaviors in order of importance,
3. ranking behaviors in order of importance,
4. assessing the changeability of each behavior, and
5. prioritizing behaviors in order of importance and changeability.

Behavioral diagnosis may be especially useful for clients with diabetes and weight management concerns in order to achieve specific behavioral changes.

Assessing what information the individual is interested in learning is equally important. Starting with what the client wants to know is recommended even if that information is not what the nutrition counselor feels is most important for the client to know. Client questions may relate to what they believe is of immediate use. If these questions or concerns are not addressed at the onset, an individual may not hear important information being given by the counselor. Providing information that is important to the individual first acknowledges the client's independence in decision making. Meeting the clients' learning needs keeps their interest better and motivates them to stay involved.

The stress of illness can interfere with the ability and motivation to learn. Frustration may result from such factors as lack of experience with the health care system, unfamiliarity with medical terms, and the inability to grasp concepts as rapidly as in the past. Denial of illness is a common defense mechanism, especially in the older adult and in parents of a sick child. Before nutrition counseling can begin, the adult must acknowledge the health problem. The client must believe that learning and changing behavior will have positive results.

Assessment is not complete until data have been interpreted. In making a counseling need diagnosis, the specific illness, physical attributes and environmental influences must all be considered. Gaining knowledge about a client's strengths, limitations and coping patterns is fundamental to setting priorities and planning counseling goals, methods and approaches. Assessment also serves to establish a baseline of data for therapy interaction and conversation, and future evaluations.

Planning

Once a counseling relationship has been established, the nutrition counselor must remain nonjudgemental, regardless of the client's feelings, and coordinate a counseling plan of care. The counseling plan is based on the outcome of the assessment and the diagnosis of an individual's learning needs. The plan should contain learning goals/objectives, content to be covered, and counseling strategies to be utilized. An individual implementation plan, formulated with the client, takes into account any barriers previously identified. The plan's final stage is evaluation.

Goals And Objectives. Danish suggests that the terms "goals" and "objectives" should be reinterpreted to make them more consistent with today's emphasis on smaller steps and permanent changes, especially in weight control. (31) He believes that to "lose 30 pounds" is the *result*, not the goal. Psychologically most clients get discouraged by goals that are so "far away." He stresses that the goals should be behavioral just like the objectives and within the person's power like, "exercise three times per week for 30 minutes" or, "eat only when physically hungry and stop when just full" or, "set a boundary of 7 hours per week spent on volunteer projects." Goals and objectives would have basically the same meaning, but could be classified as "goals and sub-goals." A sub-goal could be to "make a tub of margarine last two weeks instead of one week," or to "buy new walking-type dress shoes to wear at work" so the client walks more. This new concept helps clients see change as more achievable, and they mentally recognize and acknowledge the importance of small steps in achieving lifestyle changes. Measurable goals help a client gain knowledge and develop skills. See Chapter 7 using this new approach.

Goals state, in very clear and precise terms, what the client will be able to do when the learning is completed. They define content, direct counseling strategies and learning experiences, set up the learning environment, and assist with evaluating program success. They are statements of what is to be achieved and should be clearly stated in terms of expected client outcomes, the result of the counseling process. A goal should describe both the kind of behavior expected and the content/context to which that behavior applies. Performance goals provide direction for clients, helping them understand the specific behaviors they must master to achieve a certain health status. They also allow clients to evaluate their own progress for themselves, which helps them become more independent.

Three Domains of Learning. The objectives of learning are classified into levels of behavior called the three domains of learning. (32) These domains include cognitive, affective and psychomotor skills.

The cognitive domain involves intellectual skills and refers to the specific knowledge and understanding an individual has or is given regarding a specific subject. Decision-making skills fall into this area as decisions are a cognitive process.

The affective domain relates to attitudes and feelings and is also critical in reaching the desired goals of the client. The individual may have the knowledge and the skills necessary to perform a task but is unwilling or unmotivated to carry it out. The affective domain is sometimes the most difficult to identify but can have a profound effect on the success of nutrition counseling. Responsive listening and other communication skills can assist clients in exploring their own feelings, thoughts, and behaviors to gain insights of themselves and their environment.

Psychomotor skills are the third domain and are a complex interplay of the neurological and musculo-skeletal systems. A client may have the ability to process information necessary to learn a skill but may not actually be able to perform the skill. The focus is on specific, observable behaviors rather than feelings and thoughts. Vision, perception, tactile sensation, coordination, and muscle strength are involved.

Behavior Change Techniques. Practice and the use of behavioral change techniques in counseling implies client involvement. Nutrition counselors can make suggestions to clients and give guidance, but individuals ultimately must decide what they want to do. The nutrition counselor can develop the framework by suggesting achievable goals and approaches to meet those goals, and solicit feedback from the client. Goals should be realistic so they can be achieved within the time frame available for counseling. Short and long-term strategies need to be designed to achieve the counseling objectives. Accomplishing short-term objectives as a step toward achieving the long-term plan enhances motivation and provides an opportunity for more client interaction.

Content. The second aspect of the planning phase relates to the content to be discussed with the client. A major component of most nutrition education programs is didactic in nature, focusing on disease characteristics and the relationship of nutrition to treatment and/or prevention. In traditional acute care nutrition counseling, the didactic technique is typically undertaken during a single teaching session. The underlying assumption in presentations of this type is that the more the person knows, the better off they will be and the more willing or able they will be to participate in self-care activities. There is evidence to suggest, however, that the standard presentation of medical facts and treatment regimens is relatively ineffective in fostering the desired behaviors or helping clients cope. (33) **It is presumptuous to expect major and lasting lifestyle changes on the basis of such short-term interventions.**

Counseling Strategies. Counseling strategies like participant modeling and contracting can provide for learning and when coupled with a strong helping relationship, they can expedite the client's feeling, thought and behavior changes. Counseling strategies relate to overall approaches to achieving short- and long-term goals. Instructional methods, like viewing a videotape or selecting from a menu, are another consideration of the counseling plan, incorporating specific applications of the various counseling approaches. The method of learning should correspond to the learning style of the client and relate directly to the goals and objectives.

The amount of time available for the counseling relationship is important in the selection of strategies. Some strategies can be implemented in shorter time spans as compared to others; behavioral strategies can be relatively short-term whereas psychoanalytic therapy can last indefinitely. With shortened hospital stays and the resulting limited time for counseling, media can be very useful to the nutrition counselor. Media, including both printed and audiovisual materials, can present repetitive information in an *interesting* manner as well as save staff time. Media, however, should not solely replace individualized one-on-one interaction.

To plan for a positive learning environment, several factors should be considered. When possible, extraneous noise should be minimized as such distractions can decrease concentration for both the counselor and the client and detract from the counseling session. Other aspects of the environment that should be considered include furniture arrangement, lighting, temperature, a positive climate and adequate time for counseling. (34)

Implementation. Once there is agreement on goals and objectives, opportunities to practice a behavior or skill should be provided. Practice should be integrated throughout daily activities. By having the client practice skills in your office or in the hospital, you provide a clear and precise definition of what the individual is to do at home in terms of diet, exercise or lifestyle changes. Implementation becomes more feasible. Continued practice in diet selection has been accomplished in inpatient and outpatient settings through the use of sample menus and food models. Some health care facilities have access to private dining areas in which clients have a more realistic opportunity to select foods. In this way, learning takes place in incremental steps and clients are not overwhelmed with too much change at one time.

Therapists who treat clients for weight loss admit being particularly concerned about their clients who do not stray from the guidelines and never test their boundaries because they do not develop the coping strategies necessary to handle unexpected events and stresses. It is much better for clients to experiment with eating out and being flexible at social events during counseling so they have support readily available while they learn how to handle the experiences.

Evaluation. Evaluation should be on-going from the time intervention strategies are implemented. An evaluation aids in determining whether clients have acquired the knowledge or skill to change their behavior. The ultimate evaluation of success is realized when the client has changed his behavior and is complying with the therapeutic regime. This is extremely difficult to evaluate in the hospital inpatient setting since changes in nutrition/diet behavior usually occur after the client is discharged.

Several types of evaluation methodology have been outlined in the literature: (1)

Reaction evaluation: data is collected about how the client is responding to a program or plan of care as the program progresses. This type of evaluation provides information to make program modifications while it is in progress.

Learning evaluation: data is collected about the cognitive skills the client has acquired. Performance/demonstration activities, recall or problem-solving can be used to gauge knowledge.

Behavior evaluation: observations about actual changes in what the client has done after learning versus before is evaluated. Questionnaires, self-rating scales and interviews are examples.

Results evaluation: routine records, such as admission data, costs, and lab results are reviewed for changes.

Evaluation has always been difficult because, except for behavioral strategies, there is not always observable criteria. Evaluating whether a skill has been learned may be the easiest to measure, whereas it is more difficult to measure value or attitude changes. Behavioral strategies are more specifically evaluated and easier to limit in a given time frame whereas those strategies that lean toward the affective domain can take longer to evaluate for effectiveness.

Cognitive learning may be evaluated using such techniques as:

- application of information (able to use exchanges in planning a meal),
- verbal rehearsal (rehearse through role play what to do when offered a dessert),
- verbal commitment (client states, "I know I can walk at least two miles three days a week."),
- role reversal (counselor says, "What would you tell a friend who was in this situation and needed sound advice?").

If the right questions are asked, both knowledge and its application can be assessed. Measurements of diet intake as part of an educational evaluation also may indicate diet-related goals that were or were not achieved. Based upon continual evaluations, the counselor and client may decide to utilize another strategy, revise goals, or terminate the counseling relationship.

Documentation of client counseling in the medical record is vital. It is equally important to document client response to the learning. If a brochure is given, a sheet of instructions provided, or a movie shown, the task of nutrition counseling is often checked off as complete. The emphasis has been on methodology and content not the client's response. Knowledge, skills, and behavior changes need to be documented. As Doris Derelian, PhD, RD says, "You can't write in the chart that you counseled a patient if all you did was hand out written pieces of paper. The patient must know the topic better, or be able to do something better, than before you began to call it counseling." (See Chapter 10 regarding documentation of patient care.)

SUMMARY

Nutrition counseling is an important independent function of professional dietetic practice. This overview, based on how adults differ from children in their learning focus, should form a basic philosophy for client counseling. These beliefs and assumptions can serve to help place nutrition counseling into a perspective where the client is the focus. You can facilitate learning and change by incorporating concepts of adult learning into your practice. In years past, the dietitian set the intended outcomes, made independent decisions about what to teach to accomplish the goals, and decided how to present the content. In contrast, the nutrition counselor, using the learning concepts reviewed in this book, would involve the client in setting goals and in deciding how to achieve them.

Nutrition counseling in the acute care setting is a challenge, primarily due to the lack of time available and the acuity of care levels. Using good assessment techniques, sticking to the "need to know" survival content as much as possible, simplifying instructions, streamlining programs, providing opportunities for practice, providing reference and resource materials, and referring clients for further follow up counseling will help get the process done more efficiently and effectively.

Assessment of one's own counseling strengths should be on-going. Counseling is both an art and a science. It is an "art" in that the personality, values and demeanor of the nutrition counselor are important variables that are subjective and difficult to define or to measure. Counseling can be considered a "science" in that much of what we know about human behavior and many of the helping strategies have been developed as structured, measurable objective concepts. Dietetic practitioners may be skilled in a variety of areas such as group facilitation, individual or family counseling, or the preparation of written materials. Questions nutrition counselors may ask themselves include: (35)

1. Did I help my client achieve their objectives as quickly as possible?
2. Did I use the most efficient strategies?
3. Would a referral source better serve my client?
4. Were my counseling strategies appropriate for this particular client?

LEARNING ACTIVITIES

1. Observe a family nutrition counseling session. What role does each family member play in the counseling session? What interactions between family members do you observe? What impact does the nutrition problem being addressed play on the family unit as a whole?

2. Counsel (or observe a counseling session) for a child under age eight. What counseling strategies are utilized? How does the child respond to each strategy identified? What changes would you recommend if the session was to be repeated based on your observations?

3. Participate in a group nutrition education session involving adults over age 55. What age-specific considerations should be made? How would you evaluate whethter or not learning or change would take place? How would the same program be altered if the average age of the participants was under 30?

4. Look at the photo of the counseling session below. Critique the session and describe what elements of the interaction are consistent with good body language and building rapport. What could you change to improve the counseling setting?

REFERENCES

1. Knowles MS. *The Modern Practice of Adult Education.* Chicago: Follett Publishing Company; 1970.
2. Erickson EH. *Childhood and Society.* New York: Norton; 1963.
3. Phone interview with Carl Greenberg, MS, Behavior Science Faculty, Family Medicine, U of Washington, Seattle, WA, January 1995.
4. Peck MS. *The Road Less Travelled.* London, England: Arrow; 1990.
5. Ellis A. Rational-emotive psychotherapy. In: Arbuckel D, ed. *Counseling and Psychotherapy.* New York: McGraw-Hill; 1967.
6. Lipkin GB, Cohen RG. *Effective Approaches to Patient's Behavior.* New York: Springer Publishing Company; 1980.
7. Sedlacek KK. Patient Teaching in a pediatric unit. In: Bille DA, ed. *Practical Approaches to Patient Teaching.* Boston: Little, Brown and Company; 1981.
8. Hornby G. *Counselling in Child Disability: Skills for Working with Parents.* London: Chapman and Hall; 1994.
9. Ivey AE, Ivey MB, Simek-Morgan L. *Counseling and Psychotherapy: A Multicultural Perspective.* 3rd ed. Boston: Allyn and Bacon; 1993.
10. Mink IT, Nahira K. Directions of effects: Family lifestyles and behavior of TMR children. *Am J of Mental Deficiency.* 1991; 91 (11): 1418-1422.
11. Mellin L. Child and adolescent obesity: The nurse practitioner's use of the SHAPEDOWN method. *J Ped Health Care.* 1992; 6: (4): 187-193.
12. Morton A, Ringles S, Christakis G. Social factors affecting participation in a study diet and coronary heart disease. *J Health and Social Behavior.* 1967; 8: 22-31.
13. Andrew GM, Oldridge NB, Parker JO, Cunningham DA, Rechnitzer PA, Jones NL, Buck C, Kavanaugh T, Shepard RJ, Sutton JR, McDonald W. Reasons for dropout from exercise programs for post-coronary patients. *Medicine and Science in Sports and Exercise.* 1981; 13: 164-168.
14. Knowles M. Program planning for adults as learners. *Adult Leadership.* 1967;16: 267.
15. Johnson DW, Johnson RT. Nutrition education's future. *Journal of Nutrition Education.* 1985; 17: 20-24.
16. Sandoval W, Heller K, Wiese W, Childs D. Stages of Change: A model for nutrition counseling. *Topics in Clinical Nutrition.* June 1994, vol. 9: 3; 64-69.
17. Prochaska JO, Norcross JC, DiClemete CC. *Changing for Good.* New York: Wm Morrow; 1994.
18. Prochaska JO. *Systems of Psychotherapy.* 2nd ed. Homewood, IL: Dorsey Press; 1984.
19. Bell LR. Nutrition counseling the critically ill and terminally ill patient. *Topics in Clinical Nutrition.* 1986; 1 (1): 16.
20. Maslow A. *Motivation and Personality.* New York: Harper and Row; 1970.
21. Williams SR. *Nutrition and Diet Therapy.* St. Louis: C.V. Mosby Company; 1989.
22. Peterson DA, Eden DZ. Cognitive style and the older learner. *Ed. Gerontology,* 1981, 7: 51-66.
23. Yeo G. "Eldergogy": a specialized approach to education for elders. *Lifelong Learning: The Adult Years,* 1982, 5(5): 47.
24. Billie DA. Educational strategies for teaching the elderly patient. *Nursing and Health Care,* 1980; 256-263.
25. Hicks LH, Birren JE. Aging, brain damage and psychomotor slowing. *Psych. Bulletin,* 1970; 74: 390.
26. Arenberg D, Robertson-Tchabo E. Learning and aging. In: Birren J, Schaie K, eds. *Handbook of the Psychology of Aging.* New York: Van Nostrand; 1977.
27. Alywahby NF. Principles of teaching for individual learning of older adults. *Rehabilitation Nursing.* 1989; 14 (6): 330-333.
28. Chown SM. Age and rigidities. *Journal of Gerontology.* 1961; 16: 353-362.

29. Kicklighter JR. Characteristics of older adult learners: a guide for dietetic practitioners. *J Amer Diet Assoc.* 1991; 91(11): 1418-1422.

30. Green LW. *Health Education Planning: A Diagnostic Approach.* Palo Alto: Mayfield Publishing Company; 1979.

31. Steve Danish, PhD, speaking on "Advanced Counseling Skills" at Annual ADA Convention, Orlando, FL, 1994.

32. Bloom BS, ed. *Taxonomy of Educational Objectives: The Classification of Educational Goals, Handbook 1: Cognitive Domain.* New York: David McKay Company; 1956.

33. Mazzuca SA. Does patient education in chronic disease have therapeutic value? *Journal of Chronic Disease*, 1982; 35(2): 521-529.

34. Hoffman SE. Planning for patient teaching based on learning theory. In: Smith CE, ed. *Patient Education: Nurses in Partnership with other Health Professionals.* Philadelphia: W.B. Saunders Company; 1987.

35. Snetselaar LG. *Nutrition Counseling Skills: Assessment, Treatment and Evaluation.* Rockville: Aspen Publications, 1989.

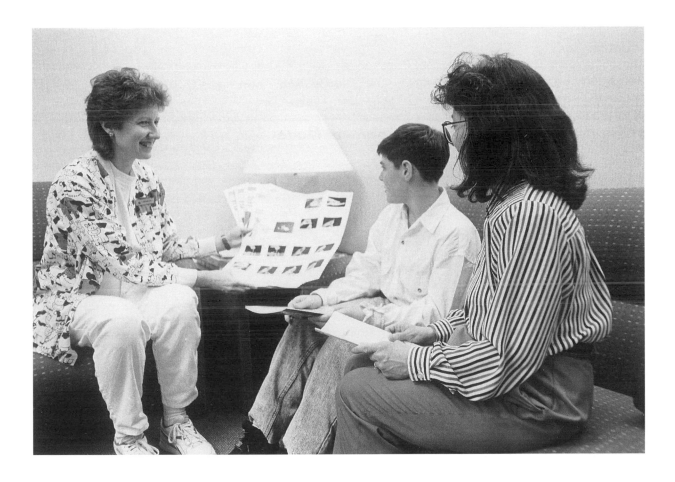

FOR YOUR INFORMATION

Personal Styles and Relationship Strategies

Ruth B. Fischer, MS, President, NutriSmart, Inc., Rochester, NY

Would you like to increase your credibility and compatibility with others? Would you like to know more about how others think and why they act as they do? Do you wish you were better able to empathize and communicate with others? Can you envision how these skills might be useful for you both personally and professionally? By taking some time to learn more about the concepts of personality development and personal style, you can learn to "read" others better.

Personality

Just as DNA provides a distinctive genetic framework for each individual, a person's personality provides a unique behavioral framework. A person's personality develops based upon the six major factors described in the Personality Development Model (Figure 2-1). (1)

FYI Figure 2-1 Personality Development Model

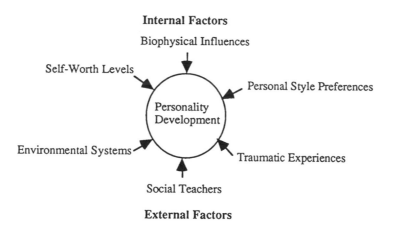

Internal Factors

Biophysical Influences

Self-Worth Levels

Personal Style Preferences

Personality Development

Environmental Systems

Traumatic Experiences

Social Teachers

External Factors

Used with permission. Copyright 1994, Robinson ET. *Why Aren't You More Like Me?* Amherst, MA: Human Resource Development; 1994.

The Personality Development Model divides factors into internal and external categories.

Internal Factors

Self-worth levels are the part of the personality that governs how a person feels about him or herself. It governs how you evaluate your behavior, appearance, feelings, thoughts and abilities. It can be influenced by what others say about you and whether you agree or disagree with what they say.

Those with **high** self-worth: (2)

- are less depressed
- evaluate their own performance more positively

- are less prone to addiction
- are more flexible
- think well of others
- are more persistent at difficult tasks
- take more personal responsibility
- are more likely to admit personal faults

Those with **low** self-worth: (2)

- expect to be rejected
- display little self-respect
- are more resistant to change
- take personal criticism poorly
- are less open with personal information
- suffer more from stress related illness

Biophysical Influences are all the biological and physical influences that affect you over your lifetime. Genetics, biochemical occurances, like puberty, pregnancy and aging, and illnesses all have an impact on your view of yourself.

Personal style preferences are the naturally occurring preferences you have that influence how you perceive, approach, and interact with information and situations. The next section focuses on this factor.

External Factors

Traumatic Experiences are any experiences that produce severe stress, whether physical or emotional. It can begin as a positive or negative event; the key is whether or not the experience leaves you feeling victimized. Different individuals will react differently to similar events. Such common events as birth of a child, divorce, promotion, job termination, and even falling off a bicycle, are examples of events that may affect your personality.

Social Teachers are the people who directly or indirectly provide posititve or negative influence on your personality development. These people, often referred to as role models, have lasting effects on thinking, personality, and behavior, and may include: parents, siblings, school teachers, religious leaders, friends, mentors, supervisors, authors, artists, and so on.

Environmental systems are any other form of experience not specifically covered in the other categories, including your social environment, community, cultural, ethnic, and religious influences. See Chapter 3 on multi-cultural influences for more detail.

After becoming better acquainted with what influences and contributes to personality development, it is much easier to appreciate the complexity of your own and your client's personalities. It is apparent why nutrition counselors: work hard to boast clients' feelings of self-worth; probe to discover the client's important behavioral and nutrition-related social teachers; identify traumatic food or body image experiences faced by their clients; and have become more interested in personal styles. Counselors use all of this information and their skills to build on clients' positive experiences and neutralize or retrain the negative ones.

EXAMINING PERSONAL STYLE

Becoming more comfortable with personal style will impact on your life, both personal and professional, through building skills to better communicate and lead others. Each person has a style of thinking, behaving, and interacting that is unique. This style acts as his or her anchor or systematic framework for viewing the world. These characteristics are grouped into four behavioral styles or personality dimensions. (3,4,5) Most people have a mixture of all four dimensions in their styles, but usually one and sometimes several styles dominate in fluencing behavior.

Although this tool is not designed as an in-depth psychological examination of human behavior, it provides a simple way of observing and understanding the differences in people through their behaviors. See Table 1 on the Four Types of Personality Style on page 40.

Flexibility

Knowing the different styles, their strengths and weaknesses, helps you quickly evaluate your clients' style in a counseling setting. You will be able to adapt how you present information—the pace and degree of detail, and how you speak in order to reduce communication barriers. People feel most comfortable in communicating and interacting from their style strengths. People tend to trust and cooperate with people who respond and relate to them in the same style

FYI Table 2-1   Four Types of Personality Style

(Self- | Contained)

DIRECTOR/ BEHAVIORAL
(Action)

General Orientation: Self-Contained and Direct

To tasks:	Wants results now
To people:	Seeks authority
To problems:	Tactical, strategic
To stress:	Doubles effort, will dictate, "If you can't stand the heat get out of the kitchen."
To time:	Future and present

Typical Strengths
Acts rapidly to get results
Is inventive and productive
Shows endurance under stress
Is driven to achieve goals
Can take authority boldly

Common Difficulties
Can be too forceful or impatient
Can often think their way is best
Can be insensitive to others
Can be manipulative or coercive
Can be lonely or fatigued

THINKER/ COGNITIVE
(Analysis)

General Orientation: Self-Contained and Indirect

To tasks:	Wants quality
To people:	Seeks security
To problems:	Analyzes data
To stress:	Withdraws, "I can't help you any further; do what you want." (5)
To time:	Past and future

Typical Strengths
Acts cautiously to avoid errors
Engages in critical analysis
Seeks to create a low stress climate
Slow, steady, methodical
Complies with authority, "show me" attitude

Common Difficulties
Can bog down in details
Can be too critical and finicky
Can be overly sensitive to feedback
Can seem to be lacking in courage
Can be too self-sufficient, alone

(Direct)   (Indirect)

SOCIALIZER/ AFFECTIVE
(Expressive)

General Orientation: Open and Direct

To tasks:	People come first
To people:	Seeks to influence
To problems:	Intuitive and creative
To stress:	Will confront it, "Listen you turkey I've taken your abuse long enough." (5)
To time:	Future and present

Typical Strengths
Spontaneous, gregarious
Acts creatively on intuition
Is sensitive to others' feelings
Is resilient in times of stress
Develops a network of contacts
Is often willing to help others

Common Difficulties
Can lose track of time
Can "overburn" and over-indulge
Can be too talkative
Can lose objectivity, be emotional
Can be self-oriented, self-assured

RELATER/ INTERPERSONAL
(Harmony)

General Orientation: Open and Indirect

To tasks:	Reliable performance
To people:	Seeks to help others
To problems:	Practical solutions
To stress:	Will submit, "OK, if that's the way you must have it, we'll try it." (5)
To time:	Present

Typical Strengths
Promotes harmony and balance
Is reliable and consistent
Tries to adapt to stress
Sees the obvious that others miss
Is often easy-going and warm
Supports and "actively" listens to others

Common Difficulties
Can be too slow to make decisions
Can Allow others to take advantage of them
Can become bitter if unappreciated
Can feel low in self-worth
Can be too dependent on others

(Open)

pattern. Being able to interact with others from their strengths shows flexibility or style-shifting on your part—changing to what makes the client feel comfortable instead of insisting that the client adapt to your style. Although this sounds easy to accomplish, practice will make you more adept at shifting your style to match your client's. See Table 2-2 on flexibility or style-shifting on page 42.

Openness

Cathcart and Alessandra describe openness as the readiness and willingness with which a person expresses emotions and enters into relationships. (5) It is the degree to which you reveal *your* feelings and thoughts and the degree you accept other people's expression of *their* thoughts and feelings.

Open people are animated and "open up" right away. They are easiest to work with in a counseling setting because you don't have to work as hard to draw out information. Nonverbal behaviors also show a person's openness such as frequent eye contact, hand and body gestures, changes in posture and facial expressions. (5) These people are more casual and flexible. They are not as specific in terms of numbers or specifics; it is not that important to them. Human relationships count heavily with these people.

Self-Contained people are just the opposite of an open person. Cathcart and Alessandra describe these people as taking a while to show warmth or become involved in relationships. They are task-oriented, well organized, and enjoy the planning process. They like structure and want to know the guidelines and procedures. They are on time and expect you to start your appointments on time. They are rational, logical, detail-oriented. Small talk is not needed with this person and they don't tell a lot of personal stories.

Directness

Another behavior dimension is directness. It shows how a person deals with information or situations. (5)

Direct people are fast-paced, assertive, competitive, dominant risk-takers who want results NOW!

Indirect people, on the other end of the scale, are slow-paced, unassertive, quiet, cooperative, and better listeners than direct individuals. They do not want to "rock the boat." They are nonconfrontational and will seek roundabout approaches.

HOW TO USE CHARTS

Using the descriptions for the four personal styles in Table 1 to help you identify your dominate personal style and those of your family members, friends, and a few colleagues or clients. It is helpful to think of the characteristics aligning themselves on two axis: open versus self-contained and direct and indirect. If you can't decide, asking three simple questions will help you place individuals into their dominant style.

1. "Is the person open or self-contained?"
2. "Is the person direct (fast-paced, assertive, risk-taker) or indirect (slower-paced, quiet, nonconfrontational)?"
3. "Is the person task-oriented (well-organized, detail-oriented, self-contained) or people-oriented (opens up easily, casual, flexible)?"

By plotting your answers, you can easily determine which is the person's strongest style dimension.

A person's dominate personal style is his or her natural communication comfort zone. It is important to remember that no style is better than another. Each style has its strengths and weaknesses. However, each style may be preferable in a given situation.

Learning how to be flexible in the use of style or style-shifting is an important skill to learn. For example, an entrepreneur may be very out-going and creative (characterized by the Socializer/Affective style), but is called upon to act concretely and decisively in a business situation (a Director/Behavioral quality). A more family-oriented example might be, if you are more of a Director/Behavioral style person, who likes quick decisions and direct confrontations, and your spouse has a Relater/Interpersonal style, communication barriers may develop in the relationship. Referring to Table 2-2, what are some of the approaches that would enhance communication and emotional stability in the relationship?

On Table2- 2, three sections under each style teach you what to avoid doing and what to do more. *You should avoid doing things on this list*: "Get most upset when others." *You should try to do more*: "Wants others to" and "Responds best to."

FYI Table 2-2   Flexibility or Style-Shifting

If your client is:	If your client is:
DIRECTOR/ BEHAVIORAL Extroverted	**THINKER/ COGNITIVE** Introverted

Needs	**Fears**	**Needs**	**Fears**
Achievement	Failure	Affirmation	Disapproval
Autonomy	Restriction	Understanding	Confusion
Power	Dependency	Order	Chaos
Rewards	Poverty	Perfection	Incompetence
Stimulation	Stagnation	Respect	Humiliation

Common Personal Characteristics

Abrupt	Determined	Accurate	Indecisive
Aggressive	Decisive	Analytical	Loyal
Bold	Domineering	Cautious	Organized
Competitive	Productive	Conscientious	Perceptive
Courageous	Restless	Critical	Perfectionist
Responsible	Self-reliant	Strict	Structured
Strong-minded	Tough	Theoretical	Unsociable
Unemotional		Worrisome	

Gets Most Upset When Others:

DIRECTOR/BEHAVIORAL	THINKER/COGNITIVE
Are too slow	Move ahead too quickly
Get in their way	Don't give them enough time
Talk too much	Are vague in their communication
Try to be in control	Don't appreciate their efforts
Waste time	Are too personal or emotional

Wants Others to:

DIRECTOR/BEHAVIORAL	THINKER/COGNITIVE
Give them summarized facts	Give them detailed information
Respect their judgment	Ask for their opinions
Support them to reach goals	Not interrupt their work
Cope with unwanted details	Treat them with respect
Cooperate with them	Do quality work the first time

Responds Best To:

DIRECTOR/BEHAVIORAL	THINKER/COGNITIVE
Direct, honest confrontations	Diplomatic, factual challenges
Logical, rational arguments	Arguments based on known facts
Fair, open competition	Freedom from competitive strain
An impersonal approach	Friendliness, not personal contact
Getting results quickly	Doing tasks well and completely

FYI Table 2-2   Flexibility or Style-Shifting (cont.)

If your client is:

SOCIALIZER/ AFFECTIVE
Extroverted

Needs	Fears
Acceptance	Rejection
Attention	Exclusion
Expression	Repression
Recreation	Boredom
Variety	Routine

Common Personal Characteristics

Appealing	Flexible
Compassionate	Friendly
Convincing	Impulsive
Creative	Intuitive
Enthusiastic	Loud
Open-minded	Restless
Talkative	Undisciplined
Unproductive	

Gets Most Upset When Others:
Are too task oriented
Confine them to one place
Are not interested in them
Compete for and win attention
Seem judgmental of them

Wants Others to:
Give them the opportunity to speak
Admire their achievements
Be influenced in some ways
Take care of details for them
Value their opinions

Responds Best To:
Being challenged in a kind way
An influencing sales approach
Enjoy competitions
Affection and personal contact
Having a good time

If your client is:

RELATER/ INTERPERSONAL
Introverted

Needs	Fears
Appreciation	Ungratefulness
Harmony	Conflict
Stability	Instability
Trust	Deception
Unity	Dissension

Common Personal Characteristics

Careful	Hard working
Calm	Lenient
Dependent	Likable
Faithful	Unassertive
Slow	Stubborn
Understanding	Warm
Shares feelings	Slow to act, relaxed
Relationship-oriented	

Gets Most Upset When Others:
Get angry, blow up or are mean
Demand that they change too quickly
Take advantage of their goodness
Are manipulative or unfair
Are judgmental of others

Wants Others To:
Make them feel like they belong
Appreciate them for their efforts
Be kind, considerate, thoughtful
Trust them with important tasks
Value them as persons

Responds Best To:
A gradual approach to challenging
A factual, practical approach
Comfortable, friendly times
Respecting their boundaries
Conventional, established ways

IN COUNSELING SITUATIONS
Director/ Behavioral
As a counselor, you support their goals and keep the relationship businesslike; if you disagree, argue facts; be precise, efficient; to influence decisions provide alternatives and probabilities of their success. *To motivate: provide options and clearly describe probabilities of success. (5)*

Direct confrontation with this type client or spouse of a client may win them over to your counseling strategy, rather than turn them away, especially if they have shown some reluctance to the counseling environment. These people respond well to directness, logic and respect for his or her judgment.

Thinker/ Cognitive
As a counselor, you support their organized, thoughtful approach; give researched facts in some detail; allow plenty of time for the consultation; encourage food records or nutrient analysis of what they are eating as a way to stay on top of their progress. These people are often perfectionists and highly organized and expect the same of you. Follow-up personal contact with a letter. *To motivate: appeal to their need to be accurate and logical; avoid gimmicks. (5)*

These people thrive on planning and will like detailed handouts. They like to be intellectually stimulated, but not overworked. They can be procrastinators and fear failure.

Socializer/ Affective
As a counselor, you support their ideas and dreams; don't argue; don't hurry discussion. You need to show interest in this person not just his or her nutritional problems. Let these type people tell you about their achievements and allow both of you to have a good time in the session. *To motivate: offer them incentives and testimonials. Let them brainstorm some strategies that will meet their need for change. Remember, it is easy for them to get side-tracked. (5)* These people like creative and interactive apppproaches to learning and problem-solving. They become easily bored and like new challenges.

Relater/ Interpersonal
As a counselor, you support their feelings; show personal interest; accurately explain objectives; when you disagree, discuss personal opinions and feelings; move along in an informal manner; provide assurances that actions or decisions will involve minimum risk. *To motivate: appeal to how it will make them and others feel better. These people like personal warmth and friendliness in relationships and enjoy sharing "war" stories.*

As a professional, applying the information learned from understanding style to foster credibility and empathy with others is appropriate and powerful. It should not be used for manipulate others, but for enhancing human relationships.

REFERENCES
1. Robinson ET. *Why Aren't You More Like Me?*. Amherst, MA: Human Resource Development Press, Inc; 1994.
2. Robinson ET. *Self Worth Inventory*. Abbotsford, BC, Canada: Consulting Resource Group International, Inc; 1990.
3. Anderson TD, Robinson ET. *Personal Style Indicator*. Abbotsford, BC, Canada: Consulting Resource Group International, Inc; 1988.
4. Anderson TD. *The Therapeutic Style Indicator*. Amherst, MA: Microtraining Assoc; 1987.
5. Cathcart J, Alessandra T. *Relationship Strategies*. Palo Alto, CA: Cathcart, Alessandra and Assoc; 1984. (Audiocassette program through Nightingale-Conant Corporation)

BALLARD STREET
By Jerry Van Amerongen

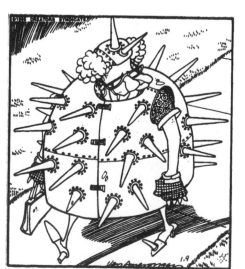

Harmony is no longer a part of Gloria's belief system.

(Used by permission Jerry Van Amerongen and Creators Syndicate.)

Appendix 2-A

Counseling the Pediatric Patient

Lyllis Ling, MS, RD, CDE, Director, Dept. of Nutr. Serv., The Children's Mercy Hospital, Kansas City, MO and Margo Murray Humenczuk, MA, RD, Clinical Nutrition Specialist

Counseling the pediatric patient presents a multitude of special situations requiring the dietetic practitioner to combine the skills of a detective, diagnostician, psychologist, advocate, educator, and nutritionist. In few other populations are the health beliefs, practices, and skills of so many intertwined and the role of the patient so varied. In this section we will attempt to present the range of counseling experiences encountered in a major pediatric hospital. The cases span the age range from newborn to adolescent on the brink of adulthood. Although many of the cases presented are those involving chronic medical and nutritional problems, the case study vignettes will provide examples which can easily be adapted for use in the acute care setting as well.

It is often valuable to use the books by Ellyn Satter as tools for families to develop appropriate feeding practices for their families. In *Child of Mine: Feeding with Love and Good Sense* (see end of article), Satter guides parents through principles of good nutrition and age appropriate feeding practices. *How to Get Your Kid to Eat . . .But Not Too Much* (full reference at the end) expands on the child-centered approach to feeding and helps parents determine the appropriate intervention, if any, for their child's feeding needs. Just as important, this book guides parents and practitioners in knowing when not to intervene. Satter emphasizes the parents' responsibility for deciding what is served and when it will be served and the child's responsibility for choosing how much will be consumed and even whether anything will be eaten. By using Satter's techniques, parents and practitioners can help children learn eating habits which will promote lifelong health and weight management.

Case Study

Many times the health beliefs of the parents and extended family affect the feeding practices employed and the acceptance of nutrition information from health care providers. These practices may not be initially apparent but can be discovered by taking time to do an in depth nutrition history. Maria was seen at the age of five months in the out patient craniofacial clinic for absent muscles in the left side of her face. She had gained 11.1 grams per day. The expected gain is 16.1 grams per day. The growth grid for linear growth was also beginning to flatten. Initially the mother reported the infant was taking 46 ounces of Enfamil with iron every three to four hours. She reported adding cereal to the bottle over the past month. Although Maria initially had difficulty drinking from a bottle she was doing well with a Haberman bottle as long as she was allowed to drink with her neck hyperextended or lying flat on her right side. When the dietitian observed the baby feeding she noticed the liquid in the bottle looked more like breastmilk than formula. When the parents were asked about the formula they explained the feeding was a Mexican health drink made from dry milk, cinnamon, sugar, and rice water. Since the parents believed this to be a health promoting supplement and baby preferred this to formula they had been using it for two feedings per day. The nutritionist acknowledged the taste preference and comfort value of traditional ethnic foods, then explained why the feeding was inappropriate for a child this age. The growth grid was reviewed with the parents with an accompanying discussion of appropriate types of protein and potential dangers of using the rice water mixture for a child of this age. The parents' belief in traditional foods to promote "health" were not initially evident but were affecting the growth and development of this child.

Case Study

Parents of children with a major medical problem or chronic illness may be resistant to change, especially if the child is currently doing well. Robert was born with a cleft palate and significant cardiac anomalies. He grew very little until after his cardiac surgery was performed at the age of three months. He was discharged on a 30 calorie per ounce formula at a volume calculated to promote catch up growth. Robert grew and gained well and started to develop some subcutaneous fat stores, especially in his extremities. His feeding of infant formula with macrolipid was delivered via gastrostomy feeding tube. When the child was seen in cleft palate clinic at the age of 11 months the dietitian advised an increase in the volume of the feeding to enable to child to continue to grow. Solid foods were reported to cause gagging and were deferred until a swallow study could be performed. The mother was very reluctant to change the volume of the feeding as the child was doing so well, and she had been cautioned about the dangers of obesity by her cardiologist. In order to get this mother to accept the change in formula, she needed to be reassured that she was right to be concerned about obesity and that the dietitian recognized the development of subcutaneous fat stores significantly changed her child's appearance which was inconsistent with the mother's perception of her child's body image. The mother verbally acknowledged that she herself was very thin and that although she knew her son's face remained very thin and that he was still less than 50% weight for height, she still feared the added weight would put undue stress on her child's heart. By contacting the cardiac dietitian the mother had seen previously for affirmation that the formula change was indeed appropriate, reviewing and explaining the child's growth on the growth grid, and encouraging the parent to voice her concerns, the change in formula was accepted.

Case Study

In working with children, it is very important to make the child the focus of attention. Even as early as four years of age, a child knows what he or she wants to eat. Shannon is a six-year old who has had insulin-dependent diabetes mellitus since she was 16 months old. As early as four years of age, she came to the clinic with her own list of questions about diet. Of course, her parents encouraged her to participate in the clinic visit by helping her remember the questions that had occurred since the previous visit. It is important to remember that sometimes a child wants to assume responsibility for his or her disease and at other times the child wants to have help. Asking the child if there are any changes to be made in the meal plan lets the child feel more in control of his or her care. Quite often the parent has never asked the child this question and can't answer for the child. If the child doesn't want to answer, he or she will defer to the parent.

Case Study

Charlie, age 12 years, was diagnosed with hypercalcuria and a diet was prescribed with low protein, low sodium, the RDA for calcium and high potassium. With so many nutrients being modified, it was important to get Charlie involved in the decision-making process early. A diet history and a list of favorite foods was obtained with the reassurance that he could help decide what changes would be made. To start on a positive note, he was given a list of potassium-rich foods and asked which ones he was willing to add to his regular food intake. Because he was using school breakfast and lunch program, the grandmother was asked to secure the appropriate school menus and to alert the cafeteria manager of Charlie's diet recommendations. In a follow-up conversation with the cafeteria manager, she was very willing to make additional fruits and lower-sodium cereals available.

Charlie wanted to be able to eat pizza when it was on the school menu and to have canned beef stew weekly. With a 1200 mg sodium limit, he learned to eat low-sodium foods at the other meals. Fortunately he became fascinated and challenged with reading labels and figuring out which food selections worked for him. He wasn't happy changing from canned to frozen vegetables until he realized how many more food choices he could have. A computer printout gave him more information about the nutrients in foods. Because he was bright, open to change, involved in developing new skills and had support from his grandmother and the school, he did well with his diet restrictions.

Flexible, Practical and Livable

Practitioners can promote acceptance of feeding changes by involving parents and children in making the changes, helping everyone involved to be as comfortable as possible with the feeding decisions, and by leaving themselves open to suggestion. People will best follow advice which makes sense to them. If the practitioner senses their advice is not being accepted, encourage the child or family to ask questions. "Help me to understand why you feel this is the best choice," is a good phrase to teach any child or family. The practitioner may want to ask, "This seems to me to be the best choice, but will this work for you?" This phrase can help bring out perceived disadvantages which the parent may otherwise be reluctant to share. Be alert to signs that parents or kids do not truly buy into the nutrition care plan. Children are frequently taught not to disagree with adults and may be reluctant to indicate a suggestion is not workable for them.

Case Study

Adolescence is a time of variable acceptance of advice from adults and of follow through on the part of the child. Developing a rapport may take time and an accepting attitude on the part of the nutritionist. Jackie is a child with spina bifida who has always had to consume a diet lower in calories than her peers to remain at an appropriate body weight. As she entered adolescence she started to gain too quickly and was counseled by a nutritionist. Jackie was able to make enough lifestyle changes to lose weight and receive praise from the medical team. At a later follow up appointment she was surprised to learn she had regained her lost weight and more. She was seen by a different nutritionist at this appointment as the previous practitioner had moved. Initially Jackie did not want to engage in conversation of any kind. Her grandmother answered for the teen at first but the dietitian continued to talk directly to Jackie, accepting all information without judgment, and acknowledging how common it is for people slip back into previous eating habits. The teen continued to give little or no response until the grandmother made a statement with which she strongly disagreed. At this point Jackie started to converse with the nutritionist and several mutually acceptable strategies were identified to help her get back on track again. What started out as an uncomfortable meeting evolved into a positive problem solving session with the teen as the leader and the grandparent and nutritionist taking supportive roles. The grandparents were able to change some established food preparation methods and work on portion control themselves which in turn assisted the adolescent in meeting her goals.

RESOURCES FOR FURTHER READING:

Satter E. *How to Get Your Kid to Eat...But Not Too Much*. Palo Alto, CA: Bull Publishing Co.; 1991.

Satter E. *Child of Mine: Feeding with Love and Good Sense*. Palo Alto, CA:Bull Publishing Co.; 1987.

Ivey AE, Ivey MB, Simek-Morgan L. *Counseling and Psychotherapy A Multicultural Perspective*. Boston: Allyn and Bacon, 1993.

Appendix 2-B

Family Counseling: The SHAPEDOWN Approach to Adolescent Weight Loss

Laurel M. Mellin, MA, RD, Director, Center for Child and Adolecent Obesity and Asst. Clinical Prof., Family and Community at the School of Med., Univ. of CA, San Francisco,CA.

(Adapted from Mellin LM, Frost L. Child and Adolescent Obesity: The Nurse Practitioner's Use of the SHAPEDOWN Method. J Ped Health Care: 6, 187-193, 1992.)

The prevalence of obesity in children and adolescents has increased 54% in children and 39% in adolescents in the last 20 years and now affects more than one in four young people. (1) Although family-based approaches to the problem recently have shown weight losses maintained at 5-year and 10-year follow-up, this care is unavailable in many communities because of an insufficient availability of trained providers.

Although diet, exercise, and behavioral strategies previously had proved ineffective in decreasing obesity in children and adolescents (2), using these modalities in a family-based approach has yielded significant and sustained decreases in relative weight. In 1983 researchers Brownell, Kelman, and Stunkard demonstrated the effectiveness of a family-based pediatric obesity intervention at l-year follow-up. (3) Subsequently, other studies substantiated these findings and showed that the maintenance of weight loss persisted (4, 5, 6) even at 10-year follow-up using this family approach.

The purposes of this article are to describe a method of care for obesity in children and adolescents in which dietitians can assume an important role and to suggest that widespread implementation of this method may have a significant impact on the prevalence and severity of obesity in the young. The program involves both preventive care by primary care providers and theraputic services by interdisciplinary pediatric obesity specialist teams.

THE SHAPEDOWN METHOD

The SHAPEDOWN program began to be developed at the University of California, San Francisco in 1979 as part of a Bureau of Maternal and Child Health interdisciplinary adolescent health training program. It is currently in its fifth edition. It has been standardized (7) and validated (6). Participation in SHAPEDOWN was associated with significant improvements in relative weight, weight-related behavior, depression, and knowledge. It has been disseminated to more than 400 clinical sites nationally.

Step I. Identification

Dietitians identify children and adolescents with disproportionate weight-for-height percentile ratios, especially those whose weight percentile has increased or who have a family history of obesity. They briefly assess the weight problem and develop a preventive care plan.

The identification of obesity alone can be a major contribution of the dietetic practitioner because a significant barrier to the primary prevention of the condition is the failure to identify the problem. Parental denial of the obesity is common. Health professionals may ignore the presence of obesity in children for a variety of reasons, most particularly, fear of identifying a problem they perceive as not treatable or anticipation of prompting negative feelings in the child or parent. In addition, clinicians may sense the family's denial of the problem and may be reluctant to confront it. Now that the long-term effectiveness of family-based approaches has been supported by research and that programs that are delivered by interdisciplinary pediatric obesity teams are more available in the community, concern about identifying an untreatable problem is less valid. Confronting a family's distress or denial about the problem of pediatric obesity is difficult but therapeutic. By doing so, the child who is teased at school about weight is no longer alone with the problem. The family's confusion, guilt, and fear about the problem can be directed toward acknowledging the child's experience and mobilizing to support the young person's weight management.

Techniques for stimulating parent awareness of the problem include reviewing their child's height and weight percentile during well child check-ups and eliciting their reactions to it, such as asking them ''Are you concerned about your child's weight?'' Should the parent of a severely obese child respond negatively, dietetic practitioners can express their concerns about the medical and psychosocial significance of the weight and discuss with the child and parent the consequences of delay in responding effectively to the problem. Negative sequelae of postponing intervention in childhood include less parental influence during adolescence, the entrenchment of unhealthful behaviors, the protraction of peer ridicule, and the rapid proliferation of adipocytes that accompanies puberty.

Step 2. Preventive Care

Obesity in children is complex and diverse in cause; however, the dietetic practitioner can conduct an initial brief assessment and develop a preventive care plan. During the review of systems, nurse practitioners can elicit a broad range of psychosocial, biomedical, and behavioral information and begin to uncover the possible origins of the weight problem: genetics, lifestyle, emotional overeating, the too-comfortable child, the too-uncomfortable child, and/or medical factors. The next step is to develop care plans that correspond to these factors (see Table 1).

FYI Table 1: Cause of Child and Adolescent Obesity: A Simplified Model for Preventive Counseling

CONTRIBUTOR	DESCRIPTION	TREATMENT/GOAL
Genetics	A genetic predisposition to fat deposition	Acceptance of one's genetic build
L ifestyle	High caloric density diet	Improve family food environment
	Inactivity	Increase physical activity
		Decrease television viewing
Emotional overeating	Hyperemotional state eating	Eat in response to hunger & satiety
		Improve communication skills
		Increase physical activity
Too-comfortable child	Indulged child	Decrease child's "comfort"
	Overprotective/permissive	Strengthen parental limit-setting practices
	Parent/child enmeshment	
Too-uncomfortable child	Deprived child, removed parents	Increase child's comfort
		Strengthen parental nurturing
	Parent/child disengagement	Improve parent/child communication
Medical problems	Conditions that affect obesity, diet or activity	Improve management of medical conditions

Typically more than one etiologic characteristic is present in a chlld or adolescent.

Genetics. Body build and, to some extent, body fatness are inherited. If the weight history of parents or grandparents indicates obesity, particularly childhood obesity, a genetic predisposition to obesity in the young person is likely. The goal of treatment, given this factor, is to increase the child's and family's acceptance of the young person's genetic body build. Because weight loss in the genetically obese may be biologically obstinate, failure to accept one's genetic body build can result in restrictive dieting, binge eating, psychological distress, and weight gain.

Lifestyle. Adipogenic behaviors (a high-fat diet, meal irregularity, and inactivity) can lead to the onset or exacerbation of obesity. Eliciting information about habitual food behaviors, such as the fat content of the milk consumed and obtaining a 24-hour dietary recall, can provide data on the caloric density of the diet and on meal regularity. Irregular eating patterns, particularly the obese pattern of skipping breakfast, skimping on lunch, and consuming large quantities of food in the afternoon and evening, can be detected. A 7-day recall of physical activity and information about the child's after-school activity is helpful. Treatment goals include decreasing the caloric density of the diet (for example, increasing consumption of nonfat milk products, fruits, vegetables, grains, and low fat meats and decreasing high-fat foods and added fat), consuming regular meals, increasing activity levels (for example, structured after-school sports, household chores, walking, and family physical activities), and decreasing sedentary activities such as television. (8)

Emotional Overeating. Disregarding internal cues of hunger and satiety can result in excessive adipogenesis. Eliciting information about the cues that trigger a child to eat when not hungry can be helpful in evaluating emotional overeating. Common cues are boredom, loneliness, sadness, and anger. The therapy for emotional overeating involves improving emotive states through psychological counseling and physical activity, increasing skills in emotionally expressive and assertive communication, substituting adaptive responses to difficult emotions, and learning to initiate and conclude eating in response to internal signs of hunger and satiety. Improving the quality of the diet and the quantity of food consumed are not primary goals but are expected to improve as the emotional overeating abates.

We teach families to express their needs, communicate, and request attention or help by saying:
1. **I need . . .**
2. **I feel . . .**
3. **Would you please . . .**

The Too-comfortable Child. The indulged child typically has overprotective, permissive parents. Parental expectations are low, and the child has too much power in the family. Often the child has a special place in the family, such as that of surrogate spouse. Parent-child enmeshment is common. The falseness of the relationship impairs parent-child intimacy, creating a sense of isolation in the child that excessive food, television, or reading diminish. In addition, the permissiveness is usually associated with indulgent food and inactivity behaviors. The treatment is to decrease the child's apparent but not actual comfort by altering the functioning of the family (for example, support one parent in separating from the child and the other in becoming more engaged and improving parental limit setting skills). Family therapy may be indicated in order to do this.

The Too-uncomfortable Child. Children who have been neglected or the victims of unusual stresses may respond to their difficult emotive responses with compulsive eating or excessive inactivity (for example, protracted television viewing or reading). The child often has a depressive affect or expressions of anger at one or both parents. The recommended treatment is to increase the child's comfort by improving family relationships and nurturing. Often psychotherapy or family therapy is required.

Medical Problems. A variety of medical problems can trigger the onset of obesity or contribute to its exacerbation. The mechanism most often induces inactivity; such conditions include congenital heart defects orthopedic problems, and exercise-induced asthma. Various medications, such as insulin and steroids, can stimulate weight gain. Treatment often focuses on improved management of the condition.

After discussing the probable factors with the young person and his or her parent, the dietetic practitioner provides them with the program books and directs them to the content that corresponds to the identified contributors to the problem. During the next three months, the family implements the intervention program, with or without periodic visits with the dietetic practitioner. At the three month follow-up visit, if insufficient progress has been made, the family may be referred to a SHAPEDOWN pediatric obesity specialist team. Indications that the guided self-care program is sufficient include an average weight loss of one-half to 1 pound per week for most young people. However, during periods of rapid growth in adolescence or for children or adolescents who had been rapidly gaining weight before the intervention, weight maintenance to a mean of one-half pound per week weight loss is sufficient. If progress with weight management is sufficient and the child or adolescent is satisfied with the guided self-care program and does not express interest in obtaining the services provided by a pediatric obesity specialist team, such as a more in-depth assessment and participating in more intensive individual and group care, then the continuation of the guided self-care program is appropriate.

Step 3. Comprehensive Assessment

When primary preventive interventions have not decreased or resolved the obesity, care by an interdisciplinary team specializing in pediatric obesity is indicated. This care involves a comprehensive, biopsychosocial assessment and includes the availability of a broad range of treatment options. Alternatives range from a group or individual application of the SHAPEDOWN program to managing the underlying causes of the obesity, such as medical, psychological, and family functioning factors before or instead of entering SHAPEDOWN.

In addition to the primary care role of dietitians described, dietetic practitioners function as members of interdisciplinary teams specializing in pediatric obesity care. The minimal disciplines represented on these teams are medicine, nutrition, mental health, and exercise. Often one or two team members deliver direct service and the remaining disciplines provide consultation.

Y.E.S. Assessment Instrument. The SHAPEDOWN method assists the dietetic practitioner in delivering truly interdisciplinary assessments without the resources required for all team members to assess each young person and family. This is done through the Youth Evaluation Scale (9), a computerized assessment instrument for eating disorders and obesity in children and adolescents. YES is composed of questionnaires for the youngsters and their parents that are compilations of standardized measures of a broad range of biopsychosocial variables related to weight and eating. As a result, for example, all children do not require assessment by a psychologist. Instead, YES provides several standardized measures of psychological functioning, so the dietitian can refer only those children whose YES results include abnormal scores on those tests.

To administer YES, the dietetic practitioner records on the questionnaires certain information obtained during a clinic visit: height, weight, triceps skin fold, fitness test results, blood pressure, waist-hip circumferences, and total serum cholesterol. The young person and parents complete the questionnaires and mail them to a central processing service. Several days later, the dietetic practitioner receives by mail from the processing service two YES reports, one for patient education and the other for the provider. The patient education report displays all the testing results including:

percent overweight	self-esteem	body fat patterning
anxiety	serum cholesterol	body image
blood pressure	physical fitness	weight management knowledge
lifestyle	family functionig	parental attitudes and behaviors
depression	motional overeating behaviors	parent-child communication

In addition, it evaluates the extent of the medical and psychosocial risks of the obesity. The provider report summarizes demographic, historic, and sensitive information (for example, sexual activity, substance use) for review by the dietetic practitioner.

On the second visit, the dietitian reviews the YES results with child/adolescent and parents to describe the extent of obesity, its medical and psychosocial risk, and potential contributors to its onset and exacerbation. With this information, the young person and family can identify their healthful characteristics and those characteristics that are not, which may be the focus of obesity intervention. For instance, Jack, a 14-year-old, learned through his YES assessment that his obesity was a medical risk because he was severely obese and had a central fat deposition pattern and family history of hypertension. The psychosocial disadvantage of his weight was significant because his self-esteem about his weight was low; he was ridiculed about his weight by peers. Correlates of his obesity were genetics, inactivity, emotional overeating, anxiety, poor knowledge of weight management, parental limit-setting deficits, an enmeshed relationship with his obese mother, and a disengaged relationship with his father who reportedly drank heavily. Those factors were explored as potential contributors to the problem.

The family develops a care plan that leads to individualized treatment. By the conclusion of the YES assessment, families have developed a care plan that is individualized according to the contributors to the problem and the medical and psychosocial risk of the obesity. Treatment plans range from other therapies (for example, family therapy, psychotherapy, medical treatment) to group obesity treatment. In Jack's case, the family was reluctant to identify the father's substance use as a problem. The provider suggested that family factors associated with substance problems can be major contributors to obesity in the child. The family elected to participate in the family-based teen SHAPEDOWN program. During the parent sessions, the father's substance-related cognitive difficulties were apparent; by the conclusion of the initial 10-week program, the father identified his substance use as a problem, and the family entered Alcoholics Anonymous programs. One of the most important benefits of this assessment and treatment process is that it often identifies problems underlying the obesity, based on standardized, computerized tests results. By doing so, families that could become stuck on the symptom (obesity) and scape-goating the child, often reframe the problem as related to family variables. Many families are surprisingly open to the computerized information and, in response to it, demonstrate a willingness to address the underlying disturbances.

FYI Table 2 SHAPEDOWN Children's Program Parent Guidelines

1. I understand clearly my child's weight, including its medical and psychosocial risks and the factors contributing to it.
2. I am aware of your feelings about my child's weight.
3. I let go of weightism and accept my child's natural body build.
4. I create a healthy but not depriving food environment at home.
5. I develop a family lifestyle that is physically active.
6. I structure an active and enriching lifestyle for my child that includes daily exercise.
7. I support each family member in openly and effectively expressing his or her feelings and needs.
8. I give my child direct messages that I accept and value him or her.
9. I set limits with my child and follow through consistently.
10. I am a good role model because I am improving my own weight, eating, or inactivity problems.

Step 4. Treatment

The orientation of SHAPEDOWN is to view obesity as a symptom with diverse biopsychosocial contributors and consequences. Rather than narrowly focusing on the excess adipose tissue, the program addresses the obesity within the context of the overall development of the child and in relation to the family and social systems as reflected in the parent guidelines (Table 2). Program goals are to normalize the child's or adolescent's weight within his or her genetic potential, to develop risk reduction diet and physical activity behaviors, and to facilitate the identification and treatment of psychosocial and biologic contributors to the problem.

The program is designed for children and adolescents aged 6 to 18 years and is comprised of workbooks and parent guides that are on four developmental levels (6 through 8 years, 9 through 10 years, 11 through 13 years, and 14 through 18 years), an instructor's guide, and support materials. The program can be applied in group sessions or in individual counseling. The duration of the initial group program is 10 weeks; it provides introductory training in SHAPEDOWN skills. Continuing care options include individual follow-up counseling and/or entering an Advanced SHAPEDOWN support group. The duration of care ranges from 3 months to several years.

FYI Table 3: The SHAPEDOWN Tasks

I solve my weight problem by accomplishing these tasks:

1. I love and value myself.
2. I accept my genetic body build.
3. I am aware of my feelings so I know what I need.
4. I recognize my needs and am committed to filling them.
5. I fill my life with pleasure from people and activities.
6. I create for myself a physically active lifestyle.
7. I eat when I am hungry and stop when I am satisfied, not full.
8. I choose a diet that is healthy but not depriving.
9. I connect with others by sharing with them my true feelings and thoughts.
10. I receive from others by asking them for what I need from them.
11. I say 'no' to people, places and things that aren't good for me.
12. I let go of things over which I have no control.

Copyright 1992, L Mellin

Training. Criteria that are designed to ensure a high quality of care have been established for becoming a provider. These criteria include:

a. delivery by an interdisciplinary team,
b. the completion of introductory (1-day) and advanced (3-day) pediatric obesity training by videotaped self-study course or by on-site course participation,
c. membership in the Center for Child and Adolescent Obesity (CAO) to receive clinical and research updates, and
d. the use of program materials and the avoidance of combining other treatments with SHAPEDOWN, specifically, restrictive diets or very low-calorie diet formulas. All costs are low. (Program and training information can be obtained from Balboa Publishing or Laurel Mellin—see reference at the end.)

Case Study

The following case study shows the four components of the SHAPEDOWN method. Rebecca, a 14-year-old, visited the dietitian who evaluated Rebecca's weight as above the 95th percentile, and her height at the 25th percentile, and identified the obesity (step 1). The dietetic practitioner began to provide preventive care with a brief assessment (step 2). Rebecca was asked if her weight was a concern. Rebecca responded that she hated her weight and burst into tears. At the conclusion of the interview, the dietitian concluded that this adolescent's obesity appeared to be related to emotional overeating and genetic factors. She described her impressions to Rebecca, and they identified the goals of accepting her genetic body build, eating when she was hungry and participating in an exercise program to decrease stress. Rebecca returned monthly for counseling with the support of program materials. Her parents did not participate in the sessions, although they received program materials.

At the three month follow-up visit, Rebecca had increased her physical activity but still engaged regularly in emotional overeating. She expressed an interest in a more intensive, group approach. The dietitian had become increasingly concerned that Rebecca may have a subclinical eating disorder. She referred the adolescent to the SHAPEDOWN interdisciplinary pediatric obesity specialist team.

Rebecca and her parents completed a YES assessment (step 3), which showed a middle adolescent with a pattern of emotional overeating and a genetic predisposition to obesity. Rebecca resembled her paternal grandmother, who was portly and large-framed. Rebecca's depression, anxiety and self-esteem scores were normal, and her family was functional. The obesity appeared to be secondary to genetic factors, conflict about body type, emotional overeating, inactivity, and lack of parenteral acceptance of the adolescent's weight. Rebecca was not bulimic.

The care plan involved a group program because Rebecca was in middle adolescence, a time when peer sameness is important. A group would allow her opportunities to be the same as others who were also struggling with accepting their body type. Moreover, it would provide structured parental support.

Rebecca enrolled in the group program (step 4) and learned to use stimulus control techniques (identifying the cues she used to start and stop eating and developing strategies for managing those cues) and binge prevention strategies (emotionally expressive communication, stress reduction techniques, physical activity) to control her eating. With support from her peers, she addressed the 12 SHAPEDOWN tasks of Adolescence (Table 3). Rebecca began exercising, a combination of walking to school, cheerleading, and aerobic classes. Slowly, she moved toward accepting her body build.

In the parent group, Rebecca's parents began to express their sadness about their daughter's body build and to come to terms with the possibility that Rebecca's body may always be somewhat rounded. This freed them to stop trying to control Rebecca's eating and weight, which, in turn, resulted in marked improvement in Rebecca's emotional overeating. After the 10-week group, Rebecca came to individual sessions bi-weekly for 5 months and achieved a moderate weight loss. Her emotional overeating subsided, and she became active in school sports. Rebecca's body image improved significantly. She had the option of participating in an ADVANCED SHAPEDOWN support group but did not feel the need for frequent sessions because weight and eating had receded as issues.

SUMMARY

Dietitians are uniquely qualified to take a leadership role in providing pediatric obesity care, which not only addresses the symptom of excessive body fat but also supports the strength of the family and the well being of the child. Although developing liaisons with other team members and acquiring additional training require effort, should dietitians take up the challenge and focus a portion of their clinical efforts on pediatric obesity care, the benefits to the health and well being of the obese young could be highly significant.

REFERENCES

1. Gortmaker SL, Dietz WH, Sobol AN, Wehler CA. Increasing pediatric obesity in the United States. *Am J of Diseases of Children*. 1987, 141: 205-215.
2. Coates T, Thorenson C. Treating obesity in children and adolescents: A review. *Am J of Pub Health*. 1978. 68: 143-148.
3. Brownell KD, Kelman JH, Stunkard AJ. Treatment of obese children with and without their mothers: Changes in weight and blood pressure. *Pediatrics*. 1983. 71: 515-523.
4. Epstein LH, Valoski A, Wing RR, McCurley J. Ten-year follow-up of behavior, family-based treatment for obese children. *J of Am Med Assn*. 1990. 265: 2519-2523.
5. Epstein LH, Wing RR, Koeske R, Valoski A. Long-term effects of family-based treatment of childhood obesity. *J of Consulting and Clinical Psychology*. 1987. 55: 91-95.
6. Mellin LM, Slinkard LA, Irwin CE. Adolescent obesity intervention:Validation of the SHAPEDOWN program. *J of Am Diet Assn*. 1987. 87: 333-337.
7. Mellin LM. *SHAPEDOWN Weight Management Program of Children and Adolescents* (5th ed.). San Anselmo, CA: Balboa Pub.; 1991.
8. Dietz WH, Gortmaker SL. Do we fatten our children at the television set? Obesity and television viewing in children and adolescents. *Pediatrics*. 1985. 75: 807-812.
9. Mellin LM. *The Young Evaluation Scale*. (2nd ed.). San Anselmo, CA: Balboa Pub.; 1987.

For SHAPEDOWN program information: Balboa Publishing, 11 Library Place, San Anselmo, CA 94960.

3

Empathy and Multicultural Sensitivity in Counseling

Rosie Gonzales, MS, RD, LD, Research Dietitian,
MD Anderson Cancer Center, Houston, TX

After reading this chapter, the reader will be able to:
- ☐ identify one's own cultural values and beliefs
- ☐ identify the single most important factor in achieving a successful counseling relationship
- ☐ identify culture-specific characteristics that may impact counseling strategies
- ☐ list communication skills that are of benefit in the multicultural setting

---

We live in a society which is growing more culturally diverse at a very rapid rate. According to U.S. Census projections, by the year 2000, more than one-third of the population will be racial and ethnic minorities, and by 2010 these population groups will become a numerical majority. (1) As our society continues to change and become more diverse, it is essential for the counseling professions to develop a multicultural perspective. (1) We must realize that every ethnic and racial group has a unique system of values and beliefs which influences behavior either directly or indirectly. This means that a "standard" approach to counseling is no longer appropriate. This standard system does not account for the differences and unique needs of diverse populations. In order to meet these needs, we must take responsibility in becoming competent and skilled in working with the culturally different client.

The purpose of this chapter is to help you develop an awareness, understanding, acceptance and the communication skills necessary for becoming a culturally skilled counselor. Although the chapter will discuss several ethnic groups, the goal is not to provide in-depth information about any one group. Rather, it is to make the reader aware of the uniqueness of each culture, and the importance of understanding the barriers to effective multicultural counseling and communication.

The Professional Standards Committee of the Association for Multicultural Counseling and Development produced a basic set of competencies and standards which define the attributes of a culturally skilled counselor. This chapter will outline these criteria by discussing three essential elements for effective multicultural counseling: 1) awareness of your own values and beliefs, 2) understanding and knowledge of the clients' world-view, and 3) acquiring appropriate communication skills. (1)

AWARENESS OF YOUR CULTURAL VALUES AND BELIEFS

Before you can work successfully with diverse populations, it is essential that you become aware of your own culture. It is not simply your ethnic heritage, but it is everything that influences what you believe, such as your religion, language, social status, level of education, gender, age, family, and ethnic group. (2) Dillard defines culture as the sharing of belief systems, behavioral styles, symbols, and attitudes within a social group. (3)

Depending on each person's background experiences and the culture to which he or she belongs, both the counselor and the client have a variety of characteristics and values that are brought to a counseling session. These influence communication and learning. Understanding your own set of values and beliefs will help you know your limitations and can assist you in becoming more aware of certain biases and prejudices which can affect your abilities as a multicultural counselor. In order to begin thinking about how your background may affect your abilities as a counselor, Ivey, et al. (4) suggests that you ask yourself the following questions:

1) What is your ethnic heritage?
2) Are you monocultural, bicultural, or more?
3) What messages do you receive from each racial or ethnic group you have listed?
4) How might your cultural messages affect your work as a counselor?

The last question will be most helpful in making you aware of your limitations as a multicultural counselor. For example, let's assume you view thinness as a desirable and healthy goal and cannot understand how anyone would want to be overweight. Now, assume that you are counseling a Native American client on diabetes, and part of your diabetic instruction promotes weight loss. However, your client considers thin people to be in poor health and overweight people to be very happy and healthy. If you are unable to accept your client's views about body size without mixing them with your own thoughts and feelings, there will be much conflict in the counseling session, and you can expect very little behavior change. Once you understand your own views, they must remain separate from those of your clients. It is not your job as a counselor to agree with your clients, but to empathetically understand their world-view without placing judgment. (4)

UNDERSTANDING AND KNOWLEDGE OF CLIENTS' WORLD-VIEW

You do not have to be of the same ethnic background as your client in order to provide effective counseling. (3) In the same respect, belonging to a particular ethnic group does not automatically make you a culturally skilled counselor. (1) To be most effective, you must be able to understand the world-view of your client and to communicate this understanding to him or her. (2) American Indians call this "walking in another man's moccasins," and psychotherapists describe this as an empathetic relationship. (4) Research suggests that establishing an empathetic relationship is the single most important and necessary factor to identify successful counseling. (2)

As implied in the previous section, knowledge about your clients' culture is a key attribute in the empathetic relationship. You do not need to know everything there is to know about their culture, but it is important to acquire basic knowledge of the cultural groups you will be counseling. Referring back to the example of the Native American diabetic, it would be helpful if you had some knowledge about this client's values, such as the traditional value of harmony with nature. This particular value may provide an incentive for weight loss, since some tribes consider overweight a condition which conflicts with the laws of nature. (5)

Ivey, et al. (4) suggests that a counselor working with diverse groups have knowledge in the following areas: specific knowledge about the client's culture; understanding of the sociological role of minorities in the U.S.; knowledge of the generic counseling literature; and knowledge of barriers that prevent minorities from using mental health services appropriately. The most common way to learn about your clients' culture is through books and audio/visual media. However, you will not fully understand them unless you also make a commitment to listen to and learn from other groups. (4) This may mean becoming actively involved with individuals from other cultural groups through friendships, projects, community events or social gatherings. (1)

Since it is beyond the scope of this chapter to discuss all ethnic groups in great detail, the author has outlined in Table 3-1 some of the fastest growing minority groups in the U.S. (1) The author has also summarized a few characteristics that she believes are important for you to understand. It should not be assumed, however, that every individual of a group has the same characteristics. Although clients belonging to one of the ethnic groups listed may share common values and experiences, you should keep in mind that acceptance and practice of these values will vary according to a client's acculturation, socialization and identification with the culture. Thus, the information in Table 3-1 should act only as a guide to enhance your awareness of cultural differences.

MULTICULTURAL COMMUNICATION SKILLS IN COUNSELING

Awareness, understanding, and knowledge of your clients' views as well as your own will be most effective if appropriate skills are also learned. (1,2) When there are cultural and ethnic differences between the counselor and the client some of the most important skills you can acquire are effective verbal and nonverbal communication skills. Without good communication between you and your client, little, if any, progress toward behavior change can be expected. (3) Understanding what your client says, how he or she says it, and even what he or she doesn't say, are all very important factors that a multicultural counselor must be aware of.

Language

If you have ever been in a foreign country, you know just how frustrating it is for clients for whom English is a second language. The ideal situation is for the counselor to be bilingual, but of course, this is not always possible. In order to overcome the language barrier with clients who have trouble expressing their thoughts in English, counselors need to have extra patience and time for a successful counseling relationship. Counselors must also avoid several language barriers to effective multicultural communication, such as the use of complex vocabulary, technical jargon, and an unnatural communication style. (5,6,8)

Table 3-1 Multicultural Characteristics and Values

ETHNIC GROUPS	HISPANICS *(Mexican-Americans)	BLACK AMERICANS	ASIAN AND PACIFIC AMERICANS *(Chinese Americans)
VALUES	o Identify with family, community, & ethnic group o Status/role in family & community	o Ethnic Identify o Kinship bonds o Strong work incentive o Strong religious ties o Adaptable family roles	o Obedience to parents o Respect for authority o Self-control of strong feelings o Praise of others o Individualism discouraged
FAMILY RELATIONSHIPS	o Highly valued o Primary source of emotional, physical, psychological support o Authority with eldest male	o Extended family in rural/urban communities o Important support system o Authority with mother or father	o Structure varies o Traditional stresses kinship with conformity to family & elders o Authority with mother or father o Obedience to parents very important
HEALTH BELIEFS	o Traditional include folk medical beliefs folk practitioners, & rituals o Hot-cold theory organizes illnesses	o Traditional include folk medicine: supernatural phenomena, herbal remedies o Family responsibility	o Yin-Yang philosophy: a hot-cold classification of foods & diseases with the goal being to create a balance of Yin and Yang.
DIETARY PRACTICES	o Staples are rice, beans, tortillas o Other common foods: chicken, lard, eggs, chili peppers, tomatoes, squash, & herb teas o Lactose intolerance common	o Similar to Anglo American o Depends on region o Lactose intolerance common	o Traditions ancient and complex o Diet associated with health & linked philosophically to other aspects of society. o Common foods: rice, wheat, pork, chicken, vegetables, eggs, soy, tea o Lactose intolerance common
RELIGIOUS ATTITUDES	o Illness is result of punishment from God o Medical care can not change outcome o Mexican-Catholic ideology	o Important part of culture o Church is central meeting place in the community o Illness viewed as punishment from God	o Traditionally Buddhist and Taoist o Many have adopted Western religions
LANGUAGE/ COMMUNICATION	o Spanish speaking o Several dialects among sub-cultural groups	o Varies from standard American English to several Black dialects o Nonverbal behavior important	o Many Chinese dialects

*Due to limited space, information is primarily for the following sub-cultural group (Sources: 3, 5, 6, 7, 8, 9, 10)

Table 3-1   Multicultural Characteristics and Values (cont.)

ETHNIC GROUPS	AMERICAN INDIANS	ARABS
VALUES	o Harmony with nature o Sharing/cooperation o Interdependence between individuals o Respect for another's rights o Noninterference with another's personal life o Peacefulness, strength, self-control, wisdom	o Family ties o Family name o Friendship o Hospitality
FAMILY RELATIONSHIPS	o Extended family with strong kinship ties o Respect opinions of family members o Important source of support o Respect elders	o Important source of support o Authority publicly seen with male, but decisions made mutually by male & female in private o Respect family and elders
HEALTH BELIEFS	o Closely tied with religion o Holistic concept of health care o Herbal remedies common o Sacred foods for tribal rituals common	o Depends on sub-culture o Folk medicine (Al-teb Al-shaebe) common with Beduins (desert Arabs) o Closely tied with religion o Female sees a female doctor and male sees a male doctor
DIETARY PRACTICES	o Varies across regions o Game, fish, fruits, berries, roots, & wild greens highly valued	o No pork o No alcohol-allowed in some countries o Cannot eat anything that eats meat: no animals with long nails or a sharp beak
RELIGIOUS ATTITUDES	o Based on belief in almighty Mother Earth o Illness seen as sign of disharmony with nature	o Islam is predominate religion o Follows Holy Koran o Religion is the government and sets the rules for living o Flexibility varies with country-Saudi Arabia most strict
LANGUAGE/ COMMUNICATION	o Numerous languages and dialects o Nonverbal communication important	o Numerous Arabic slangs, depending on country. o Basic Arabic spoken in countries close to Mediterranean o Body language/hand gestures very common o Direct eye contact considered disrespectful o Left hand or "non-dominant" hand considered dirty

(Sources: 3, 5, 6, 7, 8, 9, 10)
No reproduction without written permission from the author

It is important to speak slowly and clearly, use simple vocabulary, and avoid the use of slang, or technical jargon. However, you must also be cautious not to treat your clients as if they are uneducated. Just because your client does not speak English well, does not mean he or she is not intelligent. Adults should be treated as adults, just simplify the terminology. It is also important to know that your client may understand English much better than he or she can speak it, and he or she may be able to speak English better than he or she can read the language. (6)

The use of medical jargon and complex ideas can cause much confusion for multicultural clients. For example, there was the case of a doctor who gave a diagnosis of gastroenteritis for a ten year old Hispanic girl. However, the little girl's mother understood that her daughter had swallowed an entire cat. The doctor did not realize that "gastro" sounds like gato (cat) and "enteritis" like entero (whole) in Spanish. It is important to explain things in easy-to-understand language, and take time to be sure the client understands. (5)

Do not try to imitate an ethnic group's communication style, which is not natural for you. For example, a Black American client may find it patronizing and disrespectful if an Anglo-American counselor unnaturally tries to use Black slang in order to show that he or she understands the client. As one Black American once put it, "anyone who tries too hard to show that he understands Blacks doesn't understand them at all." (8) It is important to be yourself and act natural because clients can see through unnatural behavior.

It may be necessary to have an interpreter if you and the client do not speak the same language. Remember to allow more time for the counseling session and realize it may be difficult to translate certain concepts. Some tips for effective communication with an interpreter include the following:

- use a bilingual staff member, community volunteer, or adult family member or friend if a qualified interpreter is not available;
- be sure the interpreter understands the goals of the counseling session;
- maintain visual contact with the client and address him or her instead of the interpreter; and
- use language your interpreter can understand and translate. (6)

Rapport

When you begin a counseling session with a culturally different client, establishing rapport may take a little longer than you are accustomed to in your own culture, but it is very important. The goal is to earn your client's respect and trust by showing him or her that you understand his or her cultural viewpoint. (2) Using "small talk" is a good way to begin communication and to show genuine concern for the client. For example, you might start by saying, "How may I help you?" (6) Another important factor for developing rapport is patience. You must be able to patiently listen and observe your client carefully in order to learn about his or her communication patterns. (2)

Subject

It is important for the counselor to be aware that certain subjects may not be acceptable to discuss with some cultural groups. Some common areas which may be considered inappropriate for discussion include personal matters, family, spouses, and religious beliefs. (6) It is important to know which subjects may be unacceptable for your client. For example, in the Arab culture, family issues are inappropriate to talk about in a counseling session because they should be resolved within the family. Actually, families often meet with elders, not counselors, in the community to resolve problems. Coffee is often served during these meetings, and it is used as a symbol of peace. If the coffee is drunk, then the problems were resolved, but if the coffee is not drunk, then the situation remains unchanged. (10)

Positive Regard

Positive regard means that, as a counselor, you are able to find strengths and values in your clients even when their attitudes are opposite from your own. For example, let's assume you are counseling a client who has made several attempts to lose weight, but has failed. If you cannot find some positive attributes in this client, it will be very difficult for the client to change his or her behavior. (4) In this case, you might reinforce positive habits by pointing out some changes the client has already made. This should be done before you recommend other suggestions for losing weight. (5)

Body Language

Crossed arms or legs, tightened lips, and a firm handshake, are all forms of body language which may be interpreted differently depending on the culture. The use of the hands varies among the different cultural groups. For example, the Arab culture considers the left hand to be dirty and should not be used during a meal. Anglo-Americans prefer a firm handshake while Native Americans view this as a sign of aggression. (6,10) Hispanics are very affectionate and do not have a problem with touching. A light kiss on one or both cheeks is a very common greeting among most Hispanics. However, being touched by a stranger may be considered very inappropriate for many Asians. (6) It is important for the counselor to be aware of appropriate uses of body language within a cultural group. It may help to carefully observe the client and see how he or she interacts with you and others. When uncertain about body language, a counselor should be conservative, and remain natural, relaxed, and attentive. (2,6)

Eye Contact

In some cultures, direct eye contact is desired, but in other cultures it is not. For example, Black Americans do not find it necessary to always look at another person while talking. He or she may be actively involved in a conversation with another person while doing other things. A counselor who does not understand this style of communication may interpret this client as being uninterested or fearful. (8) Some groups, such as Asians, believe that staring is impolite. (6) The eyes are seen as a powerful tool by Native Americans and Arabs, and they do not make direct eye contact as a sign of respect for the speaker. (5,10) It is believed, among Arabs, that staring limits the speakers freedom to talk. (10) It is important to understand that the eyes are used by all cultures to convey meaning and understanding. (2) The key is to know what it means within a particular culture. It may help to observe your client during the counseling session, watching for signs of appropriate eye contact.

Distance

The most comfortable physical distance between the counselor and the client varies among cultures. If the counselor is not aware of the client's preference, he or she may offend the client. (3) Hispanics usually have a smaller personal space than Anglo-Americans, and Asians usually prefer the most distance from another person. (6) In the Arab culture, personal space depends on an individual's gender. Personal space is small when talking to someone of the same gender, but more distance is appropriate with someone of the opposite gender. (10) Asking the client to select where he or she would like to sit may help you determine the preferred distance for your client.

Emotions

Each culture has their own way of showing emotions. Hispanics are very expressive while Asians typically show very little expression. (11) Self-control of feelings is viewed by Asian Americans as a very important behavior. (3) Even within a culture, you might find much diversity. Some Indian tribes encourage expressing emotions while others discourage it. (11) The counselor must remember that visible signs of happiness, anger, or sorrow are not always an accurate indication of what a person is feeling. Therefore, you must be aware of the form of emotional expression shown by the groups you are counseling.

Silence

If your client is silent during the counseling session, it does not necessarily mean he or she is disinterested. For example, many Native Americans consider their personal lives and inner thoughts to be private and do not want to share them with others until those people are known and trusted. If a Native American client appears silent, it may seem as if she lacks interest, but actually she is carefully observing the counselor's behavior. (5) It is not uncommon for Arabs to spend up to 30 minutes together in silence. (6,10) The counselor must be prepared for silent pauses or even interruptions in the communication process with diverse cultures.

CONCLUSION

When counseling other cultural groups, it is important to realize that most people are very proud of their own values, customs, and behaviors, and they are unlikely to adopt new ideas or practices if they conflict with their current system of beliefs. Therefore, your goal as a counselor should be to work towards understanding and accepting your clients' cultures. Instead of trying to change their views and beliefs, you must build on them to develop a plan and promote positive change. To meet this challenge, counselors must develop a multicultural perspective and make an active commitment to becoming culturally competent and skilled in working with diverse populations.

This chapter outlined three essential elements which should serve as your criteria for working with racial and ethnic minorities:

- you must be aware of your own culture which will enable you to know your attitudes, values, biases, and limitations as a multicultural counselor;
- you must understand your clients' world-view by gaining knowledge and by taking a proactive role to learn about their culture;
- you must work towards developing culturally appropriate communication skills.

LEARNING ACTIVITIES

1. Spend some time writing down notes about your upbringing. Consider such factors as the socioeconomic environment, important events that occurred, your parents' philosophy about life and their aspirations for you, the importance of social and family traditions as well as the role food played in your growing up. Discuss your notes with a colleague. How does this information impact your food beliefs and practices today?
2. Observe/participate in meal preparation and the meal presentation in an ethnic setting different than your own. What do you observe? How does this insight change your approach to counseling an individual from this ethnic background? What impact does this insight have on your practice as a nutrition counselor?
3. Choose one ethnic group, and with a colleague, role-play a typical counseling session for a therapeutic diet modification (e.g. weight loss, low cholesterol). What skills and/or knowledge must you bring to the counseling session? Evaluate your counseling skills after the role-play. What were your strengths? What areas can you improve on?

REFERENCES

1. Sue DW, Arredondo P, McDavis RJ. Multicultural counseling competencies and standards: a call to the profession. *J Counsel Devt.* 1992; 70:477-486.
2. Pedersen PB, Ivey A. *Culture-Centered Counseling and Interviewing Skills: A Practical Guide.* Westport, CT: Praeger Publishers; 1993.
3. Dillard JM. *Multicultural Counseling.* Chicago, IL: NelsonHall Publishers; 1983.
4. Ivey AE, Ivey MB, Simek-Morgan L. *Counseling and Psychotherapy: A Multicultural Perspective.* Boston, MA: Allyn and Bacon; 1993.
5. *Nutrition Education for Native Americans: A Guide for Nutrition Educators.* US Government Printing Office, Washington, DC: US Dept of Agriculture, Food and Nutrition Service; Sept 1984. FNS-249.
6. *Cross-Cultural Counseling: A guide for Nutrition and Health Counselors.* US Government Printing Office, Washington, DC: US Dept of Health and Human Services; May 1990. FNS-250.
7. *Ethnic and Regional Food Practices Series: Mexican American Food Practices, Customs, and Holidays.* Chicago, IL: Diabetes Care and Education Dietetic Practice Group of The American Dietetic Association.;1989.
8. Sue DW. *Counseling the Culturally Different.* NewYork: John Wiley & Sons, Inc; 1981.
9. *Southeast Asian American Food Habits.* US Government Printing Office, Washington, DC: US Dept of Agriculture, Food and Nutrition Service; Sept 1980. FNS-225.
10. In conversation with Tariq Bakri AlAbbassi, BA. November 22, 1994.
11. *Culture-bound and Sensory Barriers to Communication with Patients: Strategies and Resources for Health Education.* Atlanta, GA: US Dept of Health and Human Services, Centers for Disease Control, Center for Health Promotion and Education; 1982. DHHS (PHS) publication 99-1572.

4

Empowerment and Weight Issues: Using the Feminist Therapy Perspective

Monica A. Dixon, MS, RD, President, Women Empowerment,
Author, Love the Body You Were Born With!

After reading this chapter, the reader will be able to:
- ☐ identify two major assumptions in counseling women using feminist theory
- ☐ describe counseling issues related to external pressures that may affect the nutrition habits of women
- ☐ identify "stuckness" in counseling a client and describe appropriate methods to address the issue

---

INTRODUCTION

In private practice, nutrition therapists counsel more women clients than men, more women with eating disorders, and a disproportionate number of clients with obesity as a primary or secondary diagnosis. As mentioned earlier in this book, the major counseling therapies commonly used were all developed by white men of Northern European heritage. Because of the limitations of their orientations, new types of therapy have emerged to better accommodate and match the needs of other segments of the population. Feminist therapy is one of the more recent therapies to evolve. It is typified by a close counselor-advocate/ client relationship, bolstering a person's self-image, and empowerment as three of its basic tenets. As counseling in general becomes more relationship-oriented, this therapy does not seem so novel as it once did. Now that traditional gender roles are less well-defined and men face many of the same pressures as women like weight biases, this type of therapy has broader application.

WOMEN AND WEIGHT ISSUES

Few Americans eat any more simply in response to hunger. We eat because the clock deems it is time, dinner is ready, we really SHOULD have that glass of milk, our friend offers us a "bite" of a new dessert, the special included "all you could eat," or the hot cookies just came from the oven.

Quietly lurking beneath our "land of plenty" hide many complicated and emotional issues involving food, dieting and feelings about one's body. The prescription of a 1400 calorie diet to an overweight person is seldom a sufficient nor effective method in attaining success in their weight loss goals. Adherence to the dietary regimen becomes difficult if not impossible for many clients in light of other more pressing needs they have that may not be getting resolved. The exploration of these needs and feelings in the nutrition counseling session can help increase the chances of success for the client, yet will demand the keenest of counseling skills.

Dietitians may feel uncomfortable or unqualified to encounter issues besides food with a client, even though these issues may be deeply woven and inextricable parts of their clients eating behaviors. Although there are areas that dietitians are not qualified to enter into in the counseling session, insight into the tenets of feminist psychology, enhancement of counseling skills and increased confidence in one's intuitive nature to determine acceptable counseling limits all can assist in empowering the client for greater success.

The first step in separating complicated weight issues with women is the perspective gained when viewing clients through a feminist view of psychology that praises the feminine in all women and does not stereotype them under the male model of psychological thought. Women have an entirely different set of life experiences from men, therefore, adopting a feminist perspective in counseling is an essential first step in empowering female clients. Feminist therapy (1) may be characterized as allowing clients to determine their own destinies without the construction of culturally prescribed sex-role stereotypes based upon assumed biological differences. This approach attempts to work toward equality in personal power between females and males. It allows women the space and skills to design a personal vision for their lives that is grounded in their unique and individual needs.

A feminist perspective of women's weight issues is essential if we are to move away from the ineffective "blaming-the-victim" approach, the endless behavioral modification treatments or the "deep-rooted psychological problems of the obese" perspective. The feminist viewpoint insists that those painful personal experiences arise from the social setting into which females are born, and within which they develop to become adult women. The fact that compulsive eating and eating disorders are overwhelmingly a woman's problem suggests that it has less to do with individual experiences and more to do with the social context in which women live their lives.

GUIDING ASSUMPTIONS OF FEMINIST THERAPY
First Assumption: Look To The Environment

There are two guiding assumptions offered by feminist therapy that closely relate to women's weight issues. The first of these is that *the primary source of women's pathology is social, not personal; external, not internal.* (2) This does not discount the woman's role and responsibility in the choices she makes as an adult in relationships, career, and so on. In your counseling, seek to be constantly aware of external forces that have brought the client to you. How has this woman's life been influenced by the social context she lives in? What external forces are influencing the decisions she has made? How independent or dependent is this woman in the context of her daily life? How connected is this woman to those passions that drive her life, offer her purpose and reason for living and provide the foundations of her existence?

External pressures to conform to the cultural model. The cultural worship of thinness in America is a significant external force on women and can hold enormous power for many. Although this value is external, it has been internalized by many American women, as is evidenced by the sky rocketing of eating disorders and obsessive dieting. (3) How many of us have seen clients who come for weight loss, yet are not considered obese by medical standards? Or clients who want to lose 10 pounds only for their class reunion or a big party coming up? Recognition and discussion of this power in the counseling session is an important first step in setting the stage for further growth for the client. There are several methods of doing this:

1) Ask the client to go back to previous stages in her life and describe the feelings she had about her body. How did she feel as a child? What types of messages did she receive about her growing body? What types of comments does she remember hearing about her body during puberty? What were the feelings she had about food and her relationship with it? How did her feelings about her body and food affect her social relationships as she grew into adulthood?

2) Help her to identify where she received the messages about how much she should weigh. Was it her parents? Her physician? A boyfriend or husband? Her girlfriends? Or was the magical number one she pulled from a hat? Have different individuals had varying effects on her weight goals throughout the years? Identifying where her weight goals have come from can aid her in beginning to see how external goals have been determined for her by others.

3) Gather a weight history from the client during the initial assessment. Find out her weight at high school graduation, during college or her early years and before and after child birth if she has children. Search for a specific picture of how the natural female life cycle has altered both her weight and her perceptions of it.

4) Have her identify a time in her life when she was most pleased with her weight, felt comfortable, happy and relatively healthy. Is this weight realistic for her now? What types of things did she have to do to maintain that weight and is she willing to do them again?

5) Ask her for specific reasons she is pursuing nutrition counseling at this time. Have her identify why she feels the time is right for her, especially if prior attempts at lifestyle change have not been remarkably successful. What factors in her life have changed that will make it work for her now? This helps to begin to put the responsibility on the client for the changes she will make in future sessions with you.

These questions and explorations can help the client to identify an internal goal that she may be happier with than an external goal that may have been influenced by someone else. She can also separate the "shoulds" regarding weight from a healthy and individual weight goal. They can also help you assess her readiness at this point to make lifestyle changes. Too often, dietitians feel obligated to continue with the counseling process, even when they have a "gut feeling" or sometimes even obvious evidence that the client is not ready to adopt the changes being recommended. Perhaps the client is initiating counseling for reasons related to external pressures to change their weight without having thought through her own preferences first. Gathering this information during the initial session can help both the counselor and client save valuable time, money and effort by assessing direction or desires clearly at the outset.

External forces to conform to cultural stereotypes. Social forces play other important roles in women's lives besides their view of how they should look and weigh. It is difficult if not impossible to get a woman to begin an exercise program if she is the prime provider of care for four young children or if she bears the burden of all the housework. It becomes important for success in the weight management process to help the woman construct a view of her present reality that will help her in defining and working toward her goals. In addition to acquiring the requisite dietary history/assessment, gather information from the woman so you can "mentally" draw a picture of her life.

1) Ask her to describe a typical day. What does she do? What responsibilities does she have? How does she spend her time?

2) Ask her about additional responsibilities. What committees does she serve on, groups she volunteers with or other situations in her life that occupy her time. This will help you begin to view her life as a complete picture and aid her in designing realistic goals that will be successful within her own framework.

3) What type of things is she doing she doesn't necessarily enjoy? Are there responsibilities she may give up in favor of completing her lifestyle and health goals?

Gathering this information will help you determine how realistic are both her weight change and personal goals. You will also gain a sense of her readiness to alter her life with the guidance you have to offer.

External forces and "stuckness" in women's lives. For many women, being caught in the trap of "to-day" and the stress of everyday life does not afford the opportunity to look to the future and envision where the treadmill of life is taking them. The term "stuckness" is a highly descriptive term coined by Fritz Perls (4) to describe the opposite of "intentionality," or purpose and direction in life. Other words used to describe "stuckness" are immobility, inability to achieve goals or limited life script. The nutrition counselor using advanced level skills will be able to help the client recognize "stuckness" and enable her to take the steps necessary to move on. Often, clients will come to the nutrition counselor because they are stuck with old eating habits, old ways of seeing their body or grown tiresome of "yo-yo" dieting and seek intentionality in their lifestyle habits.

Begin by asking the woman to draw you a mental picture of where she would like to be in five years. What will she look like? Who will she socialize with? Where will she live? How will she spend her days? What will she do for leisure? What type of work will she do? Allow her to tap into her creative powers to draw this vision. Let her relax and her thoughts flow. Do not interrupt her nor judge her. Seldom are we allowed the safety of being able to "dream." You are there to listen.

Some clients will have a very difficult time with this exercise. They may respond, "Well, gee, I never really thought about it" or "I have absolutely no idea!" Clients such as these are clearly manifesting their "stuckness" in life and are perfect candidates for help in broadening their vision of the future. Urge her on. Encourage her to begin to identify thoughts she may only have remotely sketched out for her future, such as, "I often think about returning to night school to finish my degree," or, "I would love to take a dance class and be involved in a dance group." The main goal is to allow her "mind wander" to what could be in her future. The external pressures felt by many women in our society do not always allow their thought processes to think about the bigger picture.

This exercise can be used in a variety of ways. I have often found it extremely helpful when working with an eating disordered client who may be amenorrheic or so caught up in binge/purge or dieting cycles that she can't find her way out. "How will you get from not menstruating to birthing the children you dream about?" or, "How might you graduate from college if you can't go to your classes because of your laxative use?" It is also helpful in allowing your client to begin to free herself from what her external circumstances may have dictated she follow, such as family and friends' expectations, which may not necessarily mesh with the goals your client has dreamed of pursuing.

It is important to pay serious consideration to the incredible amount of energy continued dieting demands from a woman. Constantly thinking about what to eat or not eat, when and how much to exercise, counting calories and fat grams, reading diet books and beating themselves up over their failure to have the perfect body all combine to drain a woman's soul. With weight loss maintenance recidivism rates nearing 98%, the majority of women are squandering valuable internal resources on unattainable externally defined goals. Attention to this in the nutrition counseling session can help women invest their personal resources to work toward a healthy balance of mind, body and spirit.

Counseling Skills Necessary in Changing the Paradigms

Helping a client draw a road map to their future goals requires some advanced level counseling skills. These include:

1) Observe your clients' nonverbal behavior. Watch for indicators of discomfort, as you may be treading on areas that are very sensitive to the client. Is the client crossing her arms in front of her to fend you off, or leaning toward you indicating excitement about the ideas? What kinds of expressions are on her face? Use the clients' comments to provide cues for the direction of your future questioning.

2) Note the clients' verbal behavior. Does the client sound angry and resentful when discussing her plans for the future, or excited and determined? Does she express anger at others in her life? Regrets? Happiness? The counseling skill of active listening is one of the most important. Hear what your client has to say, not just what you want her to say. Our world would be better place if more people really listened to others.

3) Your most important skill will be determining client discrepancies. Watch for incongruities, mixed messages, contradiction, and conflict throughout the interview. An effective counselor will be able to identify these discrepancies, to name them appropriately, and when appropriate, to feed them back to the client. These discrepancies may be between nonverbal behaviors (client is laughing while describing the total sense of powerlessness she feels about dieting), between two statements (client says she really wants to be thinner, but cannot give up any type of high-fat foods), between what clients say and what they do (client says she wants to lose weight, but continually misses appointments), or between statements and nonverbal behavior (client says she loves low-calorie foods, but hangs her head and looks at the floor while she talks about them). They may also represent a conflict between people or between a client and a situation (client says her family has attempted to enforce a diet on her since she was 10).

As these examples demonstrate, incongruity is common in the nutrition counseling process. Using confrontational skills appropriately can help move your client toward intentionality. While all counseling skills are concerned with development, it is the confrontation of these discrepancies that acts as the lever for the activation of human potential. It is actually a combination of skills such as open-ended questioning, confrontation and feedback that often results in a client's examination of core issues. With some clients, it may be adequate simply to identify and label the incongruity with the client. Focus on the elements of the incongruity, and not the person. Often the simple question, "How do you put these two together?" will lead a client to begin thinking about her inconsistency and possible resolution.

If this is not effective, you may need to move to summarizing the incongruity for the client. "Mrs. Jones, on the one hand you say that you really wish to lose weight, but on the other hand you say you will not eat low-fat foods" or, "Jennifer, you say that you really want to start changing your diet, but each week you come without having done your food records." Follow this with, "How does that fit for you?" Many clients are unaware of their incongruities and mixed messages; pointing them out gently but firmly can be extremely beneficial to them. For some clients, even your summarization's will be inadequate to help them recognize their inconsistencies, and only your repeated disclosure of the discrepancy over time will help them move away from denial of the problem and accept responsibility.

The Road Map to Change

Now that you have gathered your data regarding your client's perceptions of her weight, her feelings toward her goals and identified any discrepancies she may have, it is time to move her from here to there. The next step in this process is to help the client identify her resources, both external and internal. Resources can be defined as anything that will be helpful to the client in attempting to work toward her goals. It is also important to identify those forces that will hold her back or act as barriers to her goals.

Suppose that the vision your client has created involves having a healthy body one year from now that she feels proud of, buys nice clothes for and treats with respect. What type of resources will help her get there? Does she need money to join her local exercise club? Does she need to buy a set of running shoes? Does she need to go to the library and check books out about exercise programs or meet with an exercise physiologist? Does she have friends who will exercise with her? Is she the tenacious type, who will be determined to follow her goal? Does she need someone to watch the children while she is gone? Each resource that the two of you can help her identify will move her closer to her goals. Many women aren't accustomed to thinking about what they have going for them in their personal inventory.

Your client will face obstacles to her success. What types of forces will work against her? Does her best friend offer her donuts every time she attempts to begin exercising? Will her partner support her or sabotage her efforts? Does she procrastinate when given a difficult task? Is her employer accommodating to a schedule change? Is there money available to buy the things she might need to get started? If not, how will she find the money?

Helping your client identify her resources and assets will demand creativity on both your parts. Helping her to change the paradigms of thinking that have restricted her ability to see things from a variety of different perspectives will surely stretch your imagination. The more well thought out the barriers and assets are that she will meet in her endeavors, the greater her chances for success, as she will meet few obstacles she has not already thought out in her session with you.

In the goal setting and resource inventory stages with the client, it is important to allow the client to develop her own ideas. She will be unable to follow through with anything that is externally determined for her by anyone else, and MUST own the solutions to her problems. Some dietitians I have worked with often become frustrated and upset because the course of action for a client is so obviously clear "why don't they just do it?" Your position is to empower their process, not design it. The road map must be drawn and owned by the client. If not, chances for success are slim. Solving her concerns and giving her solutions only makes you guilty of exactly that which you are attempting to disassemble; pressure to conform to an external model she must live under.

Following are key concepts for an empowerment-based practice, no matter the diagnosis or gender of the client: (5)

- emphasis on the whole person
- setting negotiated goals
- transference of decision-making and leadership

- promotion of the person's inherent drive towards health and wellness
- education for informed choices about treatment options
- patient selection of learning needs
- self-generation of problems and solutions
- treatment plans viewed as ongoing experiments

Case Study

The following is a scenario that may help you in visualizing this process at work:

Audrey is a 19-year-old client who presents with symptoms of Anorexia Nervosa. She is a physician referral, due to recent weight loss and onset of amenorrhea, but has not yet been given the DSM diagnosis of Anorexia Nervosa. Audrey insists that she is eating well and is getting plenty of food. The diet history you gather reflects otherwise. Her protein and calorie intake are exceedingly low for her height and weight. Throughout your first and second session with Audrey, she continues to insist that she is eating adequate calories and does not need to eat anymore. As you develop a rapport with her, you sense that there are incongruities in her message, and that in fact she is experiencing significant hunger pains, dizziness and apathy.

Audrey: I'm really feeling better than I ever have in my life. I really don't understand why everyone is making such a fuss. (Client states denial)

Counselor: You say you are feeling quite good, yet last week you complained about feeling tired and unable to get through your work day. How does that fit for you? (Counselor points out discrepancy in information)

Audrey: Well, that is just sometimes. I usually feel almost euphoric and in control of my life. (Client again denies a problem)

Counselor: Tell me how you feel in control of your life. (Counselor uses open-ended question to gather more information)

Audrey: I am strong and I can make my own decisions about the food I eat. No one else can tell me what to do. My mom used to always try to make me eat certain foods and now I can do what I want to. (Client seeking identity through resistance)

Counselor: What other kinds of things do you want to do? (Counselor works toward moving client out of current paradigm of "stuckness" and looking at future).

Audrey: I'd like to get into college eventually when I save enough money and I would like to get married and I suppose have some kids. (Client identifies some disconnected, not clearly defined goals).

Counselor: How will you save enough money to get into college if you are missing so much work because you are weak and tired now? (Counselor identifies discrepancy between verbal statement and actions)

Audrey: Well, I suppose sometimes I don't feel I have the energy I used to, but that really has more to do with my heavy schedule, don't you think? (Client is beginning to internalize the discrepancies and seeks counselors approval)

Counselor: It has more to do with the lack of calories your body is getting to do the things you need to do today. What you eat today and tomorrow and the next day not only fuels your body to have the energy to do your daily activities, but it also affects your attitude and the way your body will perform in the future. Your menstrual cycle will not return until you provide your body enough calories for the rest of its activities, and you will probably not have children until your menstrual cycle returns. You will not have the strength to complete your studies until you eat enough calories. Only you can make the changes in your diet that will result in a healthy future for you. (Counselor confronts client with reality of her actions and behaviors and focuses responsibility on client)

Audrey: I guess I never really thought about those things. But I am pretty afraid. And what kind of food can I eat that will not make me "blimp out"? (Client identifies fear of change, but ability to begin the process)

At this point, the counselor has confronted Audrey with her inconsistencies in her statements, helped her identify a vision for her future that is incongruent with her activities today, and helped increase Audrey's awareness that the responsibility rests on her to change. Obviously, a client of this background would be much more complicated to work with, and results would never be this quick, but the confrontation and movement toward intentionality process has begun.

The Second Guiding Assumption: Each Individual Must Still Take Responsibility

Feminist therapy includes viewing a woman in the social context within which she lives her life, and using that information to help her move towards creating her own vision of the future void of the "stuckness" she may have exhibited. The second assumption of feminist therapy important for the nutrition counselor is that *the focus on environmental stress as a major source of pathology is not used as an avenue of escape from individual responsibility.* (2) Each individual, regardless of her social condition, is responsible for making the changes necessary within her own life. No one else, including the counselor, can maintain that responsibility. Feminist therapy believes that women must be free to make their own decisions. In many cases this may become work that is beyond the scope of the nutrition counselor, yet there are avenues that can begin the process necessary to help women regain power and control over their own lives in ways appropriate in the nutrition counseling session.

Since women are expected to devote enormous energy to the lives of others, often the boundaries between their own lives and the lives of those close to them may become blurred. Molding their lives to others' concerns, feeding others, or not knowing how to make time in their lives for themselves are frequent issues for women. A mother is constantly at the beck and call of others; everyone else's needs become more important. This becomes pertinent in many weight loss counseling sessions as the woman returns week after week never having found the time to complete the tasks you have jointly agreed upon. She may be having difficulty defining her needs as important in the greater family picture.

Although this may be an appropriate time for the use of the confrontation skills discussed earlier, it is also an appropriate time for aiding her in learning to set her own boundaries. For some women, this can be unfamiliar territory they are treading into. She must begin by first determining what exactly is hers in terms of time, goals and resources. Assist her in defining limits. What block of time during the day can she set aside only for herself? What must she give up in order to find the time? What benefits would she gain? Who else can she delegate responsibility to? Where does she begin and others end? In my many years of counseling women, I have found this by far the most difficult task, primarily because of societal expectations about what the "ideal" woman should be and lack of learning in the early years that our identities and needs are separate and unique from others.

Help the woman explore her uniqueness and individuality. Ask her what traits she has that make her different from others in her life. How can she use those traits as assets to alter her lifestyle and pursue her own goals? Give her homework where she establishes her needs with significant others in her life and discusses how they can be of help in her new lifestyle changes. Clients have had great success with a small assignment I have them do each morning as they gear up for the day. Answer on a sheet of paper the questions, "Today I want . . ." and "Today I feel . . ." Many of your clients will say, "I want . . .WHAT??? I don't understand what you mean." You will need to teach them how to identify their wants in life. Do they want to go out to lunch with their nagging friend? Do they want to take a short nap today to catch up on lost sleep? Do they want to clean the house, or would a walk in the woods be more desirable? The same happens with "Today I feel . . ." Help them learn to pinpoint their feelings each day. A wonderful quote I use from Alice Koller's book, *An Unknown Woman* (6) is, "Is this thing I'm doing worth being alive for?"

Most importantly, how much better could she meet the needs of others in her life if she allotted time for her own needs first? A garden left unattended in the hot sun proffers no fruit. Women, much like gardens, need frequent water, healthy, nourishing food, fresh air and adequate rest. Nurturing our own needs first and taking great care of our powerful bodies puts us far ahead when needing to nurture others.

CHANGE DOES NOT COME WITHOUT RISK
"And the trouble is, if you don't risk anything, you risk even MORE." Erica Jong

Risks to the Counselor
Empowering women to accept responsibility for their own lives, establish decisive boundaries, determine their own goals and create a vision for their future does not come without risk. There is risk involved for both the counselor and the client. Awareness of these risks will help you determine ahead of time how far you feel comfortable pushing the limits.

The risks to the counselor are that you may broach significant emotional issues the woman has had hidden for some time. Ironically, using your advanced level counseling skills to establish a unique rapport with the client can put you in the position of being the first person who really ever sat and listened to her at length. You must be prepared for numerous types of latent concerns that can provoke great emotion in your client. Remembering life goals that have been waylaid, prior sexual, verbal or physical abuse, current domestic violence at home or within the family can all come to the forefront in your sessions. You must be prepared to deal with these prior to their onset. Think through your own feelings about these issues. Many advanced counselors can benefit from seeking counseling themselves to understand where they stand on important life issues. Be sure you have resolved your own troubles with these potentially emotional traumas before you attempt to help someone else discuss them. In addition, learn to pay attention to your senses and intuition. I believe that far too much emphasis has been put on "proper" ethical counseling behavior, and not enough on the human side. For many of your female clients who become upset over emotional wounds, a hug and a shoulder to cry on may be the best immediate response you can give them. Trust your own intuition and the knowledge you gather from the client, both verbal and nonverbal, to determine when a hug might be necessary or when a referral to a specialized therapist is necessary.

I remember a client early in my career who came to me with little in her charts except notes from a frustrated physician unable to get information from her. She appeared to be significantly underweight, pale and with poor affect. She never responded verbally to me once during our entire first session. I reluctantly set an appointment for a second session with her. I spent the entire week following her visit trying to determine what the problem was and how I might help her nearly catatonic state. At her second appointment, I walked to her and held her. Again, she never uttered a word, but cried in my arms for her entire second session. Finally, on her third visit she began to slowly speak to me about the Anorexia Nervosa that was ravaging her body. Only through connecting with her on a basic human level was I able to get from her information that her physician and school counselors had been unable.

Risks to the Client

The risk to the client who is learning to empower her life can be great as well. A woman who decisively makes lifestyle changes, pursues her goals and with determination follows her dreams can be an intimidating force to a partner who is unaccustomed to seeing his mate behave this way. Her new found self, sense of boundaries and freedom to choose her destiny may be setting her up for abusive situations with her partner if he is a batterer. This is one of the many risks of being in the counseling business, yet another responsibility the client must own. You cannot take responsibility of this magnitude upon yourself. Refer her to the local Women's Shelter, found in the phone book, or refer them to the National Domestic Abuse Hotline at 1-800-333-7233. All women's shelters maintain advocates who can assist your client in a networking system of help and protection. The call must be the responsibility of your client. The social support networks can do nothing until the battered woman herself takes the first step. Even well-trained domestic abuse counselors experience the frustration of being unable to intervene. This number can be helpful to you as well in gaining information to identify potential battering revealed in counseling sessions, determining the level of danger a woman may be in or learning of other resources available in your area. Although the risk of this situation happening may be slim, it is important information for the counselor who concerns herself with the greater picture of her clients' lives.

Rethinking the Nutrition Counseling Paradigm

Feminist therapy differs from traditional therapies in that it views women's problems as being external in origin and influenced by the social setting women find themselves in. It encompasses a broader and more descriptive view of the specific world women exist within and the life span issues that women face that are unique to being a woman in our society. The social stresses that women live under are not viewed as an exemption from personal and individual responsibility. Every woman is entitled to learn to establish her own boundaries, create her own vision for her life plan, determine her future goals, and choose healthy lifestyle choices to empower her body to seek her goals. Nutrition counselors will find that adapting a feminist perspective to counseling women can enhance their chances for success. The nutrition counselor is the woman's ally in her unique and individual process, gently challenging, prompting, prodding and supporting her growth in changing her current paradigms.

To see how this theory can be adapted to counseling men and women clients with disordered eating and gross obesity, read the FYI article by Bob Wilson that follows on pages 69-72 called, "What Works Best For Gross Obesity: From a recovered patient's perspective."

> "The symptoms people come to me with are really their deep emotional
> process work and they are asking me to shut it off so they can continue
> to live their busy, rushing lives and avoid their process."
>
> *Anonymous Physician*

LEARNING ACTIVITIES

1. Attend a group weight management session of your choice where the majority of participants are women. Listen closely to conversations/ discussions regarding weight issues. What do you learn? Can you identify external pressures related to culture? "Stuckness?"
2. Observe a counseling session for a woman with weight management issues, preferably with a therapist trained in counseling. How does the therapist address cultural issues? What strategies are used to identify weight issues?
3. Analyze one popular woman's magazine from the feminist therapy perspective. What issues do you identify? What impact do you suspect this has on women? How would you change the publication?

SUGGESTED ADDITIONAL READING

Dixon M. *Love the Body You Were Born With*! New York: Putnam; 1996.

An interactive workbook to use with clients that can change the way they think about and treat their bodies. By working through the entertaining, thought-provoking steps, women will gain the knowledge and the strength they need to get off the diet roller coaster, stop abusing their body, and begin appreciating themselves for the powerful and wonderful person they are! A MUST for every woman who has ever squandered her resources by dieting or beaten herself up for not being thin enough.

Bordo S. *Unbearable Weight: Feminism, Western Culture and the Body*. Berkeley: University of California Press; 1993.

In this provocative book Bordo untangles the myths, ideologies, and pathologies of the modern female body. Likening the womanly form to the image of a voracious animal of "unbearable weight," Bordo explores our tortured fascination with food, hunger, desire, and control and its effects on women's lives. A fascinating read for anyone involved in counseling women with weight issues.

Pinkola Estes C. *Women Who Run With the Wolves: Myths and Stories of the Wild Woman Archetype*. New York: Ballantine Books; 1992.

Within every woman there is a wild and natural creature, a powerful force, filled with good instincts, passionate creativity, and ageless knowing. Her name is Wild Woman, but she is an endangered species. Though the gifts of wildish nature come to us at birth, society's attempt to "civilize" us into rigid roles has plundered this treasure, and muffled the deep, life-giving messages of our own souls. This book stretches the current paradigms of thinking about being a woman in our society; not only a useful tool for counselors of women, but a thought provocative book for every woman who seeks to understand her own individuality and uniqueness.

Orbach S. *Fat is a Feminist Issue*. New York: Berkley Group; 1978.

Orbach's book pioneered the field of compulsive overeating and its relationship to the cultural stereotypes and roadblocks women find themselves trapped in. Orbach's classic book details many methods of implementing feminist psychology into therapy with women suffering with compulsive overeating or eating disorders.

REFERENCES

1. Rawlings E, Carter D. *Feminist and nonsexist psychotherapy*. In: Rawlings E, Carter D, eds. Springfield, IL: Charles C. Thomas; 1977.
2. Gilbert L. *Feminist therapy*. In: Brodsky A, Hare-Mustin R, eds. New York: Guilford; 1980.
3. Fontaine KL. *The conspiracy of culture: women's issues in body size*. Nursing Clinics of North America. 1991; 26: 669-676.
4. Perls FS. *Gestalt Therapy Verbatim*. Moab, UT: Real People Press; 1969.
5. Funnell MM, Anderson RM, Arnold MS. Empowerment: A winning model for diabetes care. *Practical Diabetology*. 1991: May-June: 15-18.
6. Koller A. *An Unknown Woman: A journey to self-discovery*. New York:Bantam; 1983.

FOR YOUR INFORMATION

What Works Best For Gross Obesity: From a Recovered Patient's Perspective

Bob Wilson, BS, DTR, Weight Counselor, Kaiser Permanente,
Computer Nutrition Analyst, and Private Wellness Practice, Portland, OR
(Adapted from his presentations to obese clients about his experiences and successful program)

ROOTS PARABLE

From our earliest experiences after birth, we all are conditioned to have certain thoughts, attitudes, emotional response patterns and learned coping behaviors. These conditioned responses form our inner unconscious "computer program" from which we create our lives and evaluate input from our environment.

Getting to the "root" causes of a specific behavior pattern or symptom (for example, being overweight) is quite a challenge. Frequently, there are many "tangled roots" that are all knotted together (see photo). You can cover up the problem by keeping the tops trimmed and neat so other people are not aware that such deep roots and problems exist. It may take many years and lots of soul-searching hard work to get to and change root causes of problems. Examples of common root problems include the need to please everyone else in order to feel self-worth (being yourself isn't enough), feeling shame or low self-esteem (which may stem from comments someone once made to you), or experiencing relationship, drug, or alcohol addiction. To change you must learn to become a "healthy caretaker" to your inner emotional self. You must learn how to nurture yourself.

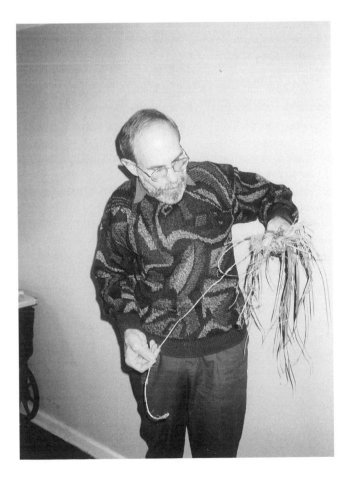

To begin the process of taking care of yourself, it is important to evaluate the relationships in your life: family, work/career, friends, material things, your feelings about yourself, and see how these things effect your relationship with food. Seek support from a nutrition therapist, mental health counselor, or support group like the 12-step program, which provides terrific support in the evaluation process. If you are depressed, having difficulty relating to people, or feel manipulated and unable to cope, psychotherapy can be invaluable.

I found that as I honestly looked into each of these areas and made plans to change each area of imbalance, my relationship with food became healthier and healthier. My relationship with myself also improved. I've come from a space of total self-hatred and disgust with myself, to a place of being a loving compassionate friend to me! I've come to accept me for who I am and who I am not. It has been a very gradual process as I've pruned and nurtured my roots as I untangled them and released their influence on my life.

MY BACKGROUND

I weighed somewhere between 320-400 pounds in the eighth grade. There were cruel jokes and mockery of me and my size, and I believed them all. I came from what would be called a dysfunctional family with multiple addictions. I was a lover, not a fighter. I wanted everyone to be happy, so I tried to take care of everyone elses' needs.

Food was my outlet for stress and coping. I followed the "see-food diet." Whenever I saw food, I ate! I ate lots of fast foods, convenience foods, huge portions, lots of candy, pastries, ice cream and sweets. I never preplanned any meals or snacks. My exercise was watching TV and playing the stereo.

Psychologically, I hated and loathed myself. I believed I was worth nothing. I did not associate food with my problems; it was my friend and the only comfort I had in life.

Finally, in 1972 when I was 21-years-old, I decided I was tired of being fat and out of control. I wanted to make a permanent change in my life. I accomplished it through the support of Weight Watchers, a 12-step program, psychotherapy, and extensive reading, gut-wrenching soul searching and work on my part. I lost over 200 pounds, which I have maintained at about 153 pounds for over 23 years.

I discovered that weight management requires developing a comprehensive set of lifeskills that perhaps others learn as they grow up, but they were new to me. Even today, I find it is difficult to be healthy in our culture because of the availability of high calorie foods. It requires thought and planning to maintain my present weight.

What Worked For Me

Following is a listing of what has made my weight loss permanent. It helps to know the crucial pieces that fit to make a person whole and healthy when he or she comes from a background and weight as mine. Of course, everyone is an individual, but this is a frame of reference.

- Basic nutrition for my needs and where to get it; I had to learn how to feed myself "right."
- How to cut back on calories and fat, yet still have enough volume of food to feel mentally and physically satisfied.
- The art of simple, healthy shopping and cooking with tasty substitutes for many of my favorite foods; I learned to plan menus.
- How to set up my home and work environment to help me out, rather than hinder me; I wasn't that strong, especially when I was stressed.
- Self-management and new ways of problem-solving; I couldn't rely on "will power." I had to make major changes in how I handled life and its choices.
- Keeping food records so I could practice problem-solving and benefit from each experience; the records reminded me how well I had done in the past.
- To become a compassionate observer of my lifestyle patterns, and acknowledge which ones worked and those that didn't; I learned to evaluate without flogging myself with guilt.
- To discover "healthy movement" or exercise; I found ways to make it enjoyable and at an appropriate level for my abilities at the time.
- How to set up a support network that provides encouragement and constructive feedback instead of the negative reinforcement of my youth.
- Patience. Patience. Patience. Practice. Practice. Persistance. The process of change goes much slower than I wanted it to go; I had to give it time.
- And finally, the most difficult thing to learn and change was my relationship with myself. Initially, the tone of my relationship was one of self-disgust and disrespect. To change my self-image required extensive work as mentioned earlier. Today, I love myself and take very good care of me. I apply developmental and lifeskills. I find ways to nurture myself like gardening, hiking, entertaining friends, and so on. I learned to set boundaries and limit my caretaking of others, which caused me some guilt. But I had to realize that I was not responsible

for other adults in my life, just me. I learned to separate their needs and problems from my own. I channeled my energy into more constructive relationships and ventures.

My Approach as a Weight Loss Counselor

From the depth of my personal transformation, I share practical, positive, and permanent solutions with all my clients. I use an eclectic approach—many parts of this and that: humor, positive feedback and encouragement, role playing, visual aids, relaxation, self-nurturing techniques, nutrition concepts, menu planning, food tasting and more. Whatever the client and I think will work for his or her particular situation. I see myself as a trainer and guide.

I try to convey to my clients an overall way of viewing and relating to themselves—one which focuses on compassion rather than contempt. I learned another approach from Stephen Schwartz in *The Compassionate Presence*. (2)

> To step beyond the examination of patterns, we must begin to notice the tone of our relationship to ourselves. We begin to notice the feeling tone in which we approach our own lives. Every experience that we meet is a proposition. "Which way am I going to experience it? Which way am I going to greet it?" All of this has to do with the tone of our relationship to ourselves. "How do I greet myself each day? Am I afraid of this being? Do I belittle this being? Do I call it names? Do I wish it were some other way? Do I have plans for it that involve manipulation and control? Do I motivate myself out of punishment, fear, and rewards by belittling myself unless I get clear? Or is my motivation an impulse of respect that comes from the depth of my heart . . ."

We each create our lives differently, so just watch, observe the results of the way YOU do it. Learn the skill of compassionate observation. Become more aware of how your body, mind, and emotions respond to the way YOU CHOOSE to create your life. Do your choices bring you towards greater peace and harmony? Balance? Health? Or towards dis-ease? Just notice. (See two handouts: 82 Ideas for Self-Nurturing Activities and Rules for Being Human.)

I mention to my clients that "If you continue to do what you've always done, you'll continue to get what you've always got!" This is why so many people are unsuccessful. They don't realize they can't continue to do the same thing and get different results. If you want different results, then you must be willing to do something different!

Permanent weight management requires lifestyle adjustment:

> If you keep the same commitments,
> the same relationships,
> the same thought patterns,
> the same food,
> the same ways of nurturing yourself,
> you'll get the same RESULTS!

The key to simplifying your life is to S. . . L. . . O. . . W it down.

1. Observe what you do. Use recordkeeping and mental awareness.

2. Evaluate what you are presently doing (or not doing) contributes to overweight, peace of mind, compulsive patterns, etc.

3. Make plans and alter your present actions. Plan different actions and DO them! Make changes "big enough to matter, but small enough to achieve." (3) From what you learn about yourself, modify your plans.

4. Practice new actions. Practice doesn't make "perfection," it makes "permanent."

A major obstacle to success is being over-busy, over commitment to others and under commitment to your self (codependency). The result? No time or energy to care for yourself. I mention to clients, "don't just try harder or push harder trying to out run your human limitations. What your life might need is pruning."

It's essential to discover when helping you is hurting me. Notice when your commitments push you out of your zone of being healthy. Not just occasionally, but on a chronic basis. There is an excellent book and workbook by Carment Berry that deals with this topic, *When Helping You Is Hurting Me: Escaping the Messiah Trap*. (4)

I know that each of us is committed to many very important relationships and "things" in our lives. Even too much of really good things. . .is still. . .too much! Balance in life is achieved by pruning commitments.

The whole focus of my counseling is on self-empowerment. Empowerment is defined as, "a process by which people gain mastery over their affairs. In this model, patients are seen as experts on their own lives. . .The role of the patient is to be well-informed, equal, and active partner in the treatment program." (1)

REFERENCES

1. Funnell M, Anderson R, Arnold M. Empowerment: A Winning Model for Diabetes Care. *Practical Diabetology*. May/June 1991; 15-18.
2. Schwartz S. *The Compassionate Presence*. Piermont, NY: River Run Press; 1988.

3. Kaiser Permanente weight loss program, Freedom From Fat.

4. Berry CR. *When Helping You Is Hurting Me: Escaping the Messiah Trap*. New York: Harper & Row; 1988.

Other Helpful Books

Hay, Louise L. *You Can Heal Your Life*. Santa Monica, CA: Hay House; 1985.

Helmstetter, Shad. *What to Say When You Talk to Yourself*. New York, Pocket Books; 1982.

Hendricks, Gay. *Learning to Love Yourself*. New York: Prentice-Hall Press; 1982.

Hollis, Judy. *Fat Is A Family Affair*. San Francisco, CA: Hazelton Foundation; 1985.

Munter, Carol and Hirschmann, Jane. *Overcoming Overeating*. New York: Ballantine Books; 1988.

Roth, Geneen. *Breaking Free From Compulsive Eating*.Riverside, NJ: Bobbs-Merrill Co/ McMillin; 1984.

Rules For Being Human

YOU WILL RECEIVE A BODY.

You may like it or hate it, but it will be yours for the entire period this time around.

YOU WILL LEARN LESSONS.

You are enrolled in a full-time informal school called "life." Each day in this school you will learn lessons. You may like the lessons or think them irrelevant or stupid.

THERE ARE NO MISTAKES, ONLY LESSONS.

Growth is a process of trial and error, experimentation. The "failed" experiments are as much a part of the process as the experiment that ultimately "works."

A LESSON IS REPEATED UNTIL IT IS LEARNED.

A lesson will be presented to you in various forms until you have learned it. Then you can go on to the next lesson.

LEARNING LESSONS DOES NOT END.

There is no part of life that does not contain its lessons. If you are alive, there are lessons to be learned.

THERE IS NO BETTER THAN HERE.

When your "there" has become a "here," you will simply obtain another "there" that again looks better than "here."

OTHERS ARE MERELY MIRRORS OF YOU.

You cannot love or hate something about another person unless it reflects to you something you love or hate about yourself.

WHAT YOU MAKE OF YOUR LIFE IS UP TO YOU.

You have all the tools and resources you need; what you do with them is up to you. The choice is yours.

THE ANSWERS LIE INSIDE YOU.

The answers to life's questions lie inside you. All you need to do is look, listen, and trust.

Source: Bob Wilson, DTR. Original source unknown.

82 Ideas For Self-Nurturing Activities

Listen to favorite music
Enjoy a long, warm bubble bath
Go for a walk
Share a hug with a loved one
Relax outside
Physical activity (of my choice)
Say or read a spiritual prayer
Attend a caring support group
Practice deep breathing
Do stretching exercises
Reflect on positive qualities "I am..."
Write my thoughts and feelings in a
    personal journal
Laugh
Concentrate on a relaxing scene
Create a collage representing the "real me"
Receive a massage
Reflect on "I appreciate..."
Watch the sunrise or sunset
Attend a favorite athletic event
Do something adventurous
Read a special book or magazine
Sing, hum, whistle a happy tune
Go dancing
Play a musical instrument
Meditate
Garden and work with plants
Learn a new skill
See a special play, movie or concert
Work out with weights or small hand weights
Ride a bicycle
Make myself a nutritious meal
Draw or paint a picture
Swim and relax at the beach or pool
Do aerobics to neat music
Visit a special place I enjoy
Smile and say "I love myself"
Take time to smell the flowers
Go horseback riding
Sit in front of a fireplace and watch the fire
Read a cartoon or joke book
Listen to my favorite kind of music
Reflect on "My most enjoyable memories"

Enjoy a relaxing nap
Visit a museum or art gallery
Practice yoga
Relax in a whirlpool or sauna
Enjoy a cool, refreshing glass of water
Count my blessings "I am thankful for.."
Enjoy the beauty of nature
Play as I did as a child
Star gaze
Window shop
Daydream
Tell myself the loving words I want to
    hear from others
Attend a special workshop
Go sailing or paddleboating
Reward myself with a gift I can afford
Take myself on vacation
Create with clay or pottery
Practice positive affirmations
Pet an animal
Watch my favorite TV show
Reflect on my successes "I can..."
Write a poem
Make a bouquet of flowers
Watch the clouds
Make myself something nice
Visit a park, woods, forest
Call an old friend
Read positive, motivational literature
Reflect on "What I value most in life."
Go on a picnic in a beautiful setting
Enjoy a cup of herbal tea/ decaf coffee
Participate in a favorite card game
Practice relaxation exercises
Practice the art of forgiveness
Treat myself to a nutritious meal at a
    favorite restaurant
Enjoy a my favorite hobby
Walk in the warm rain
Watch snowflakes fall or rain drops
Put out wild bird seed and watch the
    birds
Create my own list of self-nurturing activities

by Bob Wilson, DTR

Appendix 4-A

Nondiet Counseling: Empowered Clients Make Healthier Choices

by Linda Omichinski, RD, Counselor and Author of "You Count, Calories Don't"
(Adapted and reprinted with permission of Linda Omichinski and
Healthy Weight Journal, vol.9, no.1; 1995.)

"Health is an independent, nondieting lifestyle characterized by nourishing eating and activity patterns, and self-acceptance."

The worldwide nondiet movement has given health professionals many new issues to consider in their interactions and interventions with clients. Society has begun to accept that diets don't work, yet weight preoccupation exists.

It takes courage to relinquish traditional medical models, yet considered risk taking is a hallmark of leadership. As we counsel clients to abandon diets and embrace healthy living, we must also provide new signposts to guide them in their journey. Clients have told us that health professionals often deliver counseling and education in language that diminishes self-esteem and rekindles the defeatist chronic dieting syndrome. We can identify with the diet mentality both personally and professionally.

Clients are looking for answers and direction. We can best assist them with an empowerment approach to their health issues. We adapt these client concerns into our program language.

HEALTH DEFINITIONS

A refocused definition of "health" is a starting point for this approach. A meaningful and tangible definition has been developed, which translates into the language of both health professionals and clients.

For the professional, health is defined as an independent, nondieting lifestyle characterized by nourishing eating and activity patterns, and self-acceptance.

For the client, health means putting aside the scale, calorie counting and fat gram levels. It means listening to one's body for signals that mean "enough" and "more," and discovering individual patterns for food and activity levels that keep you energized. It means finding the strength to accept yourself just as you are and get on with life. Clients can simultaneously be large, healthy and happy if they demonstrate the characteristics of this definition. These new parameters could replace weight standards and diet preoccupation in your clinical approach.

CHALLENGE THE COMFORT ZONE

The first step to offering the client an empowerment approach is to understand your new role as counselor. You are now a facilitator, adding a new dimension to the traditional role of teacher. Expertise and education are not abandoned, rather, knowledge and objectivity are redirected. It's natural for clients to want diets from us because they want to lose weight. We may think fulfilling this request is the best approach, but is it? Does the client really want a diet, or merely the sense of security that comes from a piece of paper telling them what to do? As dietitians, are we listening to the client, or staying in our own comfort zones by providing an individually prescribed weight loss diet sheet?

ESTABLISH TRUST

A facilitator explores the client's understanding of, and experience with, dieting by asking probing, open-ended questions that gently challenge personal myths and understanding. Here are the types of questions that create this atmosphere of trust:

- What makes you want to lose weight?
- Have you thought about whether you accept yourself as you are?

- How do you feel when society tells you to look a certain way?
- Do you have to feel this way?
- If you don't accept yourself, what will happen?

A recent counseling experience might further clarify this style. I saw Alma for an initial assessment of her obesity. We worked through the nondiet nutrition concepts that would enable her to stabilize her weight. A week later she called to tell me it wasn't working. She wanted to lose weight, and she needed a diet sheet. Is it appropriate now to give the client what she wanted, that is, a diet sheet? The medical model says yes. I analyzed what Alma told me.

Why didn't it work for her? Was having a diet sheet an attempt to control one aspect of her life? Then I probed further, and Alma opened up. She felt overwhelmed with the stressors in her life:

1. her daughter was always unloading her problems on her,
2. she was dependent on her husband for transportation,
3. she had lost interest in life and was bored frequently,
4. she took no time for herself, and
5. she ate to suppress these feelings; she ate for psychological hunger, not just physical hunger.

Identifying these situations enabled us to explore possibilities to break this negative cycle. Alma became aware that she was eating for reasons other than physical hunger. She could see that she needed to make her own decisions about more than just what food to eat.

BE A FACILITATOR

Move into the facilitative role, working with the client by exploring, challenging assumptions and framing open-ended questions. Explore the failure of diets with the client. The key here is to elicit acknowledgement from the client that diets don't work. Simply telling them does not allow the client to take ownership of the idea. Through their past dieting experiences, assist them in coming to the conclusion themselves. Another important step is to jointly identify weight cycling and a history of chronic dieting in the client's health profile. This will impact the client's ability to lose weight with a healthier lifestyle. However, when we focus on healthier living per se and not weight loss, improved lifestyle for the client is the desired result. The client's weight will stabilize, decrease, or slightly increase depending on the genetic profile and client's history of chronic dieting.

TRANSFER POWER

Become an enabler of healthy living by transferring power for healthy decisions to the client as discussed in Chapter 4. With the empowerment model, we assist the client in identifying what steps they are making in the process of healthy living, not what they are not doing. We, as facilitating agents in this process, desire changes to be permanent. We can assist clients in reflecting on their true lifetime goals, which yields more emotional and physical health benefits. For example, how can clients experience the enjoyment of increased activity? Possibly by experimenting with different activities to find one they enjoy. We can suggest they model others who partake in activity for the fun of it.

In our new role as facilitators, we enable the client to explore the options, but the final decision is up to the client. The type of questions we can ask are: How can you get the most enjoyment from your food? The answers you would want to draw from the client could be:

- by paying attention
- allowing myself to taste and savor food without guilt
- eating regularly so I don't come to the table too hungry
- tuning into the texture of foods

Clients begin to appreciate the flavors, textures and subtle changes in making slight shifts toward a lower fat eating pattern. The process takes time but is enjoyable, resulting in preference changes.

MATCH LANGUAGE TO INTENTIONS

Do you use words like overweight? Use the word large instead. Do you focus on weight as a measure of success? Replace with the word health. Are you able to present the educational information with a health focus? Focus on lifestyle changes, not weight loss. Do you give clients the final choice? Extract lifestyle experiences from your client. Using this information, you can identify and personalize the choices available to the client. Here is a helpful list to cue you further about the art of changing language and using positive expressions of encouragement.

DIET LANGUAGE Medical model	NONDIET LANGUAGE Empowerment model
preach	enable
compliance	examine
control	explore
adherence	identify
should	study
must	reflect
prescribe	enjoy
best for you	extract most enjoyment
approval	empower
limit	experience
regimen	delightful
will power	choice

CASE STUDY #1

Sally went on a quick weight loss program and lost 80 pounds. She eventually stopped dieting and started to gain the weight back. Now she was at a decision point. She wanted two things: to follow a nondiet program emphasizing healthier living; and to avoid regaining any more weight.

Yet, the very consequences of dieting might interfere with her desire to stop weight gain. Change in body composition occurs with dieting along with fat loss, there is loss of water and muscle mass. The effect is a lowered metabolism. So, Sally could choose to start the vicious diet cycle again with the predictable effect of weight gain, or she could choose a nondiet approach to health without any focus on weight issues.

When Sally is equipped with knowledge about how her body will react to either choice, she is empowered to take responsibility for her past actions and her own health. She can choose health goals over weight loss/ gain goals. The key here for the health professional is the parameter of models for counseling.

In the medical (diet) model, the client and health professional view weight gain as failure, noncompliance and reason to quit. In the empowerment model, the health professional facilitator guides the client through self-discovery. The client concludes that diets don't work and is empowered to focus on improved well-being, not weight loss.

The facilitator's role as an enabler makes Sally aware of her options. Sally is empowered to be in charge of her own life. As an informed client, she can make her own life choices. Results are not immediate and external goals are no longer the endpoint. Sally studies the process of identifying the factors that will allow her to improve her quality of life. She discovers her own patterns for food and activity levels that keep her energized. She learns to let go of the constant preoccupation with food and weight. She begins to listen to her body for signals of hunger and fullness.

The facilitator recognizes that this process makes an impact on Sally's life that is more likely to be long-term. Sally no longer needs people to police her progress with daily management of her eating or her life. Sally accepts the consequences of past dieting as she sets new goals for her future health. Contrast these positive results with the experiences most health professionals have with diet treatment. Perhaps we recommend exercise for 1/2 hour three times a week, using a prescribed exercise plan. Or we may prescribe a specific individualized regimen or meal plan for the individual, who attempts to follow it to seek our approval. We retain control with this method, doing what we feel is best for the individual. If they don't comply or adhere to the plan with its implied limitations, its should's and should not's, we feel we have failed, and that the client does not have enough "motivation."

This new role for the facilitator is often uncomfortable. Traditionally, he or she may be more familiar with the didactic approach of telling Sally what she should do. With practice though, the empowerment approach is reinforced through satisfying experiences.

CASE STUDY #2

Hazel is starting to sort out lifestyle situations that were affecting her enjoyment of food. She is a 43-year-old woman with arthritis. Her doctor suggested that she decrease her weight to ease discomfort. I asked Hazel about her weight history. She felt that genetically her body weight was high. Previous attempts to cut back on calories did not result in weight loss. Hazel was 114 to 120 pounds when she got married. Six children later, she was around 215 pounds.

I built an expanded profile on Hazel with further discussion using open ended questions:

- ate under stress
- craved sweets
- perfectionist tendencies
- all or nothing diet mentality
- ate for psychological hunger
- ate automatically to suppress feelings
- felt guilty when eating sweets
- frequently did not taste food
- ate more since didn't taste food due to guilt feelings
- got too hungry before eating, therefore ate quickly
- came to table too hungry
- habit of cleaning plate
- overate because she likes the food
- spent little time on self; resentment and frustration built up. (Hours spent on renovating daughter's room created a lot of frustration for Hazel, as her 18-year-old leaves room messy.)

Hazel had tangled her emotional with her physical hunger needs and needed help to establish new patterns for energizing healthy routines. The client with this type of profile is well-suited to the empowerment approach to health.

If Hazel had been put through the traditional diet with the expectation of weight loss, only one type of result is measurable. If she didn't lose weight, the outcome of diet lifestyle counseling would be failure.

However, with the empowerment model, I sent this report back to the referring doctor: "Thank you for the consult. Hazel eats automatically when under stress and when frustrated. She has a perfectionist type of behavior and places high expectations on herself. The weight is somewhat stabilized but she has increased about five pounds lately, probably due to psychological eating.

Learning to eat only for physical hunger is key to stabilizing weight. Breakfast is quick, but not substantial. I'm suggesting the addition of a protein like low-fat cheese to her usual toast and jam breakfast for more holding power. Ways to minimize frustration were explored. Will assess Hazel's progress in one month's time."

For more information on the HUGS nondiet program for health professionals call (800) 565-4847 or write HUGS Intern'l., Box 102A, RR#3, Portage la Prairie, MB R1N 3A3 Canada.

Call Healthy Living Institute at (701-)567-2646 to order *Healthy Weight Journal* @ $59.00/year; *Health Risks of Weight Loss*, 3rd ed, @ $19.95; *Health Risks of Obesity*, 2nd ed, @ $29.95.

Editorial comment: Several publishers predict the nondiet or "intuitive eating" movement will be the next major trend to hit the public market. It makes the old rigid diet regimes a thing of the past. Although we believe in empowerment, intuitive eating, self-acceptance, and have taught the physiology of dieting for years, we believe some appropriate food and exercise information (not the one size fits all or preplanned rigid regimes) can still be effective and professionally responsible, especially when there is a strong personal or family history of diabetes, cancer or hypertension along with being heavy. For other clients, we recognize many will love this nondiet approach and have been waiting a lifetime for it to arrive.

Section II
Integrating Theory, Skills, and Practice

5

Business Skills That Improve Your Communication and Success

Kathy King Helm, RD, LD

After reading this chapter, the reader will be able to:
- [ ] describe key marketing techniques to use in promoting your services
- [ ] critique the scheduling of an appointment done over the phone for effectiveness
- [ ] list key components of the outpatient chart
- [ ] discuss rationale for setting fee schedules

You can increase your chances for success by improving the way you get referrals, schedule appointments, and offer small amenities to patients and clients. It is not uncommon for patients or clients to be totally turned off by a counselor because of what was said or not said over the phone while scheduling the initial appointment. Some outpatient clinics report having as many as 25-50% of their appointments not show. This shows something is very wrong with the way patients are referred or how they are handled upon referral.

IMPROVING HOW PATIENTS ARE REFERRED

For the purposes of this discussion, assume you are a 43-year-old female office manager who just had your gall bladder removed and you are going home. This morning your physician diagnosed high cholesterol (326 mg/dl) from your routine hospital blood work. You come from a family with bad hypertension usually controlled with drugs. You have no symptoms and about 20 extra pounds for your height. When your physician told you about your cholesterol he or she said, "You are too young to have cholesterol this high. It has to come down. I don't want you to eat any eggs and have red meat just twice a week. If you can't bring it down with your diet, I'll give you medication. I'll make a referral to our dietitian."

What was "right" about this scenario from the physician's and your (the patient's) perspective?
1. The physician expressed concern about your cholesterol level so you would feel a need to change it.
2. The physician indicated several food guidelines to help assist lowering your cholesterol level.
3. The physician gave a backup option for cure in case the first one didn't work, so you would not worry.
4. The physician gave you a referral to the dietitian for more in-depth nutrition instruction.

Did this scenario "work" for both you and your physician? Yes, it probably did.

What was "incomplete" with this scenario from the referral dietitian's point of view? Put yourself in the dietitian's role now.
1. The physician did not explain enough about the importance of lifestyle changes on the patient's prognosis, i.e. low fat diet, exercise, and moderate weight loss. If there wasn't time for that, there should have been at least an explanation in physiologically simple terms why cholesterol is dangerous. This is especially true given her family history.
2. The physician gave incorrect and incomplete guidelines on how to eat, which will mean the dietitian has to contradict them and risk confusing the patient.
3. The physician didn't "market" the dietitian's abilities and skills. This isn't a simple referral for blood work. The physician is asking the patient to make major lifestyle changes in order to accomplish the goal of reducing her blood cholesterol level. A strong third party referral at this point is very important.
4. And finally, the physician didn't involve the patient in the discussion. Good medical practice today should involve the patient and the patient's consent for what is about to take place. The physician should have asked

if she wanted a referral to the dietitian, and if so, would she rather have the consult before she leaves or on an outpatient basis after she recuperates from surgery.

It would really help if physicians made referrals differently, but who's going to change them? You! Figure out what you want physicians and other health professionals to say when they refer their patients to you, and present the information in person at monthly hospital or clinic meetings, at their private offices, and over lunch. Have fun with it but make it short and sweet and back everything up with examples and researched information on patient compliance and behavior change.

The next time your friend Dr. Jones says, "I refer at least a half dozen patients a week to your office." You can say, "Boy, that's great. But they are getting lost some where. Tell me what you say when you refer them."

He or she explains what's said. You can then say, "Let me tell you how to market my services so patients will want to call for an appointment."

Give referral agents examples of short phrases to say to patients like, "Changing your diet and your weight are the most important things you can do to lower your cholesterol. Our dietitians on staff can help you fit the guidelines to your lifestyle, and work with you long-term on problems that make it difficult for you to change. They've had patients who lowered their cholesterol by _____mgs/dl in six months."

Look at your long-term patients and let your referring health professionals, colleagues, and employers or consultant accounts know how well they are doing, whether you work in inpatient, clinic, or private practice settings. People refer patients to professionals they trust and respect—who produce results with patients. Market your services through your patients' successful outcomes in monthly or quarterly newsletters or direct mailings, through presentations at meetings, and by writing personal letters to referral agents. (If you don't have any successful patients, work on that situation first and foremost.)

"Seamless" Dietitian to Dietitian Referrals

This discussion is not complete without mentioning that dietitians need to refer patients and clients to each other more often. In private practice when one dietitian is a specialist in allergies, vegetarian diets, or eating disorders it is common in many cities to send referrals to each other. In private practice having successful patient outcomes is so crucial for professioanl image and ultimate survival that it takes precedence over the possible loss of income from the consult. Today, dietitians in other settings are no less accountable for positive outcomes from their nutrition intervention.

Another growing opportunity for referrals among dietitians is from inpatient to outpatient clinic, home health, private practice, or long-term care and back to inpatient, if necessary, in a continuing circle. A nutrition summary (see Chapter 10) or a quick call to the next practitioner should be made in order to create "seamless" dietetic care for our patients and clients. Just as your family would expect the hospital Nutrition Support dietitian, taking care of your mother on TPN, to call the Home Health dietitian or nurse who will carry on the therapy, our other patients expect that same continuity and should receive no less.

It shows professionalism and maturity on a dietitian's part to make sure patients are referred to other practitioners when they need more long-term follow-up or more specialized nutrition therapy than you can provide.

Even if a referred patient is given your name and phone number, ask your referring colleagues to send you a note or call you with the patient's name and number. In the first few days after the referral is made, you should call and introduce yourself, show interest in helping, and send a brochure. If the patient is interested in making an appointment he or she will mention it, otherwise do not turn the call into a sales call. The brochure will reinforce your credibility and availability. This simple phone call could bring in an extra five to ten or more referrals per week.

CREATING AN EFFECTIVE PRACTICE

If you work at an office, establish office hours and days and try to follow your schedule as closely as possible to help develop an image of stability and continuity. As long as clients can leave a message for you, it is not necessary to be available in the office, in person, five days a week. When starting a new private practice at a fitness center or medical complex, try to condense your client consultations to a few days per week. The remaining days can then be used to hold down another job while you start your business, or give you time to market your business, write, take care of family, or whatever.

Telephone

Telephone coverage for your department or business is extremely important. The telephone is your clients' major link with you. During normal business hours Monday through Friday, clients should be able to either reach you by phone or leave a message with a secretary, answering service, or voice mail machine. Messages on telephone answering recorders should be well prepared—keep trying until you record a message that people will not only listen to but, most importantly, respond to. A higher level of service is perceived when calls are returned promptly.

Some hints that may be important to you concerning your telephone answering service or receptionist include the following:

Do not allow your services and fees to be given to clients unless the person is trained to properly "market" your business. Have them say, "I will be happy to take your name and number and have the nutrition therapist call you back."

Caution your answering service or secretary about giving out your private home phone number and address. Have the answering service try to reach you instead of letting them give out your number.

When you are out of town, instruct your answering service to tell people that, "Ms. Jones will be in the office to return your call on Monday, July 10; can she call you back at that time?" Or, if you have another dietitian cover your practice, you might have the answering service say, "Mary Smith, a Registered Dietitian, is covering all calls and I can have her call you if you wish." If it is an emergency in private practice, leave the number of the local hospital clinical nutrition department, or leave a number where your answering service can reach you or leave a message for you. In an outpatient clinic, have the receptionist call or page an inpatient clinical staff person who is covering clinic calls.

HOW TO SCHEDULE APPOINTMENTS

Worst case scenario is when a prospective patient calls your office for an appointment, is treated as an inconvenience by you or the receptionist, and is only asked information about scheduling the appointment. Later when a prospective patient considers the cost (time and financial) of the appointment and the apparent quality of the service, it's easy to see why he or she may decide not to keep the appointment. Why don't patients call to cancel? Because they didn't feel anyone cared if they called in the first place.

So, how can this scenario be improved? First, there needs to be an attitude adjustment. It must be remembered who is the consumer and who is the provider. Who will continue to make a living because of the other? The dietitian, of course. The dietitian must control this situation better and institute changes that will make the potential patient feel special, nurtured, and cared for from the very beginning. That means the dietitian should take the initial contact with the client more seriously.

Philomena Koulbanis, RD, the dietitian in Chapter 1 who only had four patients not show for appointments in seven years, shared her secret. She said,

> "I'm a one person office with an answering machine. I record a very pleasant message on the machine and let it take the messages when I'm with clients. I never call anyone back unless I have at least 10-15 minutes to talk. In that time I find out how they heard about my business, who their physician is, if there is a diagnosis, and most importantly, what their problems and needs are from their point of view. Then I briefly tell them what I can do for their specific problems, how I like to work long-term with clients, and that I would like to work with them. I always mention how much my services cost so they can plan better or wait to make an appointment if they can't afford it at that time."

What we can learn from Ms. Koulbanis' strategy is that clients like to feel they are special to their therapist, their needs are her priority, and money isn't much of an issue if the perceived value is high. The initial phone call also lets the two parties involved screen each other to see if they want to work together and to help the therapist anticipate barriers and problems better.

If you work in a clinic or office where someone else answers your phone first, you must train the office phone staff how to say one of two things: 1) pleasantly thank the person for calling and put the person through to the dietitian or take the phone number so the dietitian can call back to schedule the appointment and answer any questions, or if that is impossible, 2) she or he can pleasantly recite several sentences you wrote about your services, philosophies, the fee, and then ask questions about scheduling the appointment.

Even if you share a receptionist with other professionals or work in a busy clinic, you must become an advocate for professional treatment of your clients. You are not overstepping your boundaries to train the person(s) on the phone how to represent your practice because you are the one who ultimately will be held responsible for your productivity and the quality of patient interaction in your office. If there is an office manager, start by discussing your needs with this person and offer to, "work together to give the patients excellent care."

Six Keys to Good Scheduling Interaction

When a prospective client calls for an appointment there are six keys to successful phone interaction:
1. Begin to establish rapport between the client and the dietitian through showing interest, concern and undivided attention.
2. Screen each other to see if macro philosophies and expectations are compatible (this is most important in situations like when a patient is looking for a quick weight loss program that you don't offer or they think you can diagnose diabetes from their symptoms). A referral to another program or professional may be in order.

3. Find an appointment time that is convenient for both of you. You don't have to accommodate your clients by being available 7AM-7PM every day of the week. But for therapists who work with a high percentage of working clients, it often works well to open early one day each week and work later another day or two. To keep you healthy and happy, leave early on the days when you work early, and sleep in and go in later when you work late.
4. Make sure your client has your office phone number, address, directions to the office, and knows where to park. This is especially important when the office is in a large medical complex. Let clients know if there is a parking fee, or a close place to park that doesn't charge a fee.
5. Ask your clients to recite all appointment arrangements, including what to bring like food records and lifestyle questionnaire, if you mail one in advance, and to give 24 hours notice if they need to cancel or reschedule.
6. You should reconfirm appointments by postcard sent at least five days in advance, or have your receptionist or another paid person (this better assures that the calls are made) call your initial appointments the day before to remind them of the visit and what to bring. By adding this step to your practice, you should save at least two or more visits each week.

Chart System

The chart system for your dietetic or private office can be as expensive as a computer system or as simple as a manila folder for each client. Because of the importance of continuity and documentation of a client's progress, it is best to have the client's nutrition chart available for all visits.

In an outpatient setting when you must generate the chart for a client, the information to include in the chart is:

- name
- address
- work and home phone numbers
- physician's name, the referring physician's name (if different)
- copy of the diet prescription (if available)
- pertinent lab values (if available—or call referring physician's office)

You will probably add to that, depending upon your practice, a diet evaluation, health risk appraisal, food records, action plan, goals and evaluation.

Follow-up session notes should list any changes in lab values and other objective measurements, plus notations on any progress toward achieving nutritional outcomes as well as significant quotes made by the client (like, "My medicine made me sick so I stopped taking it," or "Do you have the woman's shelter number?," or "I made myself throw up every day this week." Be sure to identify clients' comments by using quotes.

Keep your remarks pertinent to the client and his or her progress instead of writing personal conjectures like, "Mother is sabotaging Johnny's weight loss efforts." Instead write what the client actually said, "My mother keeps feeding me second helpings and giving me cookies and stuff." Also, instead of writing the remark, "noncompliant," which labels the client, perhaps unfairly, write what the client did that lead you to that conclusion. For example, you might say, "Agreed to keep food records but has not kept them for 5 weeks; no change in high fat noon meal; is exercising 2x/wk for 1 hr. each." This more extensive statement states the facts as you know them instead of subjectively drawing conclusions. It may be that the client found it easier to begin exercising first instead of changing his food habits. That's his choice, and not deserving of the label "noncompliant" or any other.

After the initial instruction and when something significant happens to a client or patient, the referring physician should be notified, and the contact documented. You can use a form letter personalized on the computer, or write a cover letter on your letterhead and send a copy of the nutrition interview sheet.

Educational Materials

Educational materials for your clients enhance your service and reinforce what you teach. They may also improve the image of your practice. See the recommendations in Chapter 2 on how to make handouts appropriate to your various markets. The typeface should be easy to read, not script; some people with poor eyesight also have trouble reading small single-spaced elite type (10 pt. on computer).

Information overload is a common problem. Avoid giving clients too many publications. Start with what each client needs or wants. Patients and their families: 1) get confused by material that is not specifically for their diet, and 2) can only absorb a small amount of information on a new subject at any one time. Patients lose sight of the most important points of the diet when so many new points are made in the additional booklets. Save the less specific material and the larger number of booklets for the few clients who want them and will use them appropriately.

Impress your clients by using folders to hold take-home materials. Use a folder with pockets on the inside and the therapist's, department's, or company's name or logo on the outside for easy identification of the contents and for advertising purposes. Attach your business card to the folder to provide your address and phone number.

Diet manuals are readily available to all practitioners today. Pages should not be photocopied directly from a manual unless it was designed for that purpose or you request permission from the copyright owner. If you want to be a private practitioner and are unaware of your local medical community's nutritional biases, try to purchase diet manuals from the local hospitals or make an appointment with a hospital dietitian to discuss what she or he uses.

What To Wear

Dress appropriate for the occasion and your patient population's expectations. People are more trusting initially of others who are like themselves. At a fitness center that might mean warm ups, or shorts and a top. At a medical complex or outpatient clinic it will mean professional dress or more casual dress (depends on the area of the country) with or without a lab coat—whatever is your personal preference and the institution's policy. In private practice dress ranges from men and women in fancy suits to more casual slacks and shirts or blouses. Again, lab coats are optional but most therapists who work with the well population do not wear them.

The most important point to remember is that you should dress so that you look professional, successful, and well-groomed without distracting from the purpose of the session. The patients and clients are not coming to dwell on your appearance, so let it be a nonissue.

FEES IN OUTPATIENT SETTINGS

The most important thing to remember about fees is that the "perceived value" of your services must be equal to or higher than the actual fees you charge in order to continue attracting clients. Put yourself in their place: assume you are a physician talking to an overweight, 35-year-old woman with three kids and a modest income. Who would you refer her to: the local Weight Watcher group that costs $25 to join and $10 per week with a record of support and success, or the local private practice dietitian who charges $75 per hour but has a reputation for working miracles with clients using a client-centered cognitive-behavioral/fitness approach? It may be a toss up, but without the reputation for success by the dietitian, Weight Watchers would win every time because its perceived value is usually equal to or higher than its fees. The above example is called marketplace competition and it is moving from the private practice arena into more traditional dietetic markets.

The variables to consider when determining your fees are:
- the level of expertise your work requires,
- your reputation and image as compared to the competition,
- the amount of overhead you must cover,
- the amount of time needed for preparation, the consultation and follow-up,
- what the market will bear—fees are usually lower in rural, small town, and lower income areas than in affluent metropolitan areas.

Even with all of these considerations, the one that most institutions and practitioners use is the last one: they charge what they think their clients and insurers are willing to pay. Whatever your fee strategy, choose fees that you feel comfortable with and ones that are reasonable given the going rates for psychiatric social workers and physical therapists with similar years of education and experience in your area.

You can tell your fees are low when the majority of the prospective clients who call you say, "Oh, that's not bad." Or, when physicians and colleagues say, "Can you make a living on that?" You can tell your prices are too high for your target market when the majority of people gasp when you state the fee, or they say, "Let me call you back." Another indication that your fees are higher than the perceived value of your service is when most new clients refuse to schedule a revisit, or they say, "I don't know my schedule right now, I'll have to call you back," and they never do.

When people are comfortable with your fees or committed to the program, they ask how soon they can make the appointment or schedule a revisit. These clients also will be more interested in special prepayment offers on follow-up visits like six visits for $120 or $20 per session instead of the usual $25. They don't mind the prospect of long-term commitment.

Business-wise, you will come out ahead professionally and financially if you charge fair, reasonable fees that encourage clients to return for follow-up and send their friends, instead of charging the most that your market will bear and have clients only come once. If your contract accounts like HMOs and PPOs perceive that your fees are too high, they may limit the number of client visits to such a point that your services become ineffective. If you know your fees are equitable, don't be afraid to defend them and show documentation of your effectiveness. (See Chapter 10 for information on inpatient billing.)

Ending a Session and Collecting Fees

The end of the interview is a good time to talk about rescheduling a visit, or to discuss why it is not necessary. This is a good "ending" subject and lets the client know that the visit is over. As you are winding up, be sure to incorporate some system to collect the fee. You may simply state, "I will make out your receipt now—how do you want to pay for your instruction?" or "The fee for the initial visit is $____ and revisits are $____ . I will give you an itemized receipt that you can attach to your insurance company's form along with a copy of the referral slip from your doctor. You can try to get reimbursed for our visit." If you have a secretary or receptionist, be sure to train her or him on how to collect fees.

If a patient continues to linger after the closing of the session and you have other commitments, you can either relax and take a minute longer, or you can try standing up and walking slowly toward the door to show him out and simply state, "I want to thank you very much for coming. I am sorry to rush, but I have another client waiting."

Third party reimbursement by health insurers and coverage by managed care programs for nutrition intervention are still sporadic. Every dietitian who counsels clients should be making the effort to introduce herself or himself to all the local managed care agencies and insurers. State dietetic associations should follow the lead of Georgia and market their members' services to all the major health insurers and managed care programs in the state. Nutrition departments in hospitals can work through the person(s) on staff who market the hospital to those entities. See Chapter 15 for more discussion on managed care.

LOCATION—LOCATION—LOCATION

In real estate, they say there are only three things to remember about what to look for in a good property: location, location, and location. Whether you work in a hospital, clinic, private practice, or home health agency, where you counsel a patient or client is very important.

In outpatient settings, the appearance of the building where you work, the actual office layout, and even the color and style of the furnishings can influence your clients' and colleagues' opinions of your services. Poor location choices can make you look less than successful or organized. The goals are to have it clean, private, and comfortable. Make the effort to create a counseling space where you and your clients are relaxed and comfortable with some of your own personality in the decor.

The other major consideration in any setting is quiet. It is not a good idea to meet patients or their families in the corner of a hospital cafeteria, in a cubical in an open-plan office, or even in their homes when kids and pets are running through. The patient/client needs and deserves your undivided attention during the therapy session. Likewise, you will be more effective if you have the full attention of the patient or client. Close doors, turn off TVs or radios, negotiate for more private space, use a conference room if your office is too open, and turn your phone over to the answering machine or have the receptionist hold all calls.

In the patient's hospital room, pull the curtain for more privacy in a semi-private room, or schedule the consult, if you have that luxury, at a time when the roommate is out of the room. Offer patients the opportunity to put on a robe instead of assuming they want to sit in their hospital gown on the edge of the bed or in the hall lobby.

In an office, try to sit level with the client and at a reasonable distance apart. Avoid looking over a large, imposing desk where the client and his family feel like school kids on the other side. Make the chairs comfortable but sturdy, and not too soft. A heavy person or someone with back problems cannot easily get in and out of a too soft couch or chair. Some counselors and clients prefer working around a table while others prefer an office space with a homey living room atmosphere—either can be effective.

If you see clients at your home, the location should be easy to find, the pets should be outside or in a bedroom, the phone should be on an answering service, and the kids and spouse invisible. Extra time should be allotted between patients' visits so that the person who comes a little early doesn't have to wait in the kitchen.

Any location should be clean and safe out of respect for the client and to avoid hurting anyone and incurring liability. Edges of carpets should be secured and steps should be well lighted. After group meetings at night, encourage clients to walk out together or call the security guard to walk people to their cars. Do the same for yourself. When the weather is snowy, make sure the sidewalks and parking lot are accessible and sufficiently clear. If the weather and roads are icy and dangerous, stay home, and call clients to reschedule them before they risk making the trip to your office. Clients don't keep appointments well during tornado alerts, hurricanes, floods and after earthquakes, so call to confirm or reschedule appointments.

MANNERS

Greet your patients or clients with kind words, a smile, and handshake or other appropriate gesture, being sensitive to the client's culture and personal style. As you know by now from the discussion in this book, initial impressions are extremely important to the development of rapport with the client or patient.

A nurse friend years ago told the story about a young physician walking into a room to do a pap smear on a middle-aged woman he had never met.

He said, "Please put your feet up here and I'll do your exam." The woman reached out to shake hands and said firmly, "I'd like to introduce myself first." The physician got the message. A patient isn't "a hypertensive or a diabetic" as we commonly refer to them in medical care. The patient is a person with hypertension or diabetes. People expect respect, civility, and manners.

HERMAN

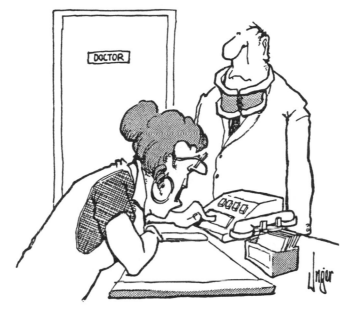

"That pain-in-the-neck's out here, doctor."

Offer Beverage or Food

Consider asking your clients if they would like a beverage like coffee or tea, or a cool beverage in the summer. In a survey of her office clients several years ago, Alanna Dittoe found that the amenity the clients like best was not her friendly manner or live receptionist, but instead it was her coffee and tea offered at the beginning of the appointment.

Another dietitian shared the secret to her success: "'Breaking bread' with my clients. I always try to offer a beverage and some tasty low-fat muffin or cookie. My clients are very loyal, and I think its because we enjoy food together instead of taking it away as they expected."

MAINTAINING COMMUNICATION

Therapists show consideration for their patients and clients (and good marketing savvy for their practice) through notes and phone calls. The note may be a simple summary of goals until the next visit, a note of encouragement, a note of appreciation for referring a friend for counseling, or a reminder.

The call may serve the same purposes, as well as establish two-way communication so you can get feedback on how well a patient or client is doing. More and more therapists are trying short phone calls in between visits for clients who need more support in the beginning or during crisis times. The call is usually made at a designated time by either party.

Many sports nutritionists maintain relationships with their clients by attending training sessions, or meets and games to see their clients compete. This extra effort shows interest and concern on the part of the therapist and can be the source of great personal and professional satisfaction, especially if nutrition intervention helped the athlete perform better.

SUMMARY

There are many noncounseling elements that contribute to the success of a nutrition therapist's practice. By evaluating your present circumstances or establishing procedures to avoid problems mentioned in this chapter and others, you will increase the number of referrals who become patients or clients, lose fewer initial appointments, and keep your patients and clients coming back for more.

LEARNING ACTIVITIES

1. With a colleague, role play scheduling an appointment with a client over the phone. What questions will you ask? How will you identify your potential clients needs? After the role play, critique your performance with your colleague.

2. Observe a counseling encounter with a dietetic professional. What business skills discussed in this chapter could you identify? Which ones were done well? What changes would you make to strengthen the encounter?

3. Look at the two counseling settings (one-on-one and "Mom & Me" good nutrition for kids) below in the photographs. Critique each setting. How could you improve it?

MOM & ME GOOD NUTRITION FOR KIDS

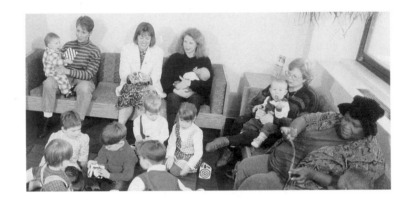

Photo courtesy of Mark Albertini. All Saints Healthcare System, Inc., Racine, WI

ONE-ON-ONE COUNSELING SETTING

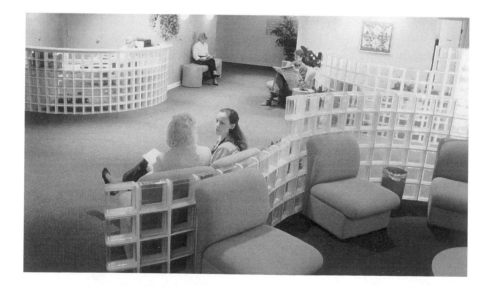

Photo courtesy of Mark Albertini, All Saints Healthcare Systems, Inc., Racine, WI

FOR YOUR INFORMATION

Counseling in Long-Term Care

Ann P. Hunter, PhD, RD, LD, Private Practitioner and Professor, Wichita State University

Dietary counseling in long-term care is similar to counseling a resident at home if the person is alert and compliant. When counseling in long-term care, it is important to be warm and cheerful because even if a resident can't hear or see you too well, she or he still can perceive genuineness and respect. Always tell the resident your name and your position and say something like, "Hello, Mr. Fermon, how are you? I'm Jane Jones, the dietitian, and I've come to talk to you about how we can improve your appetite." Speak slowly and clearly. Unless he is hard of hearing, and that should be in his chart, there is no reason to raise your voice and yell. If it is early in the morning, orient him by saying something like, "Today is Tuesday and it's snowing outside. The streets are a little icy but it seems to be melting." Keep your food discussion uncomplicated and practical. Treat the resident as you would a beloved, respected grandparent, not as a child.

There are times as a consultant in long-term care when institutionalized residents require creative strategies. This may happen for several reasons. Residents may feel angry at restrictions and they may not want to take responsibility for their health and lives. Also, they tend to be more frail with more severe health problems. Since there are many "caregivers" to a resident, there needs to be a collaborative effort to assure adherence to dietary regimes.

CASE STUDY

This case study deals with an 87-year-old female resident, whom we will call Sadie, with poorly controlled Type II (NIDDM) diabetes and obesity. She had been instructed several times as an outpatient and resident on the diet ordered for her: 1500 kcal diabetic diet with three meals and mid-afternoon and bedtime snacks.

In the residence center, Sadie's cognizance ranges from very alert and ambulatory when her blood sugars are controlled to hazy and confused when they are not. Sadie loves sweets and goes to great lengths to manipulate other residents, staff and her family into sharing their desserts or bringing her cookies. Her daily blood sugars at mid morning and afternoon are consistently high. Her physician wants to avoid insulin therapy due to Sadie's high blood insulin levels. On admission two years ago, Sadie weighed 180# at 5'3", but now she is stable at 174#. Two attempts to put Sadie on a lower calorie diet failed when she became very agitated, and started stealing food from other residents, which caused her to actually gain weight.

After repeated attempts of trying to work with Sadie, the dietitian tried two new strategies: a more liberalized diet, and an inservice for Sadie, her family and staff on NIDDM diabetes. Upon recommendation from the dietitian, Sadie's physician changed her diet order to a Liberalized Geriatric diet (regular diet, minimum concentrated sweets, and medium portions ranging from 1500-1799 kcal per day). Spot checks showed that Sadie ate an average of 1500-1600 kcal per day. She was much more compliant since she was served small servings of the same foods served to everyone else.

The group session on NIDDM diabetes was open to all residents with diabetes and their families. It was mandatory for staff personnel. Sixty percent of all families of residents with diabetes were represented. This approach opened discussion on the effects of too many high sugar foods being brought to residents.

Inservice Outline
- Description of Type II (NIDDM) diabetes including complications and treatment
- Discussion of the Liberalized Geriatric diet and its use in diabetes
- Specific concerns of staff or families regarding residents with diabetes at Pleasant Manors
- Brainstorming session on suggestions for other methods of showing concern, love, and care for resident: (group suggestions given)
     Spend more time with resident
     Reward with crafts, puzzles,and other nonfood items
     Increase exercise activities to burn calories and handle stress better
     Choose any unavoidable food gifts from a list of acceptable items provided by dietitian
     Have dietitian provide one-on-one help to residents and families to work through problems
- Closing statements reinforcing the dangers extra foods pose to the resident

All employees and families not present at this meeting were contacted and given the inservice information. The results of the meeting were incorporated into the resident's care plans.

FOR YOUR INFORMATION

Counseling in the Hospital Outpatient Setting

Linda Gay, MS, RD, CDE, Yale-New Haven Hospital, Centers of Nutrition, New Haven, CT

Yale-New Haven Hospital has been providing outpatient nutrition consultation services since 1958. After working in various outpatient specialty clinics for a number of years, I joined the full-time staff of the Nutrition Clinic in 1991. Approximately 50 percent of the time our staff counsels in clinics such as Radiation Therapy, High Risk Obstetrics, or Ear, Nose and Throat Surgery. The remainder of our time is spent counseling clients in our offices or in community outreach work such as health fairs and lectures.

Maintaining a steady flow of referrals is an ongoing process. Some of our clients learn about our Centers from the Yellow Pages or from former clients, but the majority of our referrals come from physicians. Our referral base includes: Yale-New Haven Hospital physicians (57%), Yale University physicians (23%), physicians in private practice (20%).

We advertise our services in a variety of ways which include marketing letters to physicians, a monthly newsletter for Medical Center personnel, lectures to professionals and lay groups, and collaboration with the staff from the Center for Health Promotion and the office of Community and Government Relations.

Our presence in the various specialty clinics allows us to develop a rapport with physicians and other health professionals and has led to our collaboration on various research projects. Timely communication with referring physicians is essential. All referrals to our centers are acknowledged by writing a letter to the physician which describes our assessment and outlines a treatment plan. In addition, quarterly progress letters are mailed to keep physicians apprised of their patients' progress. Many physicians will refer a patient to our Centers despite the fact that the person had been seen by a registered dietitian. I have often overheard statements such as "I would prefer that you speak with 'our' dietitian." This reflects the mutual respect and rapport that we work hard to achieve and maintain. Such was the case with "Mary".

CASE STUDY

"Mary" is a 68-year-old female with a 30-year history of gastrostomy feeding. She was referred by a physician in Reproductive Endocrinology who noted an elevated cholesterol level (265 mg/dl) on routine laboratory examination. A 24-hour recall revealed that Mary took nothing by mouth and that she used blenderized food delivered in bolus feedings via syringe into a gastrostomy tube. Computer nutrient analysis of the composition of her tube feeding revealed that her caloric and protein intake were adequate; however, the tube feeding was high in total fat (41% of calories), saturated fat (13% of calories) and cholesterol (approximately 500 mg/day).

My first thought was to switch her to a commercial tube feeding, however, she was unwilling to make the change. Thirty years previous, she had a bad experience with a canned tube feeding, and she was adamant that she did not trust them. Furthermore, she wanted "real food" in her tube. On special occasions such as birthdays, she would blend a slice of cake and consume it via her gastrostomy. If she felt hungry between meals, she would prepare and blend typical snack foods and consume these in place of her usual formula. Psychologically, she equated "real food" with a "normal" lifestyle and any deviation from this pattern was unacceptable.

It was therefore decided to treat Mary as any other client with hypercholesterolemia. That is, a fat controlled diet composed of everyday foods. Mary and I formulated a new blenderized diet which was lower in total fat (32% of calories), saturated fat (6% of calories), and cholesterol (200 mg/day). I urged her to include a variety of foods from all food groups to help assure nutritional adequacy. Mary accepted the suggestions and a follow-up appointment was scheduled in one month. She returned for follow-up as scheduled and a review of her diet showed good compliance. She was able to maintain her weight during the month on the new formula. Seven months after the initial consult, Mary was still maintaining her weight and her total cholesterol had dropped to 198 mg/dl. An initial report and a progress report were sent to her referring physician (see form that follows).

This case study illustrates the importance of considering a client's preferences and lifestyle. Unless we, as counselors, can get a client to embrace our recommendations, they are useless. With the advent of cost containment in medical care, we will see more treatment, including medical nutrition therapy, shift to the outpatient areas. We must be ready to meet this challenge by maintaining an open mind. We should begin working now with inpatient dietitians and physicians to help increase our referral base in this vital area.

FYI Figure 5-1   Outpatient Counseling

NUTRITION CLINIC
Progress Report - Nutrition Consultation

Patient Name_____   Date_____

Diagnosis_____   Physician_____

Date of initial nutrition consultation_____   Medical Record #_____

Nutrition Prescription_____

NUTRITION PROGRESS NOTES:
Anthropometric data:

Height_____   Original Weight_____   IBW_____

                              Present Weight_____   Goal Weight_____
Degree of compliance with prescribed diet:

1)   excellent_____

2)   good_____

3)   fair_____

4)   poor_____

Progress:_____

_____

_____

_____

Plan:_____

_____

_____

_____

Further Information Requested:_____

_____

_____

_____

                    _____   _____
                         Consultant   Date

6
Assessment

*Michele Fairchild, MS, RD, Assoc. Dir., Clinical Nutrition, Intern-
ship Dir., and Ellen Liskov, MPH, RD, Ambulatory Nutrition
Specialist, Yale-New Haven Hospital, New Haven, CT*

After reading this chapter, the reader will:
☐ **identify at least four types of nutrition therapy assessments**
☐ **identify the basic parameters of a clinical nutrition assessment**
☐ **identify psychosocial factors that influence food intake**

OVERVIEW

Assessment is a dynamic, comprehensive and organized system of gathering information relevant to the nutritional care of your client. It should identify any red flags, which indicate a client is at risk nutritionally. It should identify, along with using good interviewing skills, contributing factors to disordered eating, starting points for therapy, and whether goals are met along the way.

The type of assessments you choose to perform will depend upon the tasks at hand. For instance, the information necessary for an outpatient at a cancer treatment center will vary significantly from that of an otherwise healthy, but overweight client. Similarly, the details collected at your initial consultation may not be repeated except at a three-month follow-up, but they may set the course for the goals for the months in between visits.

During follow-up sessions, you may investigate and assess many of the thoughts, behaviors, and developmental skills that seemed problematic during the first session, or you may expand the first session into a more comprehensive assessment and goal-setting visit. (See FYI section "Teaching Developmental Skills When Counseling Adults" at the end of this chapter, page 101.)

Assessment should be a part of each and every counseling session. Something so simple as having the client recap his or her progress and behavior or cognitive challenges since the last visit will assess more clearly where the client is and whether strategies are working. Merely looking over a person's food record at each visit is incomplete and should not be used as the only assessment. Some examples of nutrition therapy assessments include:

- evaluation of present nutritional status (looking at a typical food intake record and computer assessment of present food intake);
- evaluation of present lifestyle and health risk status;
- establishing baseline biochemical and anthropometric values and monitoring them to assess outcomes of diet changes and nutrition intervention;
- understanding psychosocial, cultural, ethnic or literacy factors, use of developmental skills, and physical limitations (e.g. illness, arthritis, poor vision, immobility, and so on) which may influence a client's food behaviors;
- identifying economic factors which may limit the client's ability to buy adequate good food;
- evaluation of client's understanding of information discussed;
- identifying the client's personal style;
- assessing motivation and readiness to change eating habits;
- evaluating success with implementing goals set during counseling.

The knowledge gained in the assessment process is crucial to developing a plan of action that is consistent with a client's nutrient needs and in helping the client see that problems do exist that need work. The future actions will have

Nutritional Assessment of the Elderly

Kaye Jessup, MPH, RD, LD, MNR-Managed Care, Ross Products Div. of Abbott Laboratories

The Nutrition Screening Initiative of 1990 developed three screening tools and a system for intervention to help prevent malnutrition. The screening tools are:

1) *Determine Your Nutritional Health Checklist* (available in English and Spanish) This screen is a public awareness tool that can be self-administered or administered by someone who interacts with older family members, friends, or clients. The screening tool questions can be appropriate for all ages. This tool is one page long and can be left in lobbies or handed to clients in physicians' offices, senior citizen centers, health fairs, home health agencies, health screening events, other community or group settings, and one-on-one with a family member.

2) *Level I Screen.* This screening tool can be administered as a follow-up to the Checklist or it can be utilized as the initial screen in the home health or other setting. It can identify people who should be more carefully evaluated for referral to other medical or community services.

3) *Level II Screen.* For someone whose Checklist or Level I Screen indicates a potentially serious nutritional or medical problem, the Level II Screen includes more specific diagnostic information. This screen must be administered by a qualified health professional to collect and interpret the information and then implement the most appropriate intervention.

To order these forms and the instruction manuals: either contact your local Ross Products representative or call the Nutrition Screening Initiative (202) 625-1662. Through NSI the Checklist is $2.00/ 25 forms, the Levels I and II forms are $3.50/ 50 forms, the Nutrition Screening Manual is $3, and the more comprehensive Nutrition Interventions Manual costs $5. See Appendix 6-B for samples of the forms.

a better chance of being realistic given the client's current eating habits, psychosocial milieu and level of understanding and motivation. Good interviewing skills are essential in order to elicit the details required in a fashion that does not bias the client's responses.

THE ASSESSMENT PROCESS

Details of assessment calculations are beyond the scope of this chapter and are very adequately covered in other books on the subject (see references 1,2,3,4,5). This chapter will cover an overview of the process, basic figures and sample forms or software that counselors use. The process may be broken down into sections including:

- Medical history, biochemical parameters, clinical examination
- Anthropometrics and fitness evaluation (see Chapter 11)
- Food intake, preferences, allergies and needs
- Psychosocial factors, family influences, developmental skills, motivation and readiness
- Lifestyle and health risk appraisal
- Personal style and preferred learning style (see Chapter 2)

As dietetic practice expands into new areas and nutrition therapy skills mature, assessments will change and the usage of the assessments will become even more foundational to the course of the therapy. Many sources are available to assist the practitioner in developing data collection forms or that offer charts, equations, and assessment tools (see references 3-7).

Screening

Nutrition screening is appropriately used in pre-admission surgical interviews, upon admission to the hospital, in private practice nutrition therapists' and physicians' offices, corporations, clinics, HMOs, senior centers, at health fairs and schools and wherever else target populations meet. See Appendix 6-A for pediatric and adult screening and assessment forms, and side bars "Nutritional Assessment of the Elderly" and "Screening Checklist for HIV/AIDS."

Screening tools can be developed for any population group. Nancy Clark, MS, RD, sports nutritionist at Sports Medicine Brookline, developed a "Nutrition Checklist" for athletes to use as they sit in the lobby waiting for an appointment with a physician or physical therapist. The tool creates awareness of possible nutrition-related problems, as well as serves as a marketing tool for Nancy's services.

In acute care settings where dietitians and dietetic technicians must prioritize care of patients, screening for nutritional risk is appropriate to identify those in need of a more comprehensive nutritional assessment.

New computer and software technology very soon will make basic screening of the client commonplace. Clients will be able to sit in front of a screen and answer questions (or a helper will sit at the screen, ask the questions, and input the information).

As more hospitals go to chartless, computer-based systems, nutrition screening will not be performed by hand by dietary personnel unless it's on a laptop or handheld computer. Eventually, all hospitals will use computers to facilitate collaboration on patient care and manage information better. It is important that dietitians recognize that tasks that do not require interpretation will be put on software and delegated to a lesser paid person. *The dietitian must work at a higher level where he or she interprets the data, makes critical assessments and calculations, works collaboratively with the medical staff, counsels with patients to improve outcomes and, with appropriate training, makes nutritional diagnoses (see Chapter 9).*

MEDICAL—BIOCHEMICAL—CLINICAL
Medical History

In the inpatient setting the medical history is readily available in the patient's chart. In the outpatient setting, when you do not have access to the client's medical record, it is recommended that the practitioner contact the client's primary care or referring physician's office prior to the initial consultation for nutritionally relevant, medical history information.

This is essential in order to identify all the factors that are influencing nutritional status or nutritional requirements. While there are many clients who can provide accurate information about their medical background, prescribing inappropriate nutritional therapy to a client can threaten your practice if he or she is a poor historian or chooses not to reveal pertinent information. After the visit, send a summary of the nutritional care to the client's physician.

Health Status. Identify any chronic or acute conditions which are affecting nutritional status, nutrient needs, food intake, digestion, absorption, or metabolism of nutrients. In the outpatient setting diabetes, hyperlipidemia, obesity, eating disorders, food intolerances, hypertension, and gastrointestinal disorders are commonly seen. Burns, infections or prolonged fever, liver or kidney disease, AIDS, complications from chemotherapy, failure to thrive, cystic fibrosis, or multiple trauma are powerful risk factors for poor nutritional status in hospitalized patients. A thorough medical history should also investigate appetite as well as dentition or other potential mechanical problems which may preclude food intake.

> ## Screening Checklist for HIV/AIDS
>
> Kaye Jessup, MPH, RD, LD
>
> Nutritional status plays a major part in the health status of a person with HIV/AIDS. It is important to identify warning signs that can lead to malnutrition and take steps to prevent it from happening. This screening form may help to identify persons with HIV or AIDS at nutritional risk in order for interventions to be implemented. A checklist is available through your Ross Products representative.

Medication Usage. Many clients will be taking medications routinely, either prescription or over-the-counter, which creates the possibility for a food-drug interaction. When a food-drug interaction is suspected or likely, be sure to incorporate information into your counseling sessions on timing of meals, food selections, or supplementation. (See drug-nutrient information references 2,9,10.)

Be sure to ask the client about any vitamin and mineral supplements currently being used as this is commonly overlooked in a medication history. Many health conscious clients self-prescribe potentially harmful doses of fat soluble vitamins, niacin, or minerals.

Biochemical Parameters

Laboratory measurements of visceral protein, immune function, or vitamin and mineral stores are used to evaluate nutritional status in the assessment process. Serum albumin is a commonly ordered test for measuring visceral protein status but it cannot detect short term changes in nutritional status due to its relatively long half life of about 21 days. Acute or short term changes in nutritional status may be detected with the use of prealbumin or transferrin due to their shorter half lives of 2-3 days and 8-10 days, respectively. Since malnutrition can depress immune function, the total lymphocyte count (TLC) can be used as a marker of nutritional status. Extreme caution must be taken with the interpretation of these parameters as they are all highly influenced by non-nutritional factors such as age, fluid status, stress, drugs, infection, AIDS, and liver or kidney disease.

Lastly, any biochemical parameters associated with a particular health condition (i.e., glucose, glycosylated hemoglobin, serum lipids, etc.) should be noted at the time of the initial consultation and then monitored during follow-up to assess the efficacy of nutritional therapies.

Clinical Examination

Physical signs of poor nutritional status may be identified by visual examination, particularly loss of somatic fat and protein stores. A very skilled practitioner may be able to detect clinical signs of protein or micronutrient deficiencies in a client's hair, skin, eyes, and mouth areas. Such physical findings, however, are often due to non-nutritional causes or are indicative of more than one deficiency state. Any suspicions about nutritional deficiencies, as detected by physical examination, should be confirmed with biochemical testing. Sources are available for further reading regarding clinical examination for detecting malnutrition (see references 1,2,11) and training is available—contact Mary Ann Kight, PhD, RD, Professor, University of Arizona (see Chapter 9).

ANTHROPOMETRICS

Anthropometric variables such as weight, circumference measurements, and skinfold thickness are commonly used to assess nutritional status and body composition. All of these measurements are relatively simple and inexpensive to obtain, but are not without error. Standardized techniques for obtaining anthropometric indices should be documented in the practitioner's standards of care so baseline values and changes in serial measurements can be accurately evaluated.

Weight. The most commonly performed type of anthropometric evaluation is weight relative to height. Many tables are available to determine ideal body weight (IBW) based upon height (see 12,13), where a percentage of ideal weight can be calculated (% IBW = Actual Weight/ IBW). Accurate use of the Metropolitan Life Insurance weight tables (12) necessitates calculation of body frame size using elbow breadth, which makes this process more complicated and prone to error. Thus, many practitioners are using body mass index (BMI) which is derived by dividing weight in kilograms (kg) by height in square meters (m $_2$). Bray (13) has defined BMI as:

- healthy 20-25,
- overweight as greater than 25-30,
- obesity as a body mass index above 30.

For hospitalized patients, evaluation of weight and weight change are simple methods of screening for nutritional risk. A patient who is 90% ideal weight and/ or has experienced a 5-10% weight loss (8) should be considered at risk for malnutrition and should undergo a more comprehensive nutritional assessment.

In children, growth charts are commonly used to identify the child's height and weight as compared to the norm. Weight-for-stature index is used to identify infants and children with obesity or acute protein-energy malnutrition (PEM). This index is calculated by dividing the child's actual weight by the 50% weight for length. Children with an index equal to or greater than 1.1 (110% of standard) require further evaluation for overweight/obesity; those falling below 0.9 (90% of standard) require assessment for acute PEM. (14)

The detriment of using weight alone as a measurement of nutritional status is that it does not provide any information on body composition such as muscle mass reserves or subcutaneous fat stores. It is also affected by the person's fluid status.

Circumference Measurements and Skinfold Thickness. Caliper skinfold measurements can be taken by a trained individual to estimate subcutaneous fat stores or total body fat. Somatic protein reserves can be determined by calculating Mid Arm Muscle Circumference (MAMC) which is derived from the upper arm circumference and triceps skinfold measurements.

Standardized techniques to perform and evaluate skinfold measurements are widely published in sports nutrition, fitness and sports medicine books, in physical assessment books and by pharmaceutical companies. (1,4) These measurements provide the most useful information when monitored over time. Skinfolds are not recommended for routine screening in children, but they may be beneficial in assessing a child's status when it is above the 90th or below the 10th percentile of weight-for-stature. (4)

Currently, waist to hip ratio (WHR) is one of the most common circumference measurements performed as an assessment of body fat distribution. A simplified technique of calculating WHR involves measuring the individual's waist at the smallest circumference and hips at the largest circumference below the waist. The waist measurement is divided by the hip measurement where a WHR of greater than 1.0 in men and greater than 0.8 in women is indicative of android obesity. Upper body, or android obesity, is associated with greater risk of diabetes, gout and heart disease. (15)

Fitness Evaluation (this is beyond scope of this chapter but see brief discussion of exercise and recommended resources in Chapter 11).

DIETARY INTAKE AND NUTRITIONAL NEEDS
Determining Current Intake

One of the more time consuming aspects of nutritional assessment is determining what a client is eating. Details about food selections, preparation methods and portions sizes can be obtained in a variety of ways and is always a challenge as factors of memory, knowledge of preparation methods for foods prepared by others, error in judgment of portion sizes, and client bias in reporting intake can negatively affect the reliability of the information. Food models are helpful when assessing portion sizes, especially when a client has not measured or weighed foods eaten. Underestimation of amounts is a common phenomenon. (16) As always, the practitioner should try to make the client feel at ease, do not act judgmental and the client will feel more like writing his or her actual intake on the food record.

It may be helpful to explain your purpose in gathering a diet history; that in order to provide assistance in identifying potential areas for change (i.e. food selections, preparation methods, or portion sizes), you need to understand what he or she is eating. Remember however, it takes multiple counseling sessions to fully understand what a client is eating and all relevant information need not be gathered in the initial consultation.

Twenty-four Hour Recall. One of the quickest ways to get a general idea about a client's eating habits is to ask the individual to recall everything he or she ate and drank within the past 24 hours. However, in addition to the inaccuracies described above with food records, the previous 24 hours may not be representative of the client's normal diet. In such cases, substitute a "typical day's" intake.

Food Records. Food records kept by a client prior to the consultation, will not only provide more information than the 24-hour recall, but will also allow more time for intervention as opposed to assessment in the counseling session. In this method, have the client complete food records, inclusive of food selections, name brands, preparation methods, and portion sizes, for at least two typical weekdays and one weekend. Bias in reporting food intake often occurs with food records when a client preferentially completes them on "optimal" eating days or based upon what he or she believes constitutes a healthy diet. Food records are also invaluable in subsequent follow-up sessions for helping both counselor and client understand the eating behavior at hand. Additional details such as location of meal or snack, hunger, mood and related thoughts can be instrumental in identifying behaviors or attitudes in need of modification during the counseling process.

Food Frequency. This type of questioning is used to identify how often specific foods or food groups are consumed by the client. Food frequency questionnaire forms can be general to all the foods commonly eaten or specially developed to quantify intake of a nutrient of particular concern, such as sodium. A food frequency can be used as a cross-check method of validating the accuracy of a 24-hour recall.

Additional information such as food preferences, food intolerances or allergies, and dining out habits can be elicited during the interview either through closed or open-ended questioning. Combined with details regarding psychosocial factors influencing food intake, the practitioner will have a reasonable understanding of what the client is eating and why.

Evaluation of Current Intake

Once you have gathered information regarding a client's intake, the next step is evaluating it in accordance with his or her prescribed diet or nutritional needs. Thus, estimating nutritional needs is a prerequisite to this step in the assessment process. The purpose of this evaluation is to assist the practitioner in identifying areas of focus in the counseling process.

Quantitative assessment of food intake for macronutrients can be accomplished using computerized nutrient analysis software, the American Diabetes/ Dietetic Associations' Diabetic Exchanges (17) or a food composition handbook (18), when sufficient details are obtained from the diet history. Semi-quantitative methods for diet evaluation have been developed for several nutrients such as fat intake. (19) The most time efficient manner of quantifying micronutrient intake is by using computerized nutrient analysis software although food composition handbooks will also be accurate. Intakes of vitamins and minerals which are consistently less than two-thirds of the Recommended Dietary Allowances (20) is a nutritional risk but does not necessarily constitute a deficiency state.

A qualitative assessment of food intake can be performed by comparing overall intake from each food group in accordance with the Food Guide Pyramid (21) or Dietary Guidelines for Americans. (22) This type of evaluation can be rapidly performed to judge the overall balance and adequacy of an individual's diet. Although counseling efforts may focus on only one or two nutrients such as saturated fat or sodium, it is important not to overlook other aspects of a healthy diet.

Estimating Nutritional Needs

Energy. Many formulas, such as the Harris-Benedict equation (23), are available for estimating energy requirements in hospitalized patients. Some simplified formulas are available to provide a reasonable estimate of caloric needs based upon level of stress for hospitalized patients and activity level and age in outpatient settings (see Table 6-1). While indirect calorimetry is likely to be the most accurate way of calculating calorie needs, it is not cost effective nor is it practical under most circumstances.

Table 6-1 Estimating Energy Needs in Adults (8)

Healthy Adults [1, 2]

Sedentary	IBW (lb.) x 13
Moderate activity level	IBW (lb.) x 15
Strenuous activity level	IBW (lb.) x 17

[1] Adjust for age by deducting 10% for ages 51-75 years and 20-25% for older than 75 years.
[2] Deduct or add 500 calories for weight loss or gain of one pound per week.

Hospitalized and Acute Treatment Outpatients

Non-stress (bed rest and nonhypermetabolic)	20 calories/ kg IBW
Mild stress (ambulatory and nonhypermetabolic)	25 calories/ kg IBW
Moderate stress (minor surgery/ ventilated surgery)	30 calories/ kg IBW
Severe stress (sepsis, trauma, major surgery)	35 calories/ kg IBW

Protein. For healthy adults, the Recommended Dietary Allowance for protein is 0.8 grams per kilogram ideal weight. (20) Protein intake for hospitalized or acute care outpatients should be estimated based upon disease state, degree of stress, unusual losses, and visceral protein status as assessed by the biochemical parameters previously reviewed. Table 6-2 summarizes protein requirements.

Table 6-2 Estimating Protein Needs in Hospitalized and Acute Treatment Outpatient Adults (8)

No deficit	*1.0*	*grams/ kg IBW*
Mild deficit	1.2	grams/ kg IBW
Moderate deficit	1.5	grams/ kg IBW
Severe deficit	1.7	grams/ kg IBW or 20% total calories
Renal failure		
Acute renal failure	0.6-0.8	grams/ kg IBW
Hemodialysis	1.0-1.2	grams/ kg IBW
Peritoneal dialysis	1.2-1.5	grams/ kg IBW
Nephrotic syndrome	0.8	grams/ kg IBW + 1 gram protein/ day for each gram urinary protein loss
Liver failure		
Encephalopathy	0.55	grams/ kg IBW
Cirrhosis	0.8-1.0	grams/ kg IBW
Hepatitis (no cirrhosis or encephalopathy)	1.5	grams/ kg IBW

Vitamins and Minerals. The Recommended Dietary Allowance (20) for vitamins and minerals are appropriate for use by healthy individuals. Recommendations for dosages can be adjusted upward for deficiency states, conditions which increase demands, or when absorption or utilization is impaired. As research identifies preventive benefits to taking additional nutrients, recommendations will change.

Fluid. Fluid intake is especially crucial for pediatric and geriatric clients, for workers or athletes in warm environments, and when a person has a fever, vomiting or diarrhea. For a child the recommendations are: (4)

1-10 kg	100	ml/ kg
greater than 10 kg	1500-1800	ml/ m2/d
greater than 20 kg	1500	ml plus 20 ml/ kg for each kg greater than 20 kg

The general recommendations for fluids are 1 cc/ kcalorie or the more common 6-8 glasses of fluid per day. Workers and athletes should drink at least the 2 quarts of fluid plus replace each pound of weight lost each day through dehydration with one pint of water. (24) Thirst is not a good indicator of dehydration in geriatric clients. (24) They should try to consume the recommended 6-8 glasses of fluid each day; more when they are in warm environments.

PSYCHOSOCIAL FACTORS AFFECTING FOOD INTAKE

One of the greatest determinants of food behaviors is an individual's psychosocial domain. (25,26) Counselors who have long-term relationships with their clients and are assisting them with changing their lifestyles should devote a considerable amount of attention to this area of assessment. One of the most challenging aspects of counseling is helping a client identify and overcome barriers to change. When these barriers are not identified in the assessment process and addressed during counseling, many clients will continue to make poor food choices, in spite of their knowledge of nutrition. These very personal details about a client's eating habits are best gathered through open-ended questioning, after rapport is established with a client. See Chapters 7 and 8 for more discussion on this subject.

Social Influence. Family and friends may have positive or negative effects on the client's eating behaviors based upon their own practices or the level of support offered to the client. (27) Also, social obligations and activities may influence dining out patterns and the food selections available. It is often valuable to gather information about other members at home, who does the majority of shopping and cooking, and social activities which necessitate a deviation from his or her normal diet.

Food Availability Issues. Poor economic resources, suboptimal preparation and storage facilities in the home, an inability to shop and prepare food due to illness, and lack of transportation to the grocery store will all impact upon the consumer food choices. After identification of these issues, referral to outside agencies may help remove such barriers. The Nutrition Screening Initiative for the elderly pointed out that 40 percent of people over 60 years in the United States live on less than $6,000 per year. (6)

Cultural and Religious Background. The environment in which we are raised will be a strong determinant of food preferences, consumption, preparation and storage behaviors. (28) Be sensitive to a client's cultural food behaviors in all counseling interventions. See Chapter 3 for more information on this subject.

Stress and Emotions. How does the patient cope with feelings of stress, anger, depression, frustration, boredom and happiness? Often, eating is in response to these external cues as opposed to hunger. The antecedent to overcoming emotional eating in behavioral counseling is identification of these triggers in the assessment process.

When a person is depressed, he or she may admit to sleeping too much, especially through the morning, or not resting well at night. The person may seem to lack enthusiasm for life in general, including interest in making or staying with behavior changes. The person may have difficulty identifying goals and strategies that he or she feels can be accomplished. Depression can interfere with a person's ability to work and maintain good relationships with family and friends. During a counseling session, a client may disclose many of these signs and symptoms to a nutrition therapist. If the person is dangerous to him or herself or to others, a referral to a mental health professional or referring physician is in order. If the person just needs small, achievable goals, enthusiastic guidance, and encouragement, the nutrition therapist is qualified to fill those functions.

Developmental Skills. When a client doesn't learn how to set boundaries or be assertive as an adolescent, he or she will often have problems with these lifeskills for the rest of their lives. By not knowing how to control their time and by allowing other peoples' priorities to become their own, clients can remain confused about their own goals and direction. Danish (29) teaches high school students how to teach junior high students how to develop developmental or lifeskills. These skills can be the missing link between many assessed nutrition-related problems and developing the behaviors to eat healthy. For example, the reason a client may overeat each evening is because work is too hectic to leave for even a short break. The more assertive person will bring this to the management's attention and request that changes are made in the schedule to allow time to eat a noon meal. For more discussion on this topic, see Chapter 2 and the FYI article by Alanna Dittoe, RD at the end of this chapter.

Motivation and Readiness. Different factors motivate individuals to change their eating behaviors. Fear of illness, feelings of improved well being due to the changes made, and the belief in one's ability to carry out the recommended actions are signs of motivation. (30) Conversely, when the client believes that there would be few benefits in making changes, that there are too many barriers which prevent him from making the changes, and his feelings of competence to do so are lacking, it is unlikely that this individual will be able to modify his diet. Motivational factors should be assessed such as client perception of self-competency, perceived threat from not taking action, and the benefits of change as opposed to the burdens. This will assist the practitioner in identifying attitudes in need of change in the counseling process. Some practitioners recommend using "Diet Readiness" tests as predictors of compliance and success in weight loss program. (31,32) (See "Weight Loss Readiness" test in Appendix 6-C.)

LIFESTYLE AND HEALTH RISK APPRAISAL

In the outpatient setting at corporations, wellness programs, fitness centers, health fairs and private practice offices, lifestyle and health risk appraisals are becoming commonplace. Through a series of questions about family and personal medical histories, food habits, stress management, exercise, smoking, alcohol intake, safety habits and so on, a client's lifestyle decisions and health risks can be determined as compared to a norm. The forms are often handed out to private clients at the first visit or they are mailed ahead of time so they can be filled out and turned in at the first visit. You can merely review the answers, or the answers can be scored by hand or by computer. Some companies that specialize in developing these tools also sell software for private offices, customized software (for large accounts), or they will run the program and mail back the results. (See sample questionnaires and feedback in Appendix 6-D.)

CONCLUSION

Assisting the client in making dietary changes requires a counselor to not only understand nutritional requirements related to both health and disease, but also the complex determinants of food behaviors. The comprehensive assessment process reviewed will enable the practitioner to better identify areas in need of modification in the client's diet and develop action plans which are considerate of the client's domain.

LEARNING ACTIVITIES

1. Select a particular type of client for nutrition counseling. Based on your assessment:
   a. What are the specific nutrition problems for this client?
   b. What are the nutrition goals for this client?
   c. What psychosocial, cultural, ethnic or literacy factors must you consider?
   d. How will you evaluate the client's motivation to learn or meet established goals?
2. Visit a medical clinic or ambulatory care setting. How are clients screened for nutrition risk? Who does the nutrition screening? What methods of assessment are used? Evaluate the effectiveness of the screening process and develop recommendations for the process if you were to make changes.
3. Interview a dietetic practitioner in private practice. How are clients screened and assessed for nutritional risk? What tools are used? How is baseline nutritional information utilized in designing the counseling sessions?
4. Compare and contrast three computer systems available for nutrition screening and/or assessment. What are the strengths and weaknesses of each? In what settings would each be appropriate for nutrition counseling?

REFERENCES

1. Czajka-Narins DM. The Assessment of Nutritional Status. In: Mahan LK, Arlin M. Krause's *Food, Nutrition & Diet Therapy*. Philadelphia, PA: W.B. Saunders Co.; 1992.
2. Whitney ER, Rolfes SR. *Understanding Nutrition*. Minneapolis, MN: West Pub. Co.; 1993.
3. White JV, Ham RJ, Lipschitz DA, Dwyer JT, Wellman NS. Consensus of the Nutrition Screening Initiative: risk factors and indicators of poor nutritional status in older Americans. J Am Diet Assoc. 1991; 91:783-787.
4. Queen PM, Lang CE. *Handbook of Pediatric Nutrition*. Gaitherburg, MD: Aspen Pub. Inc.; 1993.
5. Chernoff R. *Geriatric Nutrition*. Gaithersburg, MD, Aspen Pub. Inc.; 1991.
6. White JV, Dwyer JT, Posner BM, Ham RJ, Lipschitz DA, Wellman NS. Nutrition Screening Initiative: Development and implementation of the public awareness checklist and screening tools. *J Am Diet Assoc*. 1992; 92: 163-167.
7. Ford DA, Fairchild MM. Managing inpatient clinical nutrition services: A comprehensive program assures accountability and success. *J Am Diet Assoc*.1990; 90: 695-702.
8. Ford DF, Liskov E, Fairchild MM (eds.). *The Yale New-Haven Hospital Nutritional Classification and Assessment Manual*. New Haven, CT: Yale-New Haven Hospital; 1990.
9. Pronsky ZM. *Food Medication Interactions*. Pottstown, PA: Food-Medication Interactions; 1993.
10. Roe DA. *Handbook on Drug and Nutrient Interactions*, (5th ed.). Chicago, IL: The American Dietetic Assoc.; 1994.
11. The American Dietetic Association. Nutritional Assessment. In: *Handbook of Clinical Dietetics*, (2nd ed.). New Haven, CT: Yale University; 1992: 5-39.
12. Metropolitan Life Insurance Co., data adapted from the 1979 Build Study, Society of Actuaries and Association of Life Insurance Medical Directors of America. Phil., PA: Recording and Statistical Corp.; 1980.
13. Bray GA. Definition, measurement, and classification of the syndrome of obesity. *Int J Obes*. 1978; 2:99-112.
14. Waterlow JC. Classification and definition of protein-calorie malnutrition. *Br Med J*. 1972; 3: 566-569.
15. Vague J. The degree of masculine differentiation of obesities: a factor determining predisposition to diabetes, atherosclerosis, gout and uric calculus disease. *Am J Clin Nutr*. 1956; 4: 20-34.
16. Litchman SW, Pisarska K, Berman ER, Pestone M, Dowling H, Offenbacher E, Weisel H, Heshka S, Matthews DE, Heymsfield SB. Discrepancy between self-reported and actual calorie intake and exercise in obese subjets. *New Eng J Med*. 1992; 327: 1893-1898.
17. The American Diabetes Association and The American Dietetic Association. *Exchange Lists for Meal Planning*, 1989.
18. Pennington JAT. *Bowes and Church's Food Values of Portions Commonly Used*, (16th ed.). Phil., PA: J.B. Lippincott Co.; 1993.
19. Remmell PS, Benfari RC. Assessing dietary adherence in the Multiple Risk Factor Intervention Trial (MRFIT). *J Amer Diet Assoc*. 1980; 76: 357-360.
20. Food and Nutrition Board. *Recommended Dietary Allowances*, 10th ed. Washington, DC: National Academy Press; 1989.
21. *Food Guide Pyramid*. Washington, DC: US Dept of Agriculture, Human Nutrition Infromation service; 1992. Home and Garden Bulletin No. 252.
22. *Nutrition and Your Health: Dietary Guidelines for Americans*, (3rd ed.). Washington, DC: US Dept of Health and Human Services; 1990. Home and Garden Bulletin No. 232.
23. Harris JA, Benedict FG. *A biometric study of basal metabolism in man*. Publications No. 279, Carnegie Institute of Washington. Phil., PA: JB Lippincott, 1919.
24. Berning JR, Steen SN. *Sports Nutrition for the 90's: The health professional's handbook*. Gaithersburg, MD: Aspen Publishers; 1991.
25. Blum LS, Horbiak J. *Take the Lead. Person-Centered Counseling Skills*. Chicago, IL: National Center for Nutrition and Dietetics, 1990.
26. Stuart MR, Simko MD. A technique for incorporating psychological principles into the nutrition counseling of clients. *Top Clin Nutr*. 1991; 6: 32-39.
27. Dwyer JT. Steps to take in primary care for achieving lasting dietary change. *Top Clin Nutr*. 1991; 6: 22-31.
28. Terry DR. Needed: A new appreciation of culture and food behavior. *J Amer Diet Assoc*. 1994; 94: 501-503.
29. Danish S. *Advanced Counseling Skills*. Presentations at ADA Annual Convention, Orlando, FL, October 1994.
30. Rosenstock IM, Strecher VJ, Becker MH. Social learning theory and the health belief model. *Health Education Quarterly*. 1986; 13: 73-92.
31. Brownell KD. *The LEARN Program for Weight Control*. Dallas, TX: American Health Pub. Co.; 1990.
32. Carlson S, Sonnenberg LM, Cumming S. Diet readiness test predicts completion in a short-term weight loss program. *J Amer Diet Assoc*. 1994; 94: 552-554.

FOR YOUR INFORMATION

Teaching Developmental Skills
When Counseling Adults

Alanna Benham Dittoe, RD, Principle, Dittoe and Associates, Menlo Park, CA

INTRODUCTION

If we can successfully teach clients the lifeskills or developmental skills to change behavior, we will have exponentially greater impact than if we only instruct them on a diet pattern. Not only will our clients perceive our services at a higher level, but we will achieve more professional satisfaction by completing cases and maintaining long-term relationships with clients. Over the last 10 years, my associates and I developed and implemented a skill-based approach to counseling adults, which uses many assessment tools and visuals. We have seen continued growth in our practices from this approach because our patients are more successful and satisfied.

Our consultative services cover three treatment phases: 1) Making a comprehensive assessment and evaluation, 2) Developing food, fitness, and health plans and 3) Teaching developmental-behavioral skills and allowing for practice.

This approach can be applied to numerous conditions, including obesity, diabetes, hypercholesterolemia, eating disorders, pregnancy, sports nutrition, and family and corporate health. In designing this approach, we took into consideration overall consumer needs and trends such as the need for personalized service, the need for various options to solutions, and the need for self-management. We found these considerations increase the perceived value of our service and ensure our patient load and financial security.

PHASE 1
Identifying Needs Through a Comprehensive Evaluation Process

Assisting clients identify their needs is one of the most important tasks we can provide. It is instrumental in whether clients' acquire the ability to become independent of treatment and manage their nutrition and health on their own.

The comprehensive evaluation process is a foundation tool we use to collect and analyze data, which ultimately identifies needs at multiple levels. During this process, we are modeling for clients how the needs identification works so they can do it for themselves in the future. The depth of the process models the detail necessary to extract and clearly identify needs. Our evaluation accomplishes the following:

- identifies problems and needs;
- identifies general solutions and communicates them in a concrete fashion to the clients through dialogue and visuals;
- explores the pros and cons around various treatment options.

From this the client and therapist create a mutually agreeable treatment plan to allow enough structure for learning, but enough flexibility to experiment with ideas.

This caring process begins with the initial client contact, which is usually the phone call to schedule the appointment. We spend up to 10 minutes briefly listening to the client's concerns and discussing the need for a comprehensive evaluation. The initial consultation lasts 1 1/2 to 2 hours, depending upon the complexity of the case. The key is being flexible. No two clients give the same level of information nor do they go through the process in the same manner. (Historically, dietitians have been too anxious to educate so they abbreviate the evaluation process. This sends the wrong message to clients about the complexity of the change process. They are lead to believe that whatever preprinted diets and food lists that worked for someone else will work for them.)

After the first session a written "needs assessment" packet is sent home with the client to gather more information on:

- culinary preferences
- fitness needs
- actual food intake, including assessing hunger regulation and volume status
- 20 different eating habits

Clients feel they are active participants in the evaluation process. Following are samples of some of the forms we use. (See Figure 6-1 Culinary Assessment, Figure 6-2 Fitness Assessment, and Figure 6-3 Habit Inventory.)

FYI Figure 6-1   Culinary Assessment

CULINARY ASSESSMENT

Please identify your favorite foods. Include how much and how often you would like to have them.

Favorite Foods	How Much & How Often?
Example: *Haagen-Dazs Ice Cream - Chocolate*	*1x per week - 2 scoops*
1) _____	_____
2) _____	_____
3) _____	_____
4) _____	_____
5) _____	_____
6) _____	_____
7) _____	_____
8) _____	_____
9) _____	_____
10) _____	_____

Please list the restaurants where you eat and the types of foods and beverages you like to order. Please include to-go and delivery items.

Example: *Piatti's: Pasta, Carpaccio, Caesar Salad, Tiramisu*

American: **Indian:**

Italian: **Mexican:**

Asian: **Delis:**

Fast Food:

© DITTOE & ASSOCIATES 1994

FYI Figure 6-1   Culinary Assessment (cont.)

CULINARY ASSESSMENT
(Continued)

Please indicate **favorite** foods you enjoy having at the following meals:

<u>Breakfast or Morning Snack</u>

<u>Lunch</u>

<u>Afternoon Snack</u>

<u>Dinner</u>

<u>Evening Snack</u>

Please indicate **favorite** foods you enjoy having during the following situations:

<u>Entertaining</u>

<u>Holidays</u>

FYI Figure 6-2   Fitness Assessment

FITNESS ASSESSMENT

Please circle the exercises that sound most interesting to you:

Bicycling	Squash
Swimming	Volleyball
Dancing	Badminton
Walking - brisk speed	Basketball
Jogging	Handball
Running in Place	Judo
Mini-Trampoline	Karate
Stationary Bicycle	La Crosse
Roller Skating	Cross-Country Skiing
Tennis	Ice Skating
Aerobics Class	Snow Skiing
Low Impact	Roving (walk a block,
High Impact	
Rowing	jog a block)
Soccer	Stairmaster
Racquetball	Nordic Track

When would be the best days and times to do these exercises?

Monday   Tuesday   Wednesday   Thursday   Friday   Saturday   Sunday

Early Morning   Noon   Afternoon   Evening

How do you prefer exercising?

Alone   Class   Indoors   Outdoors   With Music

Weather conditions: Cold   Cool   Warm   Hot

© DITTOE & ASSOCIATES 1994

FYI Figure 6-3   Habit Inventory

(0875A:0039A)

HABIT INVENTORY

Put the corresponding number on the blank line next to the answer.
Answer each of the questions based on your normal eating habits (not when
you are trying to diet). For each question, answer "often", "sometimes", or
"rarely". The answer has a number correspondent with it, put the number on
the line and total the numbers.

Example: I consume bread at snacks and/or meals	2	Often	2
		Sometimes	1
		Rarely	0
Total	2		

Starch Intake

1) I consume bread at snacks and/or meals.	Often	2
	Sometimes	1
	Rarely	0

2) I consume starches at dinner like potatoes, rice, noodles, and corn, etc.	Often	2
	Sometimes	1
	Rarely	0

3) I snack on crackers, fruit, bread, pretzels, or cereal.	Often	2
	Sometimes	0
	Rarely	1

4) I eat more starch at dinner than I do the main entree.	Often	2
	Sometimes	1
	Rarely	0
Total		

Fat Intake

1) I eat proteins like beef, hamburgers and red meat at lunch or dinner.	Often	0
	Sometimes	1
	Rarely	2

2) I snack on cheese, nuts, chips, peanut butter, candy bars, chocolate, and leftovers from dinner.	Often	0
	Sometimes	1
	Rarely	2

3) I consume fast foods like fries, onion rings, fried chicken, milkshakes, burritos, or hot dogs.	Often	0
	Sometimes	1
	Rarely	2

4) I use oils, margarine, butter, sauces, salad dressing on foods.	Often	0
	Sometimes	1
	Rarely	2
Total		

(Continued)

A vital part of the evaluation is diagnosing the problems and showing clients exactly what problems are occurring, why they are occurring, and more importantly, what can be done about them. Visuals are invaluable. We use the Food Patterns sheet (Figure 4) to explain how we see people eat at three different calorie levels with the middle one (Pattern B with more moderate but adequate calories) being more realistic as they try to lose weight. Pattern A illustrates the typical pattern of a person with great fluctuations in intake from semi-starvation to bingeing (stuff and starve). Pattern C is more severe dieting with inadequate calories and deprivation.

FYI Figure 6-4   Food Patterns

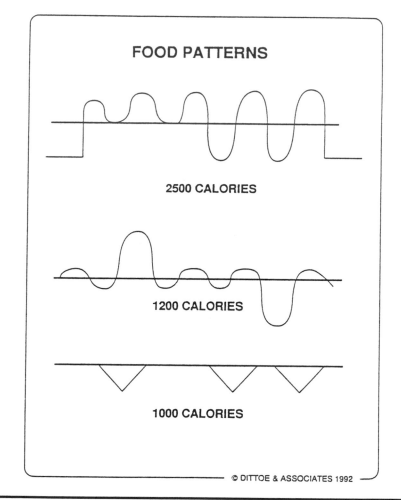

FOOD PATTERNS

2500 CALORIES

1200 CALORIES

1000 CALORIES

© DITTOE & ASSOCIATES 1992

During the evaluation we assess seven developmental-behavioral skills. The following will give a brief description of how we assess the client's ability in each skill. Overall skill levels become more apparent as treatment progresses and clients try working through problems and changes in behavior.

1. *Active listening* is easily assessed through the conversation style of the client. If clients are having difficulties in this area, they are easily distracted and interrupted. They have difficulty answering questions and following directions correctly. Although this skill is so obvious, it is easily overlooked and assumed adequate.

2. *Determines own needs* is assessed by inquiring about a client's health, family, career and personal goals. Their responses will give insight as to how in tune they are with their needs.

3. *Decision making skills* will be apparent when you ask a client what changes he or she would propose to make. The classic symptoms of poor decision making are when the client: a) has difficulty generating options, b) vacillates between options, c) becomes "stuck," d) denies there is a problem.

4. *Separation skills* will show up when clients easily take the load of others, distracting them from taking care of their own needs. Clients' thoughts and actions often are driven by external forces, or they confuse their needs with others. They generally show excessive worry about others.

5. *Delegation skills* will apparent when the client takes on too much when they could easily acquire help. Clients express feelings that are out of control or overwhelming.

6. *Assertiveness skills* can be assessed by the level and intensity of questioning by the client. A more assertive person will be more active in the counseling process. A less assertive person often will be more agreeable and accepting of any suggestions made by the therapist. A passive-aggressive person may be agreeable on the surface, but may have no intention of following through.

7. *Limit-setting skills* will be indicated if clients have a lot of chaos in their lifestyles, feel overwhelmed and show signs of just "letting things happen." Lack of the skill shows when the client can not find time for assignments and appointments designed to improve his or her health, the stated goal.

At the end of the evaluation the client will leave with a concrete idea of what is happening and what will be occurring in the future in therapy. Evaluation continues through the entire treatment process because the client's needs and skills also will evolve from analyzing and experimenting with ideas. Treatment will be adapted as the client changes. It is essential the client understands this from the very beginning.

PHASE 2
Investing Time and Money for Health

The average consumer lacks an appreciation for the amount of time, effort, and money it takes to make nutrition changes. They are clearly aggravated by health care providers who do not address this issue assertively. There is every indication in the marketplace that consumers are willing to spend time and money on health as indicated by the money spent on books, videos, weight management programs, fitness clubs, and lite food products. We need to "market" the benefits of our services to our customers and to health care insurers and managed care providers. In our practice we found that if we impress clients with how the skill-based process will meet their needs better, there is a greater willingness on clients' part to invest time, money and effort into the process.

We use the worksheet below to assist clients in creating adequate time for addressing health issues. The top of the diagram shows various steps in increasing time necessary to work on health, and the bottom half is used for figuring actual time allotments for office visits, exercise, meal preparations, or identifying problems or conflicts. Some clients have this figured out before they arrive for the first visit, but others start from scratch. (See Figure 6-5 Investing Time for Health.)

Figure 6-5: Investing Time for Health

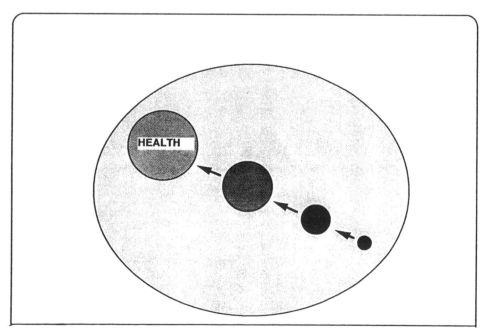

The "Phasing Treatment" visual (Figure 6-6) is used to illustrate the stages of therapy. As skills improve, treatment visits are less frequent. The phasing concept shows timing flexibility, encourages self-improvement, and shows that treatment will not go on indefinitely (some people worry about that).

FYI Figure 6-6   Phasing Treatment

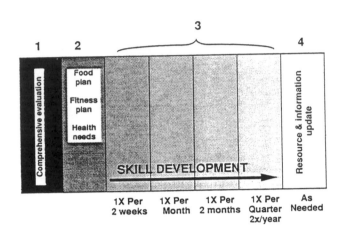

© DITTOE & ASSOCIATES 1992

Designing a Food Plan

A client benefits by helping design their own food plan. The Food Plan visual (Figure 6-7) identifies various needs to consider prior to making decisions on what to eat.

Calorie needs are self-explanatory; we use an abbreviated version of the Harris-Benedict equation.

Culinary preferences give clients permission to include all food preferences, which assists clients in moving away from the "dieting" mode.

Volume needs identify satiety and the volume of food a client's body needs to feel satisfied. Internal cue regulation will be discussed later.

Lifestyle needs are straightforward and need to be addressed in detail at this stage and in the future. More specifically, clients need to anticipate challenging situations, create solutions, and practice them in your office before experiencing them in normal living.

Transition needs like holidays and schedule changes magnify existing problems and issues. Clarity and confidence, not to mention a change in attitude, are often derived from handling an event well. One of our goals is to teach clients to "think on their feet." Experience is often the most effective facilitator and the counselor supports this through a neutral, but optimistic, attitude.

Structure is needed in food plans so that clients know what to do when they leave the office, but flexible enough to allow them to experiment with ideas. It is important to assess how much structure individual clients need.

Nutrient supplementation is based upon what the client is unable to realistically consume through his or her diet. Recommendations are not made until after the food plan is developed because we often see improvement in nutrient density.

FYI Figure 6-7   Food Plan

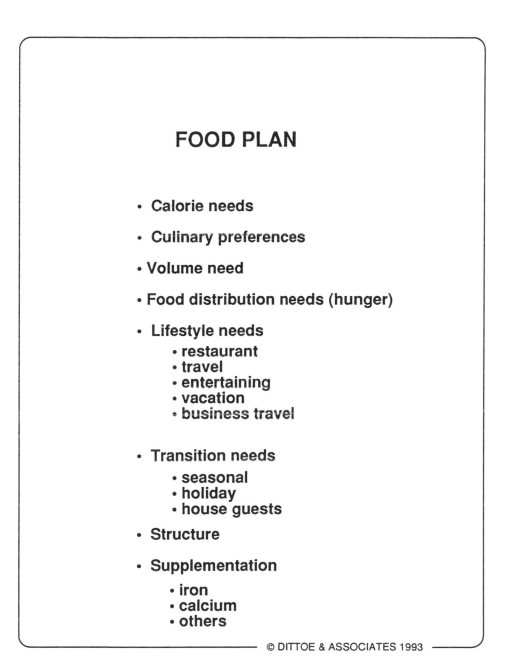

FOOD PLAN

- Calorie needs

- Culinary preferences

- Volume need

- Food distribution needs (hunger)

- Lifestyle needs
  - restaurant
  - travel
  - entertaining
  - vacation
  - business travel

- Transition needs
  - seasonal
  - holiday
  - house guests

- Structure

- Supplementation
  - iron
  - calcium
  - others

© DITTOE & ASSOCIATES 1993

The "Sample Menu" visual (Figure 6-8) illustrates a food plan draft. Please note that we incorporate the following concepts:

- structure
- food preferences
- experimenting with decreasing fat
- identifying true hunger and volume needs
- increasing nutrients through better food choices.

The overall goal is to allow adequate time to experiment with these concepts to clarify needs in all areas, which usually takes several weeks. Food plans need to be continually updated with a client.

FYI Figure 6-8   Sample Menu

SAMPLE MENU

BREAKFAST
  HUNGER LEVEL?

SNACK
  MUFFIN OR FLAVORED BAGEL

LUNCH
  1/2 SANDWICH
  MEAT?
  POULTRY?
  LITE MAYO? HOW MUCH?

SNACK
  8 OUNCES FROZEN YOGURT

SNACK
  1/2 SANDWICH

DINNER
  HUNGER LEVEL?
  MAIN ENTRE
  2 ITEMS? 3 ITEMS?
  BAKED POTATO
    OR   } HOW MUCH?
  PASTA
  SALAD OR VEGETABLE
  DRESSING?

SNACK — YES?

© DITTOE & ASSOCIATES 1992

Internal Cue Regulation: Hunger and Satiety

We have discovered that addressing hunger and satiety are two of the most effective self-monitoring tools used for long-term control. They allow clients to move away from external monitoring tools such as diet records and food plans. While working with this issue, many feelings may surface that affect food intake.

The "Volume Needs" hunger scale (Figure 6-9) represents every possible option from starvation to stuffed. Have the client take a standard sandwich and divide it into eighths. The client should begin the experiment at a comfortable hunger level, not starved as it will distort his or her volume needs. The client should eat 1/8 at a time slowly, experiencing the different levels until satiety is reached. The experiment may need to be repeated a second or third time until the client is able to internalize the appropriate volume. The majority of clients state it takes anywhere from 6/8 to a full sandwich to feel satisfied. Ninety percent of the time this is less than they commonly eat. Clients' volume needs will vary slightly from meal-to-meal and day-to-day, but this will make them consciously aware of how much food makes them feel physiologically satisfied. They will begin to distinguish between physical and psychological hunger. It is reasonable to expect hunger again in several hours, and people will vary when they feel it. Be sure to encourage clients to use this at the time they eat the food. Recall is too inaccurate.

FYI Figure 6-9 Volume Needs

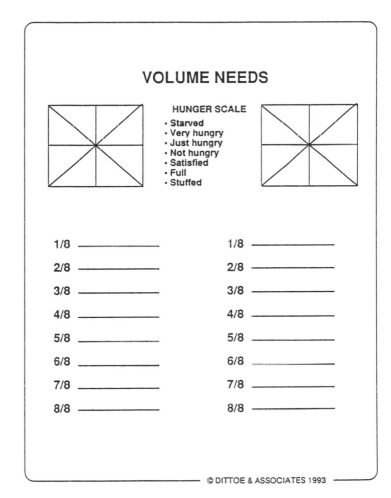

PHASE 3
Developmental-Behavioral Skills

We find the majority of our clients with eating and health problems have difficulty with some or all of the developmental-behavioral skills mentioned earlier in this article and in Chapter 2. Acquiring these skills will have an enormous impact on a client's ability to achieve more complex problem-solving. It is our experience that a dietitian's ability to teach these skills is limited by that person's own emotional growth and familiarity using the skills.

Dietitians can be taught these skills through formal education and training like getting a master's in counseling or taking Laurel Mellin's ShapeDown weight management certification (see Appendix 2-B). Another method is to experience psychotherapy supervision or therapy from a competent licensed counselor, psychologist or psychiatrist.

If a client is having continued difficulty with basic problem-solving or compulsive/ addictive behavior, it is very appropriate to refer him or her to a mental health counselor. We find that by using a collaborative approach with clients, their long-term outcomes are very successful.

Following is an overview of treatment ideas and the way we use developmental-behavioral skills to improve our clients' nutrition and food-related outcomes.

Active listening It is very appropriate to discuss this skill "head-on" with clients. Then give clients examples of how to listen more actively such as concentrating on the concepts instead of each word the other person is saying, or maintaining eye contact (when culturally appropriate), or keeping hands and feet still, or avoiding listening to or thinking about anything but the immediate conversation. There is an accumulative effect of this skill in that clients get better and better as treatment progresses, if they work on it. Poor listening skills usually stem from a deficit early in life either genetic (like Attention Deficit Disorder ADD) or a learned behavior, or it may be from a hearing impairment.

Determines own needs is assessed by inquiring about a client's health, family, career and personal goals. Their responses will give insight as to how in tune they are with their needs.

Decision making To help clients improve their ability with this skill, begin with simple decisions around scheduling appointments and making decisions on the food plan where they have guaranteed success. Ask the client to generate an option or decision first. If the client gets stuck, ask it again, rephrase it or come back to the question later. This will force the clients to start thinking on their own. For example, "It appears you have a need for quick dinners; what are your options?" Walk through the pros and cons of each option until they discover a reasonable one.

Ask, "What are your fitness options on the weekends, during the week, and during the winter?" Have clients draw from both past and projected experiences. When you walk clients through this detailed process, they will be able to create decisions, determine their needs and build on them later. If clients are coached in a gentle way, their progress is acknowledged, and if they are encouraged to do it more often, their confidence will grow.

Separation skills We help clients improve in this skill by encouraging them to become more neutral and less effected by the views of others. We ask clients to comment on others' behaviors and then walk them through the "so what" process. It allows clients to see the absurdity of the other individual's behavior, the significance of it, or how their own behavior is judgmental. This concept is called "grounding." It provides a foundation for protecting clients' own needs, and therefore separating from others. It also is effective to walk clients through the impact of their decisions, which generally translates into conflict and causes anxiety for clients. As a result, they need to learn to tolerate others' anger and inappropriate feelings in order to hold onto their own decisions. By explaining this on a practical level and using humor, it helps clients grow through the process. As mentioned earlier, if clients have a prolonged struggle in this area, a referral to a mental health professional is appropriate.

Delegation skills This skill gives considerable leverage and freedom to a client. In our world of juggling many roles, learning to delegate can relieve stress created by a pressured schedule. To help clients, have them create a list of all tasks and situations they ideally would like to delegate; discuss the pros and cons of each and determine which ones could be delegated. Often we get a better understanding why clients aren't delegating through this process. Walk the client through the list starting with the easiest task first. Clients will again build upon their successes and hopefully, continue the process after nutrition intervention is over.

Assertiveness The lack of assertiveness is a common problem for clients having difficulties with food issues. When a person is not assertive, he or she often feels lack of control except in one area—what and how he or she chooses to eat. Becoming assertive allows clients to ask for help when they need it, set limits on others' inappropriate behavior, and ultimately improve their self-esteem. We first help clients define aggressiveness and passiveness, then we explore the middle road of assertiveness. It helps to point out times when they are assertive on an issue and congratulate them for it. Role playing through "lifelike" examples suggested by the client or created by the counselor allows the client to acquire confidence and experience. Start on less emotional examples to build the client's confidence and then move on to more "emotionally charged" issues when he or she is ready. Continue to work on the skill through several sessions, if necessary. We stress that being assertive usually means speaking in a reasonable tone, stating needs in a reasonable fashion with confidence and including some room for flexibility.

Setting limits This involves setting limits on tasks, individuals and situations to allow adequate time to become healthier. Many times this process raises conflicts which are difficult for clients. By exploring these conflicts, you will get an idea of how complex the client's problems are and again, a referral may be in order.

The next step is to walk clients through past food-related scenarios that were a problem and rework them. This will give them lifelike experiences before they tackle anticipated problems. For example, doing too much on the weekend is a classic issue with many clients. Have clients set priorities so they can incorporate some fun and let less important tasks go (or delegate them)! A second common example is having too much to do after work. Have clients learn to set limits on phone calls or tasks that interfere with their ability to unwind and relax. Have them ask family members for help with dinner or run errands for them. Again, walk them through solutions so they can build confidence in this skill.

SUMMARY

The accumulative effect of learning the previous skills will now allow clients to problem-solve at a higher level. By counseling clients using the skills and visuals, the clients understand their problems better and the solutions more clearly. They get to the root of many of their long-standing behaviors and thoughts that have been complicating their lives for years. As a result, nutrition intervention becomes a major turning point in clients' lives.

Appendix 6-A

Pediatric Nutrition Assessment (Birth to 36 months)

Children's Hospital Medical Center

Diagnosis: _____

Growth History:

Previous Weights			Previous Heights			Growth Velocity: _____
date	kg	%ile	date	cm	%ile	
___	___	___	___	___	___	_____
___	___	___	___	___	___	
___	___	___	___	___	___	_____

Date				NUTRITIONAL RISK CRITERIA
Age				
Weight (kg)				< 5th %ile
%ile				
Length (cm)				< 5th %ile suggests growth retardation
%ile				
Head Circumference				< 5th %ile
%ile				
Ideal Weight for Length				
Weight/Length Index (actual weight - ideal weight for length)				80% to 90%; Mild PEM* / 70% to 80%; Moderate PEM* / <70%; Severe PEM*
Height/Age Index (actual HT ideal HT for age)				90% to 95%; Mild Chronic Malnu. / 85% to 90%; Mod. Chronic Malnu. / <85%; Severe Chronic Malnu.
Arm Circumference/ Head Circumference Ratio				.28 to .31; Mild PEM* / .25 to .28; Moderate PEM* / <.25; Severe PEM*
Arm Circumference (cm)				
%ile				< 5th %ile
Arm Muscle Circumference (mm)				< 5th %ile
%ile				
Arm Muscle Area (mm^2)				< 5th %ile
%ile				
Tricep Skinfold (mm)				< 5th %ile
%ile				
Subscapular Skinfold (mm)				< 5th %ile
%ile				

*PEM: Protein Energy Malnutrition

Date					NUTRITIONAL RISK CRITERIA
Albumin					0-6 mo <2.9 gm/dl / 6mo-3yr <3.5 gm/dl
Transferrin					<200 mg/dl
Pre Albumin					
Retinol Binding Protein					
Total Lymphocyte Count					< 1500 mm^3

Intake

    Dates _____

    Kcal/Kg _____

    gm pro/kg _____

Oxygen consumption: Date ____ REE = _____ RQ = ____ Maintenance _____ Kcal/day

    Catch Up _____ Kcal/day

NUTRITIONAL NEEDS+ ____ Kcal/Kg ____ gm pro/kg

based on _____

    (+energy needs increase 7% per degree F.)

Expected rate of weight gain for size:_____

Comments: _____

_____

_____

_____

CHMC NS #1029 5/

Pediatric Nutrition Assessment (3-18 yrs.)

NUTRITION ASSESSMENT
(3 to 18 years)

Diagnosis:

Growth History: Previous Weights   Previous Heights
date kg %ile   date cm %ile

Previous Growth Velocity:

	NUTRITIONAL RISK CRITERIA
Date	
Age	
Weight (kg)	< 5th %ile
%ile	
Height (cm)	< 5th %ile suggests growth retardation
%ile	
Ideal Weight for Height	
Weight/Height Index (actual weight - ideal weight for height)	80% to 90%; Mild PEM* 70% to 80%; Moderate PEM* <70%; Severe PEM*
Height/Age Index (actual HT - ideal HT for age)	90% to 95%; Mild Chronic Malnu. 85% to 90%; Mod. Chronic Malnu. <85%; Severe Chronic Malnu.
Arm Circumference (cm)	< 5th %ile
%ile	
Arm Muscle Circumference (mm)	< 5th %ile
%ile	
Arm Muscle Area (mm²)	< 5th %ile
%ile	
Tricep Skinfold (mm)	< 5th %ile
%ile	
Subscapular Skinfold (mm)	< 5th %ile
%ile	

*PEM: Protein Energy Malnutrition

	NUTRITIONAL RISK CRITERIA
Date	
Albumin	<3.5 gm/dl
Transferrin	<200 mcg/dl
Pre Albumin	
Retinol Binding Protein	
Total Lymphocyte Count	< 1500 mm³
Intake Dates	
Kcal/Kg	
gm pro/kg	

Oxygen consumption: Date ____ REE = ____ RQ = ____

NUTRITIONAL NEEDS+
based on ____ Kcal/Kg ____ gm pro/kg

	Maintenance	Catch Up
	____ Kcal/day	____ Kcal/day

Expected rate of weight gain for size: ____

Comments:

+(+energy needs increase 7% per degree F.)

CHMC NS #1150 5/90

Used with permission. Clinical Nutrition Services, Children's Hospital Medical Center. Cincinnati, OH.

Pediatric Outpatient Services Form

CHILDREN'S HOSPITAL MEDICAL CENTER

VISIT: RECORD OF

___ INITIAL   OUTPATIENT SERVICES

___ FOLLOW-UP   NUTRITION CLINIC

REFERRAL:

___ INTERNAL   DOCTOR NAME   DOCTOR NUMBER

___ OUTSIDE HEALTH   APPT TIME   ARRIVAL TIME   PROF COURTESY
FACILITY OR M.D.

GUARANTOR ADDRESS CHANGE:

X	DIAGNOSIS	CODE	X	DIAGNOSIS	CODE	X	DIAGNOSIS	CODE
	Anemia, Iron Def	280.9		Feeding Problem	783.3		Nutrition Deficiency	269.9
	Anemia, Aplastic	284.9		Fracture-Mandible	802.20		Obesity Exogenous	278.0
	Anorexia Nervosa	207.1		Gastroenteritis	558.9		Omphalocele	553.1
	Atrial Septal Defect	745.5		Glycogen Storage Dis	271.0		Osteogenic Sarcoma	170.9
	Biliary Atresia	751.61		Hepatoblastoma	155.0		Pancreatitis	577.0
	s/p Bone Marrow Trans	V42.8		Hepatitis	573.3		Prader-Willi Syndrome	759.8
	Bowel Atresia	751.8		Hirschprung's Disease	751.3		Pyelonephritis	690.80
	Brain Tumor, All	192.9		Hodgkin's Disease	201.90		Renal Insufficiency	593.9
	Bronchopulm, Dysplasia	770.7		Hypoglycemia	251.2		Renal Rubular Acidosis	558.8
	Bulemia, non-organic	307.51		Immunodeficiency	279.3		s/p Renal Transp.	V42.0
	Burns	949.0		Inflammatory Bowel Dis	558.9		Retinoblastoma	190.5
	Celiac Disease	579.0		JRA	714.3		Rhabodymyosarcoma	171.9
	Cerebral Palsy	343.9		Leukemia, Acute Lymph	204.0		Short Gut Syndrome	579.2
	CHF	428.0		Leukemia, Acute Mono	206.0		Sickle Cell Anemia	282.6
	Cirrhosis	571.5		Leukemia, Acute Myelo	205.0		Systemic Lupus Eryth	710.0
	Cleft Lip	749.10		Leukemia, Chron Myelo	205.1		Tetrology of Fallot	745.2
	Cleft Lip & Palate	749.20		Leukemia, Acute Undiff	208.0		Trans of great vessels	745.10
	Cleft Palate	749.00		s/p Liver Transp	V42.7		Ulcerative Colitis	556.0
	Constipation	564.0		Lymphoma, Malignant	202.80		Undiff. Sarcoma	239.2
	Crohn's Disease	555.9		Malabsorption-Misc	579.9		Ventricular Septal Def	745.4
	Cystic Fibrosis	277.0		Malnutrition, Severe	262		Well Baby/Child Care	V20.2
	Developmental Delay	783.4		Malnutrition, Moderate	263.0		Weight Loss	783.2
	Diabetes Mellitus	250.01		Malnutrition, Mild	263.1		Wilm's Tumor	189.0
	Diarrhea, chronic nonsp	558.9		Malnutrition, Unspec	263.9		Volk Sac Tumor/Male	186.9
	Encopresis	787.6		Myelomeningocele	741.9		Volk Sac Tumor/Female	183.0
	Esophageal Atresia	750.3		Nector, Entercolotis	557.0		Other	
	Ewings Sarcoma	170.9		Nephrotic Syndrome	581.9			
	Failure to Thrive	783.4		Neuroblastoma	194.0			

SERVICE PERFORMED _____   DISPOSITION: RETURN APPOINTMENT _____

REFER TO: _____

Adult Nutrition Risk Screening Form

UNIT NO.

NAME

ADDRESS

BIRTH DATE

(If handwritten record name, unit no. and birth date.)

YALE NEW HAVEN HOSPITAL

Nutrition Risk Screening Form

NUTRITION RISK FACTORS

☐ 1. Age (< 18 or > 50) _____
☐ 2. Diagnosis/ _____
   Treatment _____
☐ 3. Metabolic/Mechanical Problems _____
   _____
☐ 4. Sig. Lab Data _____
   _____
☐ 5. Diet Order/Nutrition Support _____
☐ 6. Sig. Meds _____
☐ 7. Wt/Ht _____

ASSESSMENT

☐ 1. Currently nutritionally stable/At low risk for Protein and/or Calorie Malnutrition (PCM).
☐ 2. At high risk for PCM.
☐ 3. Has PCM. Type _____ /Code _____
☐ 4. Receiving comfort measures only.
☐ 5. Unable/Unwilling to comply with medical/nutritional therapy.
☐ 6. Advanced nutrition support is indicated.
☐ 7. Other _____

Class: _____

RD PLAN

☐ 1. Will follow-up as needed or when consulted.
☐ 2. Will adjust diet to _____
   unless advised otherwise.
☐ 3. Full nutrition assessment and recommendations to follow. _____
☐ 4. Other _____

ATTENTION RN

☐ 1. No additional recommendations.
☐ 2. Obtain Wt. _____
☐ 3. Obtain Ht. _____
☐ 4. Record P.O. intake. _____
☐ 5. Recommend pt. attend _____
   _____ class.
☐ 6. Note diet adjustments (above).
☐ 7. Other _____

ATTENTION MD

☐ 1. Continue current nutrition therapy.
☐ 2. Diet adjusted to _____
   _____ unless advised otherwise.
☐ 3. Obtain the following labs:
   _____
   _____
☐ 4. Other _____

_____   _____   _____
Dietitian   /Beeper No.   Date

F-2705 (Rev. 7/92)   **Medical Record Copy**

Used with permission.

Appendix 6-B

Determine Your Nutritional Health

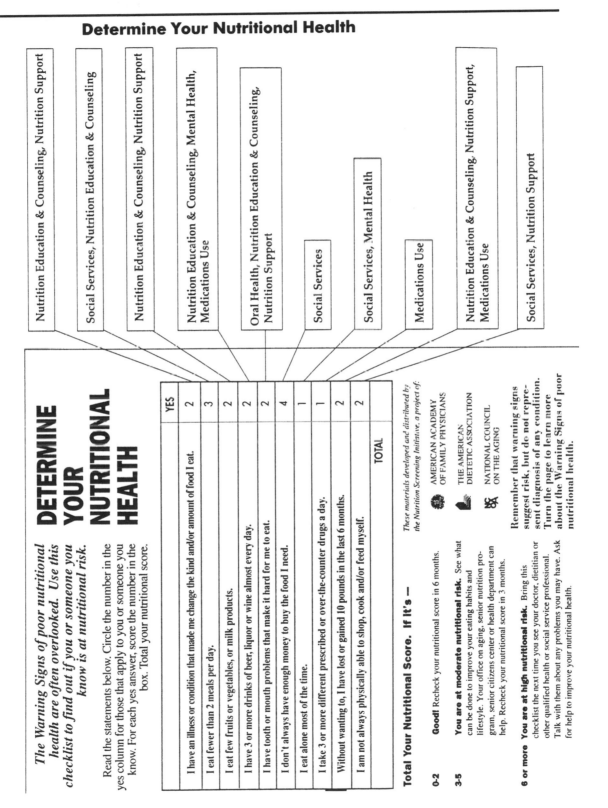

The Warning Signs of poor nutritional health are often overlooked. Use this checklist to find out if you or someone you know is at nutritional risk.

Read the statements below. Circle the number in the yes column for those that apply to you or someone you know. For each yes answer, score the number in the box. Total your nutritional score.

DETERMINE YOUR NUTRITIONAL HEALTH

	YES
I have an illness or condition that made me change the kind and/or amount of food I eat.	2
I eat fewer than 2 meals per day.	3
I eat few fruits or vegetables, or milk products.	2
I have 3 or more drinks of beer, liquor or wine almost every day.	2
I have tooth or mouth problems that make it hard for me to eat.	2
I don't always have enough money to buy the food I need.	4
I eat alone most of the time.	1
I take 3 or more different prescribed or over-the-counter drugs a day.	1
Without wanting to, I have lost or gained 10 pounds in the last 6 months.	2
I am not always physically able to shop, cook and/or feed myself.	2
TOTAL	

Warning Signs references (right side):

- Nutrition Education & Counseling, Nutrition Support
- Social Services, Nutrition Education & Counseling
- Nutrition Education & Counseling, Nutrition Support
- Nutrition Education & Counseling, Mental Health, Medications Use
- Oral Health, Nutrition Education & Counseling, Nutrition Support
- Social Services
- Social Services, Mental Health
- Medications Use
- Nutrition Education & Counseling, Nutrition Support, Medications Use
- Social Services, Nutrition Support

Total Your Nutritional Score. If It's —

0-2   **Good!** Recheck your nutritional score in 6 months.

3-5   **You are at moderate nutritional risk.** See what can be done to improve your eating habits and lifestyle. Your office on aging, senior nutrition program, senior citizens center or health department can help. Recheck your nutritional score in 3 months.

6 or more   **You are at high nutritional risk.** Bring this checklist the next time you see your doctor, dietitian or other qualified health or social service professional. Talk with them about any problems you may have. Ask for help to improve your nutritional health.

These materials developed and distributed by the Nutrition Screening Initiative, a project of:

- AMERICAN ACADEMY OF FAMILY PHYSICIANS
- THE AMERICAN DIETETIC ASSOCIATION
- NATIONAL COUNCIL ON THE AGING

Remember that warning signs suggest risk, but do not represent diagnosis of any condition. Turn the page to learn more about the Warning Signs of poor nutritional health.

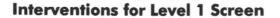

Interventions for Level 1 Screen

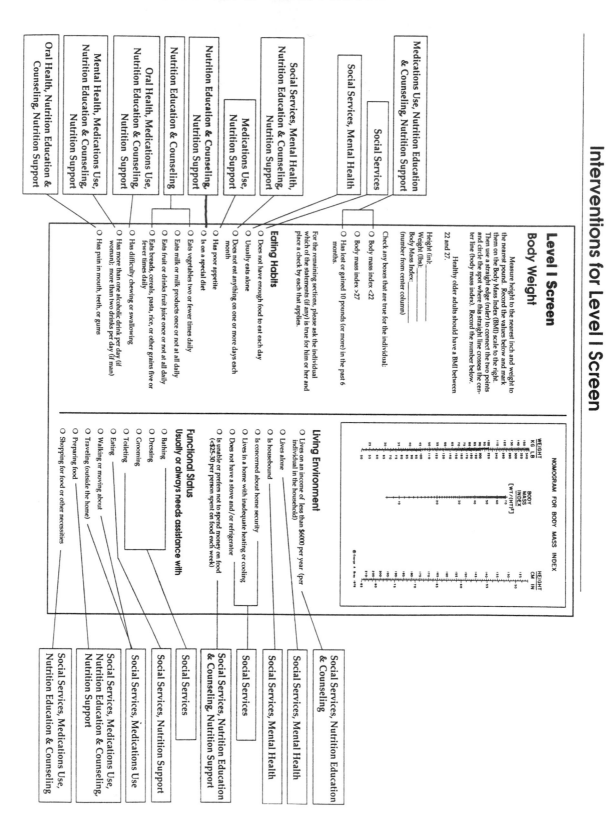

Interventions for Level 1 Screen

Level 1 Screen

Body Weight

Measure height to the nearest inch and weight to the nearest pound. Record the values below and mark them on the Body Mass Index (BMI) scale to the right. Then use a straight edge (ruler) to connect the two points and circle the spot where this straight line crosses the center line (body mass index). Record the number below.

Healthy older adults should have a BMI between 22 and 27.

Height (in): _____
Weight (lbs): _____
Body Mass Index: _____
(number from center column)

For the remaining sections, please ask the individual which of the statements (if any) is true for him or her and place a check by each that applies.

○ Has lost or gained 10 pounds (or more) in the past 6 months.

○ Body mass index <22

○ Body mass index >27

Check any boxes that are true for the individual:

Eating Habits

○ Does not have enough food to eat each day
○ Usually eats alone
○ Does not eat anything on one or more days each month
○ Has poor appetite
○ Is on a special diet
○ Eats vegetables two or fewer times daily
○ Eats milk or milk products once or not at all daily
○ Eats fruit or drinks fruit juice once or not at all daily
○ Eats breads, cereals, pasta, rice, or other grains five or fewer times daily
○ Has difficulty chewing or swallowing
○ Has more than one alcoholic drink per day (if woman); more than two drinks per day (if man)
○ Has pain in mouth, teeth, or gums

Living Environment

○ Lives on an income of less than $6000 per year (per individual in the household)
○ Lives alone
○ Is housebound
○ Is concerned about home security
○ Lives in a home with inadequate heating or cooling
○ Does not have a stove and/or refrigerator
○ Is unable or prefers not to spend money on food (<$25-30 per person spent on food each week)

Functional Status
Usually or always needs assistance with

○ Bathing
○ Dressing
○ Grooming
○ Toileting
○ Eating
○ Walking or moving about
○ Traveling (outside the home)
○ Preparing food
○ Shopping for food or other necessities

NOMOGRAM FOR BODY MASS INDEX

WEIGHT KG LB — BODY MASS INDEX [WT/(HT)²] — HEIGHT CM IN

Intervention boxes (left/top):

- Medications Use, Nutrition Education & Counseling, Nutrition Support
- Social Services
- Social Services, Mental Health
- Social Services, Mental Health, Nutrition Education & Counseling, Nutrition Support
- Medications Use, Nutrition Support
- Nutrition Education & Counseling, Nutrition Support
- Nutrition Education & Counseling, Nutrition Support
- Oral Health, Medications Use, Nutrition Education & Counseling, Nutrition Support
- Nutrition Education & Counseling
- Mental Health, Medications Use, Nutrition Education & Counseling, Nutrition Support
- Oral Health, Nutrition Education & Counseling, Nutrition Support

Intervention boxes (right/bottom):

- Social Services, Nutrition Education & Counseling
- Social Services, Nutrition Education
- Social Services, Mental Health
- Social Services, Mental Health
- Social Services
- Social Services, Nutrition Education & Counseling, Nutrition Support
- Social Services
- Social Services, Nutrition Support
- Social Services, Medications Use
- Social Services, Medications Use, Nutrition Education & Counseling, Nutrition Support
- Social Services, Medications Use, Nutrition Education & Counseling

Appendix 6-C

Weight Loss Readiness Quiz

NATIONAL CENTER FOR NUTRITION AND DIETETICS

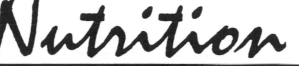

Nutrition

FACT SHEET

Weight Loss Readiness Quiz

Are you ready to lose weight? Your attitude about weight loss affects your ability to succeed. Take this Readiness Quiz to learn if you need to make any attitude adjustments before you begin. Mark each item true or false. Be honest! It's important that these answers reflect the way you really are, not how you would like to be. A method for interpreting your readiness for weight loss follows:

1.___I have thought a lot about my eating habits and physical activities to pinpoint what I need to change.

2.___I have accepted the idea that I need to make permanent, not temporary, changes in my eating and activities to be successful.

3.___I will only feel successful if I lose a lot of weight.

4.___I accept the idea that it's best if I lose weight slowly.

5.___I'm thinking of losing weight now because I really want to, not because someone else thinks I should.

6.___I think losing weight will solve other problems in my life.

7.___I am willing and able to increase my regular physical activity.

8.___I can lose weight successfully if I have no "slip-ups."

9.___I am ready to commit some time and effort each week to organizing and planning my food and activity programs.

10.___Once I lose some initial weight, I usually lose the motivation to keep going until I reach my goal.

11.___I want to start a weight loss program, even though my life is unusually stressful right now.

Scoring the weight loss readiness quiz. To score the quiz, look at your answers to items 1, 2, 4, 5, 7, 9. Score "1" if you answered "true" and "0" if you answered "false."

. For items 3, 6, 8,10, 11, score "0" for each true answer and "1" for each false answer. To get your total score, add the scores for all questions.

No one score indicates for sure whether you are ready or not to start losing weight. However, the higher your total score, the more characteristics you have that contribute to success. As a rough guide, consider the following recommendations: 1) If you scored 8 or higher, you probably have good reasons for wanting to lose weight now and a good understanding of the steps needed to succeed. Still, you might want to learn more about the areas where you scored a "0" (see "Interpretation of Quiz Items" below). 2) If you scored 5 to 7, you may need to reevaluate your reasons for losing weight and the methods you would use to do so. To get a start, read the advice below for those quiz items where you received a score of "0."

3) If you scored 4 or less, now may not be the right time for you to lose weight. While you might be successful in losing weight initially, your answers suggest that you are unlikely to sustain sufficient effort to lose all the weight you want or to keep off the weight that you do lose. You need to reconsider your weight loss motivations and methods and perhaps learn more about the pros and cons of different approaches to reducing. To do so, read the advice below for those quiz items where you marked "0."

Interpretation of Quiz Items. Your answers to the Quiz can clue you in to potential stumbling blocks to your weight loss success. Any item score of "0" indicates a misconception about weight loss, or a potential problem area. While no individual items score of "0" is important enough to scuttle your weight loss plans, we suggest that you consider the meaning of those items so you can best prepare yourself for the challenges ahead.

1. It has been said that you can't change what you don't understand. You might benefit from keeping records for a week to help pinpoint when, what, why, and how much you eat. This tool is also useful in identifying obstacles to regular physical activity.

Weight Loss Readiness Quiz (cont.)

2. Making drastic or highly restrictive changes in your eating habits may allow you to lose weight in the short-run, but be too hard to live with permanently. Similarly, your program of regular physical activity should be one you can sustain. Both your food plan and activity program should be healthful and enjoyable.

3. Most people have fantasies of reaching a weight considerably lower than they can realistically maintain. Rethink your meaning of "success." A successful, realistic weight loss is one that can be comfortably maintained through sensible eating and regular activity. Take your body type into consideration. Then set smaller, achievable goals. Your first goal may be to lose a small amount of weight while you learn eating habits and activity patterns to help you maintain it.

4. If you equate success with fast weight loss, you will have problems maintaining your weight. This "quick fix" attitude can backfire when you face the challenges of weight maintenance. It's best — and healthiest — to lose weight slowly while learning the strategies to keep the weight off permanently.

5. The desire for and commitment to weight loss must come from you. People who lose and maintain weight loss successfully take responsibility for their own desires and decide the best way to achieve them. Once this step is taken, friends and family are an important source of support, not motivation.

6. While being overweight may contribute to a number of social problems, it is rarely the single cause. Anticipating that all your problems will be solved through weight loss is unrealistic and may set you up for disappointment. Instead, realize that successful weight loss will make you feel more self-confident and empowered, and that the skills you develop to deal with your weight can be applied to other areas of your life.

7. Studies have shown that people who develop the habit of regular, moderate physical activity are most successful at maintaining their weight. Exercise does not have to be strenuous to be effective for weight control. Any moderate, physical activity that you enjoy and will do regularly counts. Just get moving!

8. While most people don't expect perfection of themselves in everyday life, many feel they must stick to a weight loss program perfectly. Perfection at weight loss is unrealistic. Rather than expecting it and viewing lapses as catastrophes, recognize them as valuable opportunities to identify problem triggers and develop strategies for the future.

9. Successful weight loss is not possible without taking the time to think about yourself, assess your problem areas, and develop strategies to deal with them. Success requires planning and takes time. You must commit to planning and organizing your weight loss.

10. Do not ignore your concerns about "going the distance" because they may indicate a potential problem. Think about past efforts and why they failed. Pinpoint any reasons, and work on developing motivational strategies to get you over these hurdles. Take your effort one day at a time; a plateau of weight maintenance within an ongoing weight loss program is perfectly okay.

11. Weight loss itself is a source of stress, so if you are already under stress, it may be difficult to implement a successful weight loss program at this time. Try to resolve other stress sources in your life before you begin a weight loss effort.

For more information, call the Consumer Nutrition Hot Line 800/366-1655 to speak with a registered dietitian.

This fact sheet is supported by a grant from Weight Watchers International, Inc.

Used with permission. National Center for Nutrition and Dietetics of The American Dietetic Association.

Appendix 6-D

Typical Nutrition Section of Health Risk Appraisal

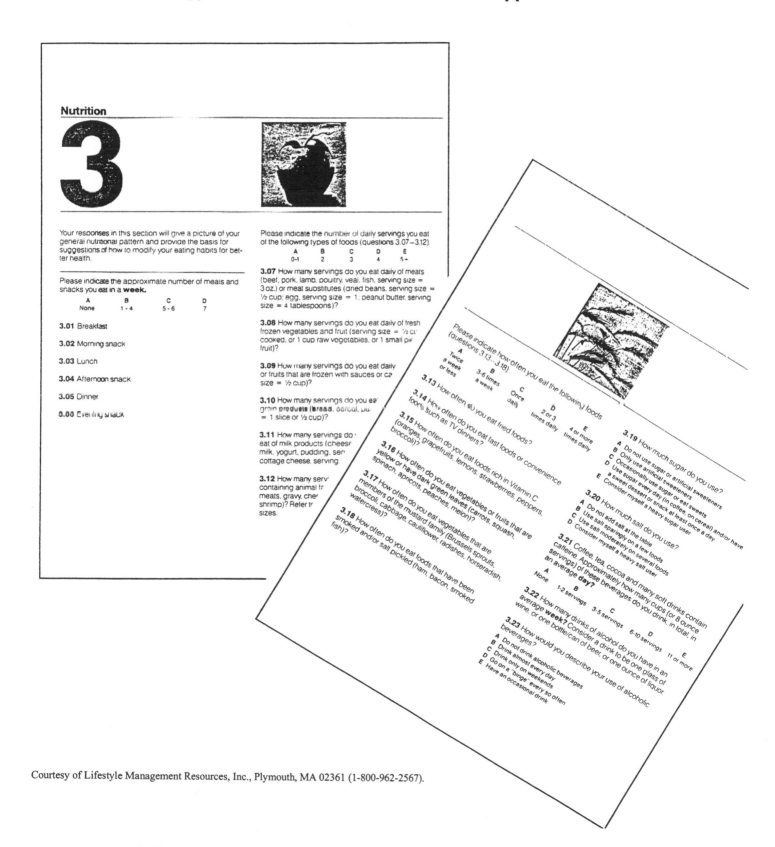

Nutrition

3

Your responses in this section will give a picture of your general nutritional pattern and provide the basis for suggestions of how to modify your eating habits for better health.

Please indicate the approximate number of meals and snacks you eat in a **week.**

	A None	B 1 - 4	C 5 - 6	D 7

3.01 Breakfast

3.02 Morning snack

3.03 Lunch

3.04 Afternoon snack

3.05 Dinner

3.06 Evening snack

Please indicate the number of daily servings you eat of the following types of foods (questions 3.07 – 3.12).

	A 0-1	B 2	C 3	D 4	E 5 +

3.07 How many servings do you eat daily of meats (beef, pork, lamb, poultry, veal, fish, serving size = 3 oz.) or meat substitutes (dried beans, serving size = ½ cup; egg, serving size = 1; peanut butter, serving size = 4 tablespoons)?

3.08 How many servings do you eat daily of fresh frozen vegetables and fruit (serving size = ½ cu cooked, or 1 cup raw vegetables, or 1 small pie fruit)?

3.09 How many servings do you eat daily or fruits that are frozen with sauces or ca size = ½ cup)?

3.10 How many servings do you ea' grain products (**bread**, cereal, pa = 1 slice or ½ cup)?

3.11 How many servings do eat of milk products (cheese milk, yogurt, pudding, ser cottage cheese, serving

3.12 How many servi' containing animal fr meats, gravy, che shrimp)? Refer t sizes.

Please indicate how often you eat the following foods (questions 3.13–3.18)

A Twice a week or less	B 3-6 times a week	C Once daily	D 2 or 3 times daily	E 4 or more times daily

3.13 How often do you eat fried foods?

3.14 How often do you eat fast foods or convenience foods such as TV dinners?

3.15 How often do you eat foods rich in Vitamin C (oranges, grapefruits, lemons, strawberries, peppers, broccoli)?

3.16 How often do you eat vegetables or fruits that are yellow, or have dark green leaves (carrots, squash, spinach, apricots, peaches, melon)?

3.17 How often do you eat vegetables that are members of the mustard family (Brussels sprouts, broccoli, cabbage, cauliflower, radishes, horseradish, watercress)?

3.18 How often do you eat foods that have been smoked and/or salt pickled (ham, bacon, smoked fish)?

3.19 How much sugar do you use?
A Do not use sugar or artificial sweeteners
B Only use artificial sweeteners
C Occasionally use sugar or eat sweets
D Use sugar every day (in coffee, on cereal) and/or have a sweet dessert or snack at least once a day
E Consider myself a heavy sugar user

3.20 How much salt do you use?
A Do not add salt at the table
B Use salt sparingly on a few foods
C Use salt moderately on several foods
D Consider myself a heavy salt user

3.21 Coffee, tea, cocoa and many soft drinks contain caffeine. Approximately how many cups (or 8 ounce servings) of these beverages do you drink, in total, in an average **day?**

A None	B 1-2 servings	C 3-5 servings	D 6-10 servings	E 11 or more

3.22 How many drinks of alcohol do you have in an average **week?** Consider a drink to be one glass of wine, or one bottle/can of beer, or one ounce of liquor.

3.23 How would you describe your use of alcoholic beverages?
A Do not drink alcoholic beverages
B Drink almost every day
C Drink only on weekends
D Go on a "binge" every so often
E Have an occasional drink

Courtesy of Lifestyle Management Resources, Inc., Plymouth, MA 02361 (1-800-962-2567).

Health Risk Appraisal–Sample Feedback Report

U. LOVELY	BIOMETRIC PROFILE SERIES 150-HR	012-31-2231
December 2, 1994		Age: 24 Sex: m

HEALTH ALERT

Blood Pressure

BIOMETRIC PROFILE

CORONARY HEALTH

	v.good	good	fair	poor	v.poor
Coronary Health Index					
Smoking (Heart)					
Blood Pressure					
Total Cholesterol					
HDL Cholesterol					
Personal Diabetes Hist.					
Blood Sugar					
Triglycerides					

CANCER PREVENTION

	v.good	good	fair	poor	v.poor
Tobacco Use (Cancer)					
Diet					

STRESS

	v.good	good	fair	poor	v.poor
General Outlook					
Physical Conditions					

NUTRITION

	v.good	good	fair	poor	v.poor
Nutrition Pattern					
Dietary Substances					

EXERCISE AND FITNESS

	v.good	good	fair	poor	v.poor
Resting Heart Rate					
Aerobic Training					
Muscle S & E Trng.					
Flexibility Training					

7

Counseling Skills for Behavior Change

Idamarie Laquatra, PhD, RD, V.P., Scientific Affairs and Training, Diet Center Worldwide, Inc. and Steven J. Danish, PhD, Dir., Life Skills Center and Prof. of Psychology & Preventive Medicine, Virginia Commonwealth University

---

After reading this chapter, the reader will be able to:
- ☐ identify four reasons for utilizing counseling skills in their practice
- ☐ discuss appropriate counseling situations for the use of confrontation
- ☐ identify influencing skills utilized in a counseling session
- ☐ identify potential barriers to client goal achievement and methods to overcome these barriers

---

BECOMING EFFECTIVE COUNSELORS

What does nutrition counseling really mean? What are you trying to achieve through your counseling? More importantly, what are the client's goals for the nutrition counseling process?

Armed with loads of nutrition facts and figures, too many dietitians flood clients with information in the hopes that their behaviors will change. How effective is giving information on behavior change? Not very. Patients forget most of what they hear during informational sessions. The more information that's given, the more that's forgotten. (1) You may lull yourself into thinking that if you can just figure out the right piece of information or point out their problems, you will motivate clients to change their behaviors. Nothing could be further from the truth. This is not to say that giving information is without merit.

The real issue is learning to understand the client and the client's problem so well that you know the obstacles clients face when trying to reach their goals.

Incorporating specific skills into your nutrition counseling demands a commitment and it often requires some significant behavior changes on your part. Just like the clients you see, making behavior changes often turns out to be quite difficult. Yet, dietitians expect clients to make incredible changes in their lives. Should you expect anything less of yourself?

Rationale For Learning and Using Counseling Skills

To change the way you counsel requires acceptance of a rationale for doing so. Specific reasons for making the effort to learn and use counseling skills are:
- the skills facilitate change,
- they empower clients to make their own decisions,
- they empower dietitians,
- they produce results.

Facilitating Change. In order to help clients change, you must first understand the problem from their perspective. The counseling skills help you zero in on the problem so you can work with clients to develop appropriate behavior change strategies.

Empowering Clients. The skills enable clients to make their own decisions and control their behaviors. A major hurdle you must face is letting clients be less than perfect. New for some practitioners is the idea of encouraging "coping" or "managing" instead of "perfection." Perfection is not necessary to be successful in life, learning to cope and manage are. For example, dietitians learn specific dietary measures for specific diseases, and unfortunately, they often teach the diet in absolutes. Clients then tend to think in absolutes and feel as though they are failures if they cannot follow the program to the letter. Steps aren't small, they are the whole problem at once.

It's almost as if counseling is backwards: the diet is given in absolutes, the client follows the diet until the first obstacle derails adherence efforts. Then the client backslides, berates his or her efforts and continues to fail to measure up to perfection. The dietitian, in an attempt to salvage the effort, suggests taking smaller steps and finally asks the client what he or she feels is possible. Wouldn't it be better to start off with a small step and then build on each success? In the long run, the client is further ahead. In addition, the client and not the dietitian would be setting the goals, increasing client participation in the process of change.

Empowering Dietitians. Counseling skills help you use your time more effectively because they help focus the direction of the counseling session. They position dietitians as more than information-givers and allow you to use all of your training in nutrition and food in new and creative ways.

Increasing Effectiveness. Using counseling skills will help clarify the problem. We must understand, however, that the problem does not exist in isolation. Counseling skills help us understand how the problem fits into the client's life. They also help clients talk about themselves and increase self-awareness.

A GUIDE TO CORE COUNSELING SKILLS

Counseling is a two-part process. (2) During the first phase, the goal is the development of a strong, trusting relationship. The second phase involves the generation of behavior change strategies. You can't bypass the first phase for two reasons. First, you can't help clients develop strategies to address a problem until you understand what the problem is from the client's perspective. Second, a good relationship is an integral part of the second phase. You don't stop listening and start changing behavior. Listening attentively while you develop behavior change strategies will keep you from putting words into the client's mouth or making erroneous assumptions. Also, as mentioned earlier, the relationship with the counselor is often as therapeutic for the client as the counseling process.

Success in counseling is based on the counselor's level of skill in both phases of counseling. To build a good relationship, counselors must hone the skills that develop the core counseling conditions of empathy, genuineness and unconditional positive regard (respect). To generate behavior change strategies, counselors must acquire the skills which promote the process of change.

PHASE I. DEVELOPING A HELPING RELATIONSHIP
Nonverbal Attending Skills

You have heard and read about the importance of "good" nonverbal skills, but how recently have you evaluated your's in a counseling session? The message you communicate involves so much more than the words you say: 55% is communicated through body language, 38% through the tone of voice you use, and only 7% through words. (3) You must ensure consistency between your verbal and nonverbal messages. The following list should refresh your memory.

Eye contact: In most cultures good eye contact without staring demonstrates that you are attending to the client and what the client says is important. It also communicates confidence.

Tone of voice: Tone of voice means inflection and loudness. You can communicate your sense of caring and your enthusiasm, friendliness and warmth.

Body language: Leaning forward with arms at your sides and hands relaxed or gesturing shows interest, openness and a calm demeanor. Head nods communicate understanding.

Practice Activity
Work with a colleague. Have him or her discuss a problem with you while you communicate your understanding with nonverbals only. Do this for two minutes, then discuss how you felt and how your colleague felt. Switch roles.

Verbal Relationship-Building Skills: Active Listening

One of the keys to developing rapport and empathy entails "active listening." You can capture the client's thoughts and feelings and communicate your understanding. Active listening requires you to reflect the thoughts and feelings of the speaker without adding your interpretations, solutions or information until you fully understand what is going on. Do not confuse active listening with parroting (repeating back what the person says). As the nutrition counselor, you must work to clearly comprehend what the problem is, let the client know you understand, and then work together to solve the problem. See Table 7-1 The Basic Listening Skills.

Table 7-1 The Basic Listening Skills

Skill	Description	Function in Interview
Active Listening Skills		
Silence or minimal response	Nod of head; "um-um"	Provides neutral feedback that the message was heard but does not indicate judgement.
Reflective responses	Statements which summarize the content or feelings of the client	Encourages elaboration, acts as promoter for discussion, shows understanding and a willingness to help, checks clarity of counselor understanding, elucidates emotions underlying client's words and actions.
Leading Skills		
Open questions	"What": facts "How": process or feelings "Tell me more" "Could you be more specific"	Used to bring out major data and facilitate the helping interaction. Elicits client response in an open-ended yet focused manner. Can be in the form of questions or open statements.
Closed questions	Usually begin with "do," "is," "are" and can be answered with a "yes" or "no" or 1 or 2 words.	Used to quickly obtain specific data. Use with caution.
Why questions	Questions which seek the reason, cause or purpose.	Can result in learning more about how the client reasons. Caution: May put the client on the defensive. Use sparingly.
Influencing responses	"That's a good idea" (encourages, "Maybe that's not the real issue (interprets), "It's self-defeating to think that" (discourages)	Encourages or discourages the client's ideas, thoughts, or course of action to change or reinforce their behavior.
Advice	Provides suggestions, instructional ideas, homework, advice on how to act, think or behave.	Used sparingly, may provide client with new and useful ideas to try.
Information	A statement made to instruct the client on appropriate nutritional practices.	Provides clients with more data to enable them to design their own solution. Note that too much information is overwhelming. Counselors must determine the amount that is really necessary to give.
Self-Referent Skills		
Self-involving responses	The counselor shares a present reaction to the client through a personal response to what the client said or did.	Can be used to provide feedback, praise or to gently confront. Gives counselors a way to use their own feelings and reactions to the client during counseling.
Self-disclosure	Counselor shares personal experience from the past or factual information about him or herself with the client.	Can build a mutual relationship with the client through similar, shared experiences.

Reflective Responses Reflective responses are basic to developing rapport, empathy and a trusting relationship. They summarize what the client said or target the feelings expressed. They serve three purposes: they help the client to continue to talk, they clarify, and they communicate a willingness to help. You must listen carefully to make an appropriate response. Following is an example of a client who is undergoing hemodialysis. He has experienced nausea and vomiting and has had problems with his appetite.

Client Concern: "I find it difficult to eat all the calories I need to. I'm finding it bothersome to keep track of my salt and fluid intake it takes so much energy. Sometimes I feel like it's all so useless. I'm not getting any better."

Reflective response that summarizes the *content*: "Sounds like you think your diet is more work than it's worth."

Reflective Response that targets the *feeling* being expressed: "You're feeling hopeless about your health right now."

Practice Activity
Tape your next counseling session (if your client agrees). Try to use at least three reflective responses during your counseling. Listen to the tape and rate your success. After you succeed in using three, try increasing the number of reflective responses you give.

Leading Skills

Some clients can profit and grow if you use only active listening skills. Many clients can work through their problems and concerns very effectively and need clarification and understanding rather than advice, direction or suggestions. (1) However, when clients are seeking direction and nutrition therapists have a clear understanding of the client's problem, they may want to use another set of skills which start the process of resolving the client's concerns.

Leading skills can be used when nutrition therapists understand the nature of the problem, have specific suggestions to help deal with the problem, and feel comfortable assuming significant responsibility helping the client work with the problem. For example, a client may not have all of the information necessary to handle a new renal or hiatal hernia regime. Or, a client is at a loss for ideas for incorporating some exercise into his daily routine. Nutrition therapists may therefore need to advise, question, influence or educate as well as coach and facilitate.

There are four different types of leading skills: questions, influencing responses, advice and giving information.

Questions Verbal responses are like tools, and there are specific tools for specific tasks. You use questions to gather new information. There are different types of questions: open questions, closed questions and ones that begin with "why." Unfortunately, dietitians overuse questions in counseling sessions. Rather than gathering significant information, dietitians often rely on questions to add more minutia to the assessment, to satisfy some curiosity or to replace silence.

To help break this habit, think to yourself, "If I already know the answer, don't ask the question!" By using a reflective response instead, you will show that you are perceptive of the client's point-of-view. This will save precious counseling time by getting to the underlying issues and it shows a higher level of counseling skill. To help you learn how to do this effectively, when you wish to ask a question of your client, first ask the question to yourself. Second, answer the question as you would expect the client to answer it. Third, make a reflective response that captures how the client would respond. Example:

Client: "I had been doing so well, and then the holidays hit. First, I started eating sweets as soon as I arrived at work. It's really hard. . .they're only available at this time of year and I hated to see the holidays go by and not even get a taste. But then, at night when I get home, I look in the mirror and ask myself what I am doing. Then, the next day comes and it's back to the sweets. Oh, I don't know. . . ."

Dietitian wants to ask: "Do you think you can break out of this cycle?"

How the dietitian expects the client to respond:" I don't know, even though I resolve to stop doing it at night, the next day, all the resolve melts away."

Reflective response the dietitian can use: "Sounds like you're frustrated about the cycle you're in right now."

Open questions put few parameters on clients, leaving plenty of room for them to respond. They allow the client to explore an issue instead of simply answering "yes" or "no." Open questions usually start with "what" or "how." Statements such as "Tell me more" and "Can you be more specific?" can be classified as open because their use elicits open-ended responses from clients.

Examples: How do you think your new behaviors will affect your family?
What obstacles will you face when you try to implement these ideas?
Tell me more about what you felt when you knew you wanted to binge?
Can you be more specific about your exercise?

Closed questions can usually be answered with "yes," "no," or in one or two words. They do not encourage exploration and they can lead to a dead-end in counseling. Closed questions pose the risk of providing little information beyond the short answer to the question. There may be times when closed questions are appropriate like to obtain specific data or close a lengthy answer; however, as a general rule, choose open questions if at all possible.

Examples: Do you understand why eating is so important when you're taking insulin?
Were you able to choose low saturated fat foods at the reception?
Do you have any questions?
Have you tried to decrease your sodium in the past?

"Why" questions can put clients on the defensive because they seem to require an excuse. Also, sometimes clients respond to "why" questions with, "I don't know." This type of answer provides little information for counselors. Questions that begin with "why" are common among friends and we usually do not think about the unintended consequences that may result when using them in counseling. Exercise caution when using "why" questions and opt

for open ones if you can rephrase the question. If you feel that you must use a "why" question, watch your tone of voice to remove any judgmental tone or threat the client may feel. (See side bar on Confrontation and when it is appropriate.)

Practice Activity
Listen to a tape of one of your counseling sessions. When you hear a closed question, stop the tape and try to change the closed question to an open one.

Influencing Responses Influencing responses are used to reinforce or discourage the client's ideas or statements. They can also offer an interpretation of what the client says or does. Influencing responses can be used to indirectly change client behavior. Following are examples of influencing responses.

Client: "I'm thinking of taking a cooking class on using herbs to try to get away from using salt when I prepare meals."
Counselor (reinforces): "That's a terrific idea!"
Client: "I want to try out that new herbal treatment for weight loss—a friend of mine said it was so quick and easy."
Counselor (discourages): "You already know that weight loss requires some lifestyle changes. Your idea really flies in the face of all we've talked about."
Client: "I know I should be eating more, but I don't like the food. I don't know anybody, they all seem so old, so I sit alone. I don't think they like me."
Counselor (interprets): "Maybe the food isn't the whole problem here."

Advice Think about your past week. Did you receive advice from anyone, even when you didn't ask for it? Did you follow the advice (even if you DID ask for it)? Advice provides clients with thoughts or behaviors they haven't tried (or at least you think they haven't tried) to help solve the problem. Good advice is specific and realistic and it's given in a tentative manner to allow the client an "out" if needed. "Perhaps you might try" or, "You might consider" are good tentative openers for advice.

You have to listen well to know what the client has tried, what has and hasn't worked in the past, and why the solution did or did not work. Unfortunately, dietitians often give advice before they fully understand the situation or before they know what was already tried. In these instances, you hear words like "Yes, but" from the client:

Client: "I'm going on vacation, and I just don't think I can follow this program while I'm away."
Counselor: "What makes you feel that way?" (Open Question)
Client: "Well, we'll be eating out and I'll be staying with friends and relatives for parts of the trip."
Counselor: "Perhaps you could do the grocery shopping while staying with friends and relatives and buy the foods you would normally eat." (Advice)
Client: "Yes, but we'll only be with friends on one weekend and I really don't feel comfortable enough with my relatives to ask that."
Counselor: "Maybe you could tell them in advance what your needs are." (Advice)
Client: "Yes, but I hate to be a bother."

This counseling session is going nowhere fast. The dietitian needs to spend more time exploring the problem before offering solutions. For example, the dietitian could ask, "What do you eat on a typical day when you are on vacation?" and then they could identify simple ways to alter the food choice or cut the volume. Or, the dietitian might say, "Imagine that you are on vacation and you are also in control of your eating habits, how would you eat?"

Not only can giving advice be a waste of precious time, but poor advice can also undermine your effectiveness. With a dependent client, advice-giving can encourage dependence on the counselor because the couselor is making the decisions.

Confrontation

Confrontation is used as an invitation and challenge to examine, modify, or control some aspect of a client's behavior. (1) It helps individuals see more clearly what is happening, what the consequences are, and how they can assume responsibility. It is hoped that clients will learn how to confront themselves and take corrective action in the future. Failure to confront when you see and hear self-defeating or unreasonable behavior implies support for the behavior.

Clients are frequently unaware of the games they play and do not realize the confusion they produce in their lives through conflicting messages. Most clients do not recognize the consequences of their maladaptive behavior. Confrontations help clients admit ownership of how they truly feel (without distortions or denial) and that they rule their own destinies. Common discrepancies include: A discrepancy between the way the client sees himself/herself and the way others see him/her; a contradiction between what the client says and the way he/she behaves; a discrepancy between two statements by the client; a discrepancy between what the client says he/she is feeling and the way most people would react in a similar situation; a contradiction between what the client is presently saying he/she believes and the way he/she has acted in the past.

The guidelines to keep in mind when formulating a confrontation response are: mutual trust and empathy must already be established in the counseling relationship; confrontation should come across as a positive, caring act, not as an attacking, judgmental one; address specific, concrete attributes of the client's behavior that the client can change; use confrontation to point out discrepancies in how client's view their assets (strengths); reponses can constructively focus on these strengths that the client may overlook.

You might try the following to gently confront clients:
"Have you ever noticed that you. . . ."
"Did you hear what you just said. . . ."
"What you are telling me now is different than what you said awhile ago about. . . ."
"You say you want to eat fewer high fat foods, but what I see you doing is. . . ."
"One of the reasons that people may respond to you that way is because. . . ."
Always remember that confrontation is an act of caring and a desire on your part to become more intimately involved with the client.
Reference
1. Tamminen AW, Smaby MH. Helping counselors learn to confront. *Personnel Guid J.* 60:1, 1981.
Used with permission. Copyright 1983 American

Practice Activity

For one week, record any advice that people give you. Keep track of whether you asked for it and whether or not you implemented the advice. See how often advice is given and how seldom it is implemented.

Giving Information Specific information about nutrition or the diet seems to be the mainstay of dietary counseling. (6) As discussed earlier, dietitians too often overwhelm clients by trying to teach them everything they will ever need to know about their diet for the rest of their lives. Clients cannot remember THAT much information. Break it up into more manageable pieces and let the client have time to review it before the next visit. Evaluate every piece of information you give. Will it really help? Does it classify as a "so what" piece of information? For example, some interesting tidbit to you may not be so interesting to a client who happens to be a novice at assessing his or her eating behavior. Use attending skills and cognitive-behavioral, psychoeducational, or other approaches to solve problems and overcome barriers.

Self-Referent Skills

Using self-referent skills provides nutrition counselors vehicles for talking about themselves and their feelings during a counseling session. Self-referent skills can increase openness, give feedback to clients, provide a model for how to talk about oneself and make the counseling session less impersonal. The focus shifts from the client to the counselor. Although these skills can be extremely effective, using them too often or too early during counseling can have some negative effects: counselors may spend more time talking about themselves than listening to the client; counselors may unintentionally offend the client; counselors may turn the counseling into "chatting" visits rather than helping sessions.

Before you use self-referent skill, you should be able to answer the following questions: What personal needs am I fulfilling by using this response? How will the client respond? What effect will my response have on the relationship? Counselors can use two types of self-referent skills: self-involving responses and self-disclosure.

Self-Involving Responses A self-involving response actively puts the counselor into the session. This response follows the format: I (the counselor) feel (this way) about what you (the client) said or did. You can use a self-involving response to gently confront or to provide feedback to the client about how you feel.

Client: "I'm sorry I couldn't stick to that program to lower my cholesterol. I know you were counting on me and I let you down."

Counselor: "I'm concerned that you're following the program for me and not yourself."

Client: "My blood sugar has been great, and I really feel like I'm starting to understand the ins and outs of the diet."

Counselor: "I'm thrilled with your progress."

Self-Disclosure This response is included because it is often used without thinking about the consequences. With a self-disclosing response, a dietitian talks about himself or herself. On the positive side, self-disclosure provides a model of how to talk about yourself and it changes the relationship from an impersonal to a personal One. On the negative side, the dietitian can end up taking up most of the time talking about his or her experiences and learning nothing about the client. For example, imagine you are working with someone who has diabetes and you have diabetes too. Dealing with restaurant eating poses a major problem for your client and it used to be a problem for you. Suppose the counseling session went like this:

Client: "I worry about eating out now. I'm not sure how to count some things and I always seem to eat more when I'm with a group."

Counselor: "Well, I have diabetes, too, and I remember how difficult I thought it was to eat out."

Client: " Really? What did you do?"

Counselor: "I asked what ingredients were in some entrees and I just asked the waiter to serve sauces and dressings on the side. I always tried to order first, so I wouldn't be influenced by someone else."

Client: "How did your friends feel?"

Counselor: "They're dietitians, too, so it didn't bother them."

Client: "Oh."

From this short interchange, you can see that the focus changed from being on the client to the dietitian, and the shared information gave little help or direction. The dietitian could have used reflective and leading skills only or the dietitian might have said the following:

Client: "I worry about eating out, now. I'm not sure how to count some things, and I always seem to eat more when I'm with a group."

Counselor: "Well, I have diabetes too, and I remember how difficult I thought it was to eat out."

Client: "Really? What did you do?"

Counselor: "I soon learned to control my portions by eating the same amount as I would at home. You know, it seems like we're talking a lot about me (reflective). Tell me more about your situation so we can design a strategy to deal with it (open question)."

Practice Activity

Listen to a tape of one of your counseling sessions. How often do you discuss your personal life? How often do you bring in your feelings? What effect does each have on the counseling session?

Practice Activity

Tape a counseling session and as you listen to the tape, record the responses you made, identify them, and rate them. If you were not happy with some responses, think of a more appropriate one. Part I and Part II of the Counselor Evaluation System in Appendix 7-A can be a helpful tool in this process.

PHASE II. DEVELOPING BEHAVIOR CHANGE STRATEGIES

To empower clients is to enable them to achieve, to take control of their lives. If you want to enable someone to do something, you have to help them develop the necessary skills to do so. Ultimately, you want your clients to have the skills they need not to diet, but to change their eating styles permanently. Telling clients what to do and simply giving information are short-term fixes; empowering offers a long-term solution.

One of the best ways to help clients gain control over their situation is to teach them how to set goals. Now this sounds simple, but it is truly amazing how few people are skilled at setting reachable goals. Setting goals involves three steps: Step 1, You help clients identify the goal; Step 2, Assess its importance; Step 3, Analyze the roadblocks which hinder goal attainment.

Let's look at each step in more detail.

Step 1 Goal Identification

In order to identify a goal, you must have a very clear picture of what the problem is. A goal is simply the flipside of the problem (if the problem is skipping breakfast and overeating in the evening, the goal is to do the opposite). *Achievable goals are positive, specific and under the goal setter's control.*

As discussed earlier in this book, the newer thinking on goals is that they should be *much smaller steps and even more achievable so that clients feel empowered.* Therefore, "losing 35 pounds" should be seen as a *result* that goals were met and achieved. In weight loss counseling when you create a very large end goal, it can seem extremely distant and overwhelming to some clients. It often fails to motivate the client after a few weeks and there are several generations of dieters who prove the approach doesn't work. It also diminishes the recognition paid to the true contributors to change like new cognitions, more mature developmental skills, healthier eating or lifestyle choices. These are the changes that must be recognized and maintained for the result to be maintained.

Goals that have the words "not" and "avoid" are negative and difficult, if not impossible to achieve. Focusing on the negative expends energy on what the client doesn't want to do. Because it's not a constructive exercise, clients start to feel frustrated or deprived, increasing the likelihood that they will give up and feel like failures. Helping clients set positive goals reveals the control and power they have in a situation.

For example, a client with diabetes may have a problem eating on a regular schedule: "I just can't seem to eat my meals and snacks regularly because my schedule is so hectic." A positive goal would be: "I want to eat my meals and snacks on a better schedule." While the goal is positive, it is vague and hard to reach. How does the client define "a better schedule?" How will the client know when the schedule improved?

Reachable goals are specific, and expressed in behavioral terms. A positive, specific goal would be: "On Monday and Tuesday of this week, I plan to eat breakfast at 8, a snack at 10, lunch at 12:30, afternoon snack at 3, dinner at 7 and an evening snack at 10." The goal is small, clear and practical. The client will know when it's achieved.

Making sure the goal is under the client's control involves two aspects:

- First, the goal must involve the *client's* behavior and not the actions of someone else. For example, a goal such as, "I want my wife to use low fat cooking methods like baking or broiling instead of frying" is an admirable goal, but it is dependent on the wife's behavior not the client's. The dietitian must help the client refocus and concentrate on *his* behaviors. In this instance, the client may decide to set a goal of asking his wife to cook using lower fat methods: "Tonight, I'll ask Joan to bake the chicken instead of frying it." Notice that the client can achieve the goal of asking regardless of whether or not Joan cooperates.

- The second aspect of control pertains to distinguishing *goals* from *results*, as mentioned above. Lowering blood cholesterol is a result; eating low saturated fat foods is a goal. Losing weight is a result; eating fewer calories and exercising three times per week for 30 minutes are goals. Goals that are achieved often lead to positive results.

Step 2 Goal Importance Assessment

Critical to the entire goal-setting process, goal importance assessment defines the motivation. The goal must be most important to the client. Goals that physicians, spouses, or nutritionists find important may or may not be meaningful for the client. Always check to see if clients feel they *should* reach the goal or if they *want* to reach it. "Want" goals are more often achieved than "should" goals. Clients say "should" to themselves so often when it comes to diet and lifestyle change that it may take time to uncover the "want" goals.

Step 3 Goal Roadblock Analysis

Four obstacles impede goal achievement:
- lack of knowledge,
- lack of skills,
- inability to take a risk,
- lack of support.

A client may have one, two, three or all four of these roadblocks.

Lack of knowledge means that the client doesn't know the "what." For example, he or she may be unaware of the calorie content of different food choices; a person just diagnosed with diabetes may not know what the consequences are of skipping meals; or an individual with kidney disease may not know what the lower potassium fruits are. If clients lack knowledge, it is appropriate to provide information or show them how to access that information.

Lack of skills means the client lacks the "how to." Ms. Jones may not know how to control her intake at a social function; Mr. Smith may not know any other way to relax besides eating; Jennifer may be unaware of rewards beyond the refrigerator; Sam may not believe he can change the way he eats. Clients often focus on their weaknesses, failing to identify strengths they already have. Teaching them to focus on their strengths will eventually help them see how they can transfer different abilities to more than one life situation. When clients lack skills, dietitians can help teach the client new skills in a systematic way (see FYI following this chapter). Skill learning requires demonstration and practice.

Inability to take risks refers to the fear associated with goal achievement. Clients may have certain costs associated with reaching their goal and their perception is that the costs outweigh the benefits. For example, Mr. Brown, who has a concern about his cholesterol level, may be afraid that he will never succeed in changing his level so he chooses not to try. Ms. Jones may be afraid her dates will feel she has a serious illness and won't want to pursue a relationship if she tries to adopt a low cholesterol eating style. As their dietitian, the focus needs to be a realistic weighing of both the real and perceived costs and benefits of changing behavior. What do they have to gain by reaching the goal? What do they have to lose?

Lack of social support may require clients to look beyond their traditional support structure to help sustain behavior changes. Sometimes, spouses or family members sabotage life change efforts. Often, the dietitian becomes the support during the initial part of counseling. The dietitian must help the client identify what support is needed, who can best or most likely will provide that support, and what is the best way for the client to ask for the support.

Using good listening skills will help you determine if the obstacles interfere with goal achievement and what they are. Once you have a clear understanding, you and the client can develop a program to achieve the goal. Make sure that the program that's designed consists of small steps so that the client will not fail during the early stages. As the client gains self-confidence, more difficult steps can be undertaken. Clients feel a sense of accomplishment when they can evaluate their progress.

Goal Setting Guide

Included in Appendix 7-A is a sample Goal Setting Guide in Part III of the Counselor Evaluation System. Feel free to use the guide, think of it as a blueprint for counseling. You do not have to ask all or any of the questions on the guide; use active listening skills to determine the answers.

APPLYING THE SKILLS IN YOUR COUNSELING

While the process of counseling described above sounds simple, the authors have found that helping dietitians change their behaviors can be just as challenging as helping clients! They've conducted numerous workshops with dietitians and the response is usually the same: there is excitement about the skills and a sincere desire to incorporate them into nutritional counseling. When the participants return to their work environments, many fall back into old habits and fail to use the skills. Why are the skills hard to implement once they return to work? Why is it so hard to change?

There are basically four roadblocks that they face when trying to implement a change (sound familiar?). They are lack of knowledge, lack of skills, inability to take risks, lack of support, or a combination of these. Note that these obstacles have nothing to do with the merits of using the skills. If you believe in the importance of the skills and have a desire to use them, the roadblocks just mentioned will be all that stand in your way.

Lack of Knowledge. If the obstacle is a lack of knowledge, you're not alone, Lack of training in this area is the primary reason for the dilemma. Traditionally, dietitians are taught about the importance of developing rapport and tailoring dietary interventions to fit the client's lifestyle without being taught the actual skills. Dietitians are also taught how essential it is for clients to accept the responsibility for change, but not taught the methods for helping clients become involved in the process. Unfortunately, most learning is through a lecture format. Your practice may occur during an internship when you observe dietitians (who may or may not know specific counseling skills) as they work with clients. You then imitate what you see. In this chapter, the authors explained the nonverbal and verbal skills needed to build an effective helping relationship and to encourage behavior change. Learning what the skills are should help you hurdle the obstacle of the lack of knowledge. Use this chapter as a reference for the counseling skills. Recognize that reading the chapter still may not be enough to cause a change in your behavior because other obstacles may stand in your way.

Lack of Skills. This is the most difficult obstacle to deal with through the written word. You may need to go through the process of skill development to increase proficiency in using the skills. There are specific steps for this and they include:

- evaluating your motivation,
- assessing your current skill level,
- setting a goal,
- practicing,
- evaluating progress.

Note that the first step is evaluating your motivation. If adopting the skills is not a priority, it just won't happen. To be actively involved in the process of learning a skill, you have to be convinced that the skill is worth pursuing. Some questions you might ask yourself include: Why bother with these skills? Why are the skills important for me? What makes me believe that I can learn these skills? Are the skills worth the trouble?

Next, assess your current skill level. Audiotape or videotape a counseling session. If you've never done this, to do so is an incredible learning process. Review the tapes with someone more knowledgeable than you (a supervisor or therapist colleague), or use the Counselor Evaluation System in Appendix 7-A. Assessing where you are will help you determine the exact skills you need to develop. If you can, have a skilled therapist model the skills so that you can observe the skills in action and then discuss their uses.

The third step in skill development involves setting a goal. Refer to the Counselor Evaluation System, Part 3. A sample of a goal might be: "I will ask an open question at least once during my counseling session with Ms. Dean." Once you set the goal, practice under supervision by having someone observe you or by making an audiotape. And don't forget to evaluate your progress on a regular basis. Compare your skills on a week-to-week basis through audiotapes to see how far you've come.

Inability to Take Risks. If this is your roadblock, you might feel afraid to use the skills because you don't know what the effects on your clients will be; you might be worried that you won't appear expert enough to your clients or you may be worried that your superiors won't accept your new approach. Whatever the problem, weigh the advantages and disadvantages of using the skills. Because the actual consequences of using the new skills in your situation are uncertain, there is a tendency to guess about the potential outcomes. In guessing, people often confuse what is likely to happen with what is probably *not* going to happen. You might want to ask yourself the following questions: What can be gained by using the skills? What can be lost? What positive outcomes will likely occur? Are there any negative consequences to consider? What is the best possible outcome and how realistic is this? What is the worst possible outcome and how realistic is this?

Lack of Support. To change the way we counsel requires a supportive environment. If we don't create an atmosphere that encourages skill use, the chances of maintaining the skills will be slim. Don't just hope that your supervisor or co-workers will see how great the skills are and support their use. If you need to, be prepared to sell them on the counseling skills. Take a win-win approach. Find out what their needs are, figure out how using the skills will fill the needs, and then tell them about it. Don't be put off by objections. Try to think of objections as a desire on their part for more information. Listen actively to the objections until you understand them so that you can provide whatever is necessary to sell your point.

CONCLUSION

As a final note, dietitians just learning this approach believe it will work well with individuals struggling with obesity. They hesitate to use the approach with clients suffering from other diseases such as diabetes, renal disease, or cardiovascular disease. Why? Dietitians may think that these diseases are more serious, or that when clients have such problems, they need to be told what to do or suffer dire consequences. Despite what you may think, dietary adherence, no matter what the problem, is notoriously poor over the long term. Also, today's recommendations for just about every disorder focus on individualizing the program to meet the client's needs and requirements. If the old approach doesn't work, why not try something new? Start with small steps and you'll see the self-esteem of clients grow as they make progress in reaching their attainable goals.

LEARNING ACTIVITIES

1. Observe a one-on-one nutrition counseling session. Identify the basic listening skills utilized by the counselor. Were they effective in moving the session along?
2. With a colleague, role play a counseling session in which the "counselor" utilizes confrontation to deal with client behaviors. What skills are needed to use confrontation effectively?
3. Observe a counseling session where the counselor is providing nutrition education information. What influencing skills did the counselor use to increase the client's knowledge level? Critique the session; what would you have done differently based on your knowledge of effective nutrition counseling techniques?
4. For one of the counseling sessions observed above, how were goals set with the client? Were the goals client-centered? What obstacles did you observe that may interfere with client goal achievement?

REFERENCES

1. Green LW. Educational strategies to improve compliance with therapeutic and preventive regimes: The recent evidence. In: Haynes RB, Taylor RB, Sackett DW, eds. *Compliance in Health Care*. Baltimore, MD: The Johns Hopkins University Press; 1979.
2. Danish SJ, Ginsberg MR, Terrell A, Hammond MI, Adams SO. The anatomy of a dietetic counseling interview. *J Am Diet Assoc*. 1979; 75: 626-630.
3. Mehrabain A. Communication without words. *Psych Today*. 1968, Sept.
4. Danish SJ, D'Augelli AR, Hauer AL. *Helping Skills: A basic training program*. New York: Human Science Press; 1980.
5. Laquatra I, Danish SJ. Effect of a helping skills transfer program on dietitians' helping behavior. *J Am Diet Assoc*. 1981; 78: 22, 181.
6. Laquatra I. Helping Skills for WIC Nutrition Education Counselors. University Park, PA: The Pennsylvania State University; 1983. Dissertation.

Appendix 7-A

Counselor Evaluation System

PART 1 EVALUATING WHAT YOU SAY

A. Counselor's Verbatim Record of Responses. From an audio or video recording write out your responses verbatim including mmhmm's, uh-huh's, etc. Use as many sheets of paper as necessary. Number each response and catagorize it: mmhmm; reflective response; open question; closed question; why question; advice-giving; information-giving; self-disclosure, and other. Rate the responses as good or effective, neutral, negative or ineffective. Responses/ Category/Rating (+,0,-)

B. Counselor's Behavior

    1. Nonverbal Behavior: Summarize your notable nonverbal behaviors. What impact did your nonverbal behaviors have on the client? Be specific.

    2. Verbal Behavior

        a. Total number of responses made:_____

        b. Percentage in each category:

Mmhmm_____	Advice-giving_____
Reflective_____	Information-giving_____
Open question_____	Self-disclosure_____
Closed question_____	Why question_____

C. Self-assessment of Verbal Responses

    1. What responses could have been better phrased? Exactly how would you re-state them?

    2. Which responses could or should have been omitted? Why?

PART 2 UNDERSTANDING THE CLIENT

A. List the most important specific topics discussed by the client.

B. What feelings does the client have about each topic?

C. Describe how these topics are related to each other.

D. Describe how the topics relate to what you know about the client; in other words, connect the client to the problem.

E. Based on the information above, what is your understanding of the client's concern?

PART 3 GOAL SETTING GUIDE

A. Goal Identification

    1. Using the client's concern/problem identified above, describe it as a positive and specific goal that the client has expressed an interest in attaining.

        a. Is the goal described stated positively? Positively stated goals describe some action the client wants to take. He/she can create a picture in his/her mind of what it is he/she wants to have happen rather than something he/she doesn't want to have happen.

        b. Is this goal stated specifically? When a client makes a specifically stated goal he/she knows when it is attained. With general goals a client may have trouble knowing when he/she has reached it; they often use words like "good," "better," "more" or "less."

        c. Is the goal under the client's control? When a client selects a goal that requires the actions of someone else rather than the client, the client does not have control over whether the goal is attained. Setting goals such as "being successful," "winning" or "being happy" are really results, not goals. Goals are the actions a client can take to reach these results.

    2. Describe the dimensions of the goal:

        a. How long has the client wanted to achieve this goal?

        b. What, if anything, has the client tried to reach the goal?

        c. Describe the specific situation in which the client came closest to reaching the goal.

        d. Describe the specific situation in which the client felt farthest from the goal.

        e. Why is it important to the client to reach this goal now?

    3. Restate the goal, if necessary.

B. Determining Goal Importance

    1. What makes the goal important to the client? Is it more important to the client than to other people in the client's life?

    2. Is the goal something the client wants to accomplish or feels he/she should or ought to accomplish?

3. From your perspective, is it worthwhile for the client to achieve the goal? Why?
4. What does the client gain by reaching the goal?
5. What does the client gain by not reaching the goal?
6. How likely is it that the client can reach the goal?

C. Roadblocks to Goal Attainment: Why has the client been unable to reach the goal?
1. Is it lack of knowledge? If so, what knowledge is needed to reach the goal?
2. Is it lack of skills? If so, what does the client need to know how to do?
3. Is it the inability to take risks? If so, what would assist the client in overcoming the fear of taking the risk?
4. Is it a lack of social support? If so, what support does the client need and who can provide it?

PART 4 IF YOU COULD. . .

A. If you could do this session over again, given your understanding of the client's concerns/problems/ goals, how would you approach the session differently, if at all, and why? Be specific.
B. What issues would you like to explore with the client in a next session? How would you pursue this direction?
C. Things I will work on related to my counseling skills:

8

Cognitive-Behavioral and Psychoeducational Counseling and Therapy

Alison Murray Kiy, EdM, NCC, RD, Counselor, Deaconess Hospital, Boston, MA Adjunct Instructor, Behavioral Sciences, Quincy College, Quincy, MA

After reading this chapter, the reader will be able to:
- ☐ distinguish between behavioral, cognitive and psychoeducational theories
- ☐ list three categories of disordered eating and potential counseling strategies
- ☐ recognize behavioral, cognitive and psychoeducational treatment strategies in given scenarios

---

One of the most important functions nutrition therapists serve is a facilitator of behavior change. Changes in eating behavior may improve your health, sports performance, or medical condition. Dietitians therefore are behaviorists. You may also be cognitivist, from the perspective that in order to bring about behavior change you might first focus on changing one's thoughts, beliefs, or attitudes with respect to food, eating, or some other dietary related behavior.

This chapter will focus on techniques used within the cognitive-behavioral category of counseling theory, including behavioral theory, cognitive theory, and psychoeducational theory, which involves both a cognitive component and a behavioral component such as hunger and fullness training. Basic premises of each approach will be explored, as well as techniques that are representative of that discipline. Subsequent to the explanation of each technique will follow a discussion of clinical utility and a case example. (See Table 8-1 Cognitive-Behavioral Techniques.)

As a practitioner, you are cautioned with regard to the use of techniques. A skilled practitioner does not merely *apply* techniques to modify a client's behavior. Instead, the skilled practitioner and client develop a caring relationship in which techniques are used in a spontaneous way to help the client. In their book on *Family Therapy Techniques*, Minuchin and Fishman describe this situation more fully. (1)

> Furthermore, technique alone does not ensure effectiveness. If the therapist (in this case, dietitian), becomes wedded to technique, remaining a craftsman, his contact with patients will be objective, detached, and clean, but also superficial, manipulative for the sake of personal power, and ultimately not highly effective. (1)

Others confirm the need to use techniques both spontaneously and ethically. (2-5) Corey outlines numerous questions a counselor might consider in monitoring one's use of techniques. (2) Some of these questions, adapted to the work of a dietitian, are summarized below.

- Do you more often give advice or do you allow clients to explore and describe their eating problems fully?
- Do you give your clients guidance and reassurance? Do you allow clients to express how they feel about their diet, circumstance and dilemmas, before giving advice? Or do you immediately tell them how to solve their dilemma?
- Do you clarify and checkout what you think clients are telling you with regards to their story, how they feel about their story, what their concerns and worries are?

Table 8-1 Cognitive-Behavioral Techniques

Behavioral Techniques	Cognitive Restructing Techniques	Psychoeducational Techniques
Classical conditioning	Decatastrophizing	Distraction
Operant conditioning	Challenging Shoulds, Oughts, Musts	Delay
Self monitoring	Reattribution	Parroting
Stimulus control	Decentering	
Imagery		
Role playing		
Real-life performance-based		
Self reinforcement		
Modeling		
Systematic desensitization		

- In what way do you use techniques? To get clients moving? Or do you wait until you have more information about what a client might need and then discuss what might help, what you see might help, and direct communication to a more personal level?
- Do you use techniques that you feel comfortable with? That you have studied, practiced, and received supervision on (a mentor has discussed your use of techniques with you)? Are your techniques mechanical or unforced? (2)

In using techniques then, dietitians must consider spontaneity as well as ethical issues. Involved in spontaneity and ethics are outcome considerations. Techniques should not be *applied* indiscriminately, but rather, with concern for the client's well-being, capacity for change, and expectations of treatment (2-4). In this regard, the client should be as much a part of the selection of techniques as the dietitian. The dietitian might ask the client such questions as, "What do you think you are capable of changing? What do you most want to change? What do you imagine the outcome might be if you change this eating behavior?" Such a discussion is illustrated in the example below.

Dietitian: "What do you imagine will help you change your eating behavior?"

Client: "I don't know. That's why I'm coming here." (This client might also be experiencing anger, which will make the application of techniques that much more difficult.)

Dietitian: "Well let us review some of what brought you here and some of your expectations for nutrition counseling. First, your doctor referred you so that you might lose weight. Your doctor thought this might help lower both your blood pressure and cholesterol level. You describe your eating as spontaneous—you just don't think about it much. We might begin by helping you understand more of your eating habits, and specifically, the triggers in your environment which may stimulate your eating. To accomplish this, you might record everything you eat and drink, and the conditions under which this takes place, for about one week. How does this sound to you?";

Client: "Well, I hate to keep records. I'm not good at doing it; but, I do want to lose weight."

Dietitian: "Let's discuss what will keep you from recording what you eat (barriers) and what will make it easier (positive reinforcements). Why don't we start with what will make it easier? Can you imagine for a moment (imagery) it is Monday morning, you are eating breakfast and you remember you should record what you eat and drink. What might help you here?"

Client: "Well, let's see. I might keep a reminder, say, on my refrigerator so that when I grab the milk for my cereal I see a note that will remind me to measure my food, and record my intake. Yes, I think a reminder note might help. Usually I don't record what I eat simply because I don't remember and then I think, 'What's the use; I already forgot. Might as well just eat. I'll start tomorrow.'"

This example illustrates a discussion between a dietitian and client which brings into consciousness, for both the dietitian and client, specific difficulties encountered by the client in the process of keeping food records (self-monitoring). It also illustrates a perspective that the dietitian will not demand that a client participate in treatment in a predetermined way; but rather, the dietitian will help the client explore the utility of a particular technique in his/her life. In doing so, the dietitian does not merely *apply* a technique. The dietitian empowers the client by providing a forum to participate in planning treatment. A client may feel encouraged because:

- more of the obstacles to reaching goals are illuminated,

- there may be greater self-understanding (that the client can make a decision; that the client has a sense of what she or he needs and wants; that the client has a sense of what will make achieving the goal difficult), and is given a measure of control over his or her problem. (2-5)

Other ethical considerations which may be useful in making the decision of which techniques to use are described below: (24)

- clients should be fully informed of the dietitian's education, training, experience, and qualifications, as these factors reflect technique selection, as well as effectiveness.
- clients should be provided with clear explanations, goals, expected outcomes, and risks (i.e. emotional, behaviorally, socially) of techniques, before techniques are used in a counseling session.
- clients should be at liberty to choose when to participate in certain activities.
- dietitians should be aware of their own values and expectations relative to eating, weight, behavior change, and other life values, to the extent that the dietitian is careful of not imposing these values on a client.

DISORDERED EATING CATEGORIES AND SELECTION OF TECHNIQUES

The example above may raise questions with regard to technique selection. Does the usage of technique vary with the degree of change required? For example, might a dietitian use a different technique for a client with an *old* eating problem, that is, established in childhood, versus a *new* eating problem, recently established with the advent of a change in one's environment? This question will be explored and answered throughout the chapter; however, a brief description of each category is further explored below.

New Eating Problems

Some clients complain of *new* problems. They struggle with dietary problems which occurred with the advent of some change in their environment or daily pattern. Perhaps this is a person who knowingly or unknowingly consumes excessive amounts of fat, sugar, or calories for reasons such as eating in a restaurant more often, change in job, or change in family status (i.e. recently married or divorced). This person may experience a change in eating simply because of a change in environment or the "rules" (cognitions) that are associated with the new environment. Further, these changes are likely reinforced by something or someone in the client's environment or value system (i.e. saved time, food tastes good, another's validation or approval).

A variety of techniques might be used to change *new* behaviors which are problematic. A dietitian and client may establish treatment goals, which change the environment, change the client's behavior in an environment, change the client's thoughts or cognitions regarding the environment, and identify methods to reinforce the learning of new behaviors and thoughts (called operant conditioning—see page 140). A combined approach is likely more effective to produce the behavior change required to sustain an improved health status.

Old Eating Problems

New eating problems may be different however from *old* eating problems. One with an *old* eating problem likely developed this problem many years earlier, perhaps in childhood. In this case, *old* eating behaviors have been well-learned and well-reinforced and may be more difficult to change. Strategies which may produce the change of *old* behaviors may include both operant conditioning and classical conditioning (see pages 138-139). For example, when the client eats some food it may reinforce a memory of a person, which yields a positive, warm feeling. In this example a certain food may precipitate a feeling of affection (classical conditioning).

Loss of Control Eating Problems

A third category of eating behaviors, different from the *new* and *old* eating behaviors described above may be experienced by a client who suffers with a sense of *loss of control* with regard to eating or weight. This is one whose degree of suffering is very intense, much beyond that of one who suffers with a change in one's environment. One who suffers to this degree may be diagnosed with a mental disorder according to the *Diagnostic and Statistical Manual of Mental Disorders (6)*, in one of three diagnostic states: Anorexia Nervosa, Bulimia Nervosa, or an Eating Disorder Not Otherwise Specified. Cognitive-behavioral therapy is also effective with this group; however, it is used somewhat differently from the two categories of eating behavior described above. Excellent summaries of cognitive-behavioral techniques for eating disorders are available in the literature (4,7-10).

It appears then that different techniques may prove more effective than others relative to the problem treated. In addition to ethical considerations and the client's expectations of treatment, two issues might be used by the dietitian to select techniques. First, you might consider how well learned the problematic eating behavior is. Second, you might consider whether the client has any degree of control over the problem eating behavior. Three categories of eating problems (old problem, new problem, out of control problem) are used throughout this chapter to help dietitians conceptualize and select appropriate treatment strategies.

Fit the Technique to the Client
One last factor, and perhaps most important, in the selection of a technique is the client him or herself. The dietitian must not forget the person. Despite the intensity of one's struggle with food or weight therein lies a person who possesses an *individual* history, *individually* prioritized needs, expectations, values, and an *individual* set of circumstances. Dietitians must not forget to explore the individuality of the client's dilemma, how the client feels about the dilemma, what did and did not work in trying to solve the client's problem. The client should be invited to explore his or her problem and should be invited to both plan and implement a treatment strategy in a personal way.

BEHAVIORAL TREATMENT STRATEGIES
This discussion starts with behavioral strategies because dietitians tend to be more familiar with these strategies; cognitive and psychoeducational strategies will follow. Behavioral strategies employed for the purpose of changing eating behavior and maintaining dietary change are not only increasingly more popular, but effective. Efficacy is well established in hypertension programs (4), smoking cessation programs (4), cholesterol lowering programs (4,11-15), diabetes mellitus (16,17), weight reduction programs (18-29), and in eating disorders programs. (30-33) The utility and value of a behavioral program extends far beyond that of producing change however. Behavioral programs offer hope, new coping mechanisms, and perhaps most importantly, an opportunity for autonomy. The provision of hope is perhaps best illustrated with clients who suffer with a sense of *lack of control* of eating behavior, as in those suffering with compulsive eating, anorexia, or bulimia. (33)

Behavioral programs offer clients new strategies for coping with difficult situations. Moreover, strategies may be used by those in all behavior categories (old, new, and out of control). Eating serves some function for a client. Perhaps some clients use food to cope with anxiety and disappointment. Perhaps food provides a source of nurturance. In some ways food itself becomes a reinforcer (stimulus—as a reward or the removal of discomfort). It is important for dietitians to be aware of the reinforcing nature of food, the function of food in the client's life, and to imagine how a client might feel if this reinforcer is suddenly removed from his or her repertoire of coping strategies. You may in some cases actively explore with the client the purposes and functions of food in his or her life. After accomplishing this, you may proceed to a second level of counseling which entails behavior change. (34)

Finally, behavior programs offer clients self-efficacy. (35) Clients learn they can indeed manage their own behavior without the assistance of a counselor. It should also be made clear to a client that it will not be frowned upon, nor is it a sign of failure when the he or she seeks continued assistance. Instead, it is seen as a high level of self-understanding. A client may merely require a "refresher course." Indeed, one study in the area of obesity management revealed that clients may actually wait too long before seeking additional help. (21) Behavioral strategies are useful and appealing to nutrition therapists. It is likely that many dietitians already employ these techniques in dietetic practice, although they may not call them by this name. The basic assumptions of behavioral theory are listed in Table 8-2; however, the following quote summarizes this approach nicely. (36)

> Most behaviorally oriented therapists believe that the current environment is most important in affecting the person's present behavior. Early life experiences, long time intrapsychic conflicts, or the individual's personality structure are considered to be of less importance than what is happening in the person's life at the present time. The procedures used in behavior therapy are generally intended to improve the individual's self-control by expanding the person's skills, abilities, and independence.(36)

You may find that as a counselor, you don't agree with all of the above premises. That is why most counselors today use many of the behavioral techniques along with other counseling theories and closer interpersonal relationships. As discussed earlier, techniques may vary with the degree and manner in which behaviors are learned (new, old, out of control behaviors). The actual differences between such problems may be better conceptualized with a discussion of classical and operant conditioning.

Classical Conditioning
> Give me a dozen healthy infants, well-formed, and my own specified world to bring them up in and I'll guarantee to take any one at random and, rain him to become any type of specialist I might select—doctor, lawyer, merchant, chief, and yes, even beggerman and thief, regardless of his talents, penchants, abilities, vocations and the race of his ancestors. (Watson, 1930)

Table 8-2 Basic Assumptions of Behavioral Theory

1. All behavior is learned, and is directly related to the events, stimuli, and reinforcers in one's environment. Therefore, all behavior can be unlearned through corrective learning experiences.
2. A personal relationship between the dietitian and client is not required for recovery to occur.
3. Symptomatic behaviors are considered nothing more than the result of learning maladaptive solutions to common problems.
4. Behavior theory relies on the principles of the scientific method; data is quantifiable and based on empirical research.
5. A client's problem can be better conceptualized by gathering precise, concrete data on the client's behavior and action.
6. Assessment focuses on current determinants of behavior; rather than historical determinants. Indeed, one need not understand historical factors to experience changes in behavior.
7. Treatment focuses on changing target behaviors; goals are explicit and well defined.

Note: summary from Corey, 1984 (3); Eysenck, 1987 (37); Ivey, 1987 (5); Wilson, 1984 (41)

Watson's quote above summarizes the ideology of classical conditioning. (38) While the assumption has been "humanized," classical conditioning continues to consider environmental factors as more important than other factors (i.e. intrapsychic, contextual, maturational) in the shaping and influencing of behavior. The validity of this assumption may be observed in the context of eating. That is, eating may indeed be conditioned. This includes those with diabetes mellitus who eat too much sugar, those trying to lose weight who eat excessive calories, and those with heart disease who smoke. Their problem is not one of insufficient knowledge, but rather, the learning or conditioning of unhealthy and problematic behaviors.

Classical conditioning may provide one framework by which to understand this phenomenon. *It refers to involuntary processes (i.e. blinking, security, fear, preferences).* These processes of conditioning were first described by Pavlov in the early part of the twentieth century. With this technique Pavlov taught his dogs to salivate at the sound of a bell instead of the presence of meat. To accomplish this, Pavlov first presented a dog with an *Unconditioned Stimulus* (US)—the meat. This US produced the *Unconditioned Response* (UR)—salivation. Pavlov then paired the US with a *Conditioned Stimulus* (CS)—the sound of a bell. The result of this pairing, when the pairing occurred at the same moment in time, was a *Conditioned Response* (CR)—salivating at the sound of a bell and the presence of meat. In time, Pavlov's dogs learned to salivate only with the sound of a bell, without the presence of meat.

Classical conditioning has been used by others to condition fear, as with little Albert and his fear of white mice, rabbits, and men with white beards. (38) Watson's research demonstrated that *conditioned responses* can be generalized by the object of such conditioning. That is, one can *autocondition* oneself. (39,40) The process of generalization occurs when the object of conditioning responds to similar stimuli in a predetermined way. That is, many stimuli may yield a certain conditioned response. For example, one may learn to eat other foods, in addition to chocolate, and drink alcohol, and smoke cigarettes when experiencing anxiety, with the goal of producing a conditioned response of security, nurturance, and peace. Other examples of classical conditioning are listed below.

Table 8-3 Examples of Classical Conditioning

Unconditioned stimulus (US)	produces	Unconditioned response (UR)
flash on a camera	produces	blinking
mother's affection	produces	security, nurturance
US + Conditioned stimulus (CS)	produces	Conditioned response (CR)
flash on camera + camera	produces	blinking
mother's affection + eating	produces	security, nurturance
Conditioned stimulus (CS)	produces	Conditioned response (CR)
camera	produces	blinking
eating	produces	security, nurturance

Extinction

In light of the examples above, classical conditioning may be used successfully in changing a client's dietary behavior. The therapeutic process is known as *extinction*. Through extinction a person that is conditioned unlearns the conditioned response. That is, with time and the intentional omission of pairing the UCS with the CS, one can unlearn that the CS produces a CR (merely seeing the camera doesn't cause blinking). After this is learned by a client, a new, more adaptive behavior can be learned. For example, if a client learns to eat when anxious to feel security, the first step in unlearning would be to avoid eating when anxious. Then you can help the client learn new ways of handling anxiety that don't involve eating. For example, a client may begin learning relaxation techniques to the extent that relaxation is paired with anxiety to produce a new response, security.

Operant Conditioning

Operant conditioning refers to voluntary processes, and is based on the premise that behavior is controlled mainly by consequences in the environment. (4,17,42) Thomdike demonstrated this principle with mazes. Thomdike placed cats in a puzzle box and rewarded, with food, only those cats who learned to solve the puzzle. Thus he used *positive reinforcers*.

Positive Reinforcers increase a desired behavior—the more frequently the cats solved the puzzle the more they were rewarded with food. Dietitians likely hear many examples of how clients reward "good behavior" with food. A client might reward himself with chocolate cake because he met an important business deadline. A different client might reward herself with pretzels for enduring a tedious afternoon at the office. A man might reward himself with a cigarette for having endured a fight with his wife. When a client engages in such behaviors, operant conditioning is at work.

Negative Reinforcers Like positive reinforcers *negative reinforcers* produce a similar outcome; however, negative reinforcers work on a different principle. A certain behavior is increased to avoid a negative outcome. For example, one may learn to eat chocolate to avoid the unpleasant situation of doing homework. Or, one might take aspirin to avoid a headache. The degree to which one participates in an activity (eating, taking aspirin) increases because one learns that homework and headaches can be successfully avoided when a particular behavior is increased. Conditioning through negative reinforcers implies that a client may be aware of how a particular behavior is reinforcing. For example, one is aware aspirin stops or decreases headaches.

Diets work off the principle of negative reinforcement. One might diet, that is, consume fewer calories, to avoid gaining weight. Thus, the incidence of dieting behavior increases to avoid the negative outcome. One might vomit to avoid gaining weight. Thus the incidence of vomiting, in a client who suffers with bulimia, may increase in frequency. There is danger in such thinking however, while effective, one is at risk of thinking irrationally. For example, a dieter might starve to avoid the negative outcome, weight gain. Moreover, this behavior may become cyclic, frequent, and result in significant health problems. While at times they are adaptive and useful, negative reinforcers may also prove harmful.

Punishments A final consequence which influences behavior is punishment. *Punishment* yields a different behavioral outcome from both positive and negative reinforcers. Punishment serves to *decrease* the frequency of a particular behavior. Many parents are familiar with this phenomenon. Time out may be sufficiently negative to correct the inappropriate behavior of a child, as it removes a child from an enjoyable activity. Thus a child may learn, through punishment, to avoid the undesired behavior (i.e. hitting, yelling). This principle is also applicable to dietary behavior. For example, a client might eat cake less frequently to avoid requiring the use of diets. One might smoke fewer cigarettes to avoid the dizzy sensation that accompanies them.

In review then, eating behavior may be influenced by both classical conditioning (involuntary behavior) and operant conditioning (voluntary behavior). The difference is teased out through the process of assessment. During assessment a nutrition therapist will determine how food is used, and the outcome of using food. Other assessment procedures may include an interview with the client and/or significant others, client self-monitoring, observation of a client's behavior *in vivo*, role playing, self-report measures, and through testing (i.e. the eating attitudes test, self-esteem scales, etc.). (4)

Assessment Procedures

During the initial interview, the dietitian should first question the general nature of the client's problem and then itemize specifics of the client's problem. It is important to proceed slowly to allow trust and rapport to develop. When you sense trust from the client, you may move to deeper material. Trust is enhanced when the dietitian engages in four activities (4):

1. Attends closely to a client's message, focuses on the client's verbal and non verbal messages, encourages the client's discussion of the problem, and withholds bias, judgment, and purposeless conversation.

2. Avoids allowing one's own values and biases from influencing the client's discussion of the problem; listens objectively.
3. Listens and responds empathically. It is important for the client to know that his/her feeling will be validated and acknowledged. For example, when hearing one's struggle with losing weight a dietitian might respond, "I can really hear how you have suffered with your weight and in your attempts to lose weight."
4. Ensures client confidentiality. Clients must know that their stories are safe and will not be repeated carelessly to other staff, other clients, and/or the client's family, without prior approval.

Simple questions, regarding the nature of one's work, place of residence, and educational experience, may be used during the first interview to ease a client's anxiety. (4) You might then proceed to questions which relate to reasons for referral. O'Leary and Wilson outlined several questions (4), listed below, to interpret the exact nature of the problem.

1. When did the problem begin?
2. How frequently does it occur?
3. When and in what situations does it occur?
4. What occurs before and after it?
5. What has been done to change the problem?

Once the nature of the problem is conceptualized, the dietitian may then inventory both the strengths and vulnerabilities of the client. Concluding this first visit with strengths may encourage the client and help him/her to feel good about himself/herself, to the extent that the client may leave the counseling session with a positive feeling. It may be this positive feeling which may keep a client in treatment.

During the second assessment appointment, you may again inventory the client's dietary problem. A functional analysis is often used to further clarify the client's problem. With this assessment technique, you identify how the client behaves in his or her *natural environment*. (4, 5, 34) A functional analysis reveals the ABCs of one's behavior. That is, more information is revealed about the target problem: the *antecedents* of behavior (triggers, what leads to eating, i.e. seeing cookies on the counter), the *resultant behaviors* (what occurs after eating, i.e. exercise, vomiting, more eating), and the *consequent behaviors* (system of positive reinforcers, negative reinforcers, and punishments, i.e. losing weight, avoiding discomfort, gaining weight, feeling full). An example is outlined below.

Dietitian: "Can you help me understand your problem more fully? It may help us both to know what happens before you eat, after you eat, and what reinforces your eating. It may help to recall a specific example when you experienced trouble controlling your eating. Tell me about the last time this happened to you."

Client: "Well, let's see. Today is Monday. Friday I got home from work. I was really tired and anxious. It was a Friday and I had a difficult week. First I hung up my coat, then I went into the kitchen for a drink. As I opened the refrigerator I saw the cookies. Then I felt the craving. So I ate some. Then I ate some more. Then I ate some more. Before I know it, I ate half the package. I couldn't stop!"

Dietitian: "Let me see if I understand you correctly. You arrived home from work feeling tired and anxious (antecedent). You hung up your coat, walked to the kitchen, opened up the refrigerator, ate some cookies (resultant behavior). Then you ate some more; but, you did not really describe what happens after eating. Am I understanding you so far?"

Client: "Yes, you got it. Then I feel just terrible. I feel depressed. Then I don't eat dinner because I'm too full and feel really bad. Sometimes I just go and read."

Dietitian: "So the consequence of eating for you is really severe. You feel depressed, overfull, and really 'bad.' Sometimes you just go and read (consequent behavior)."

In this example, the dietitian effectively engages with the client, inviting the client to tell her story. Without significant prompting, the client sufficiently delineates the details of her experience, to the extent that antecedents, resultant behaviors, and consequent behaviors are identified. Not depicted in the example however is information regarding how the target behavior is reinforced in the client's natural environment.

A final part and critical aspect of the assessment interview is to ascertain what maintains the problematic behavior in question (4, 5). If a client is aware that an eating problem exists, understands, and is not happy with the ramifications of this problem, how is it that the problem continues to exist?

From a behavioral perspective, life problems take on a life of their own. Problems are maintained by the reinforcers in one's environment. Relative to the example above, one might presume that eating is maintained through the taste of the food. A second hypothesis might be that the client receives more attention after eating than before. Perhaps the client calls a friend and commiserates about how terribly her diet is going. A third hypothesis relates to the experience of the client. Perhaps the positive feeling this client experiences after eating relates to contracting to begin a diet "tomorrow," and buy new dresses after losing weight. Indeed, reinforcers may not be rational.

Through assessment the dietitian experiences and conceptualizes the depths of a client's problem. With this information the client and you may proceed to treatment planning. As discussed earlier, clients should be involved in treatment planning. Appendix 8-A represents a sample format which might be used by you and client to achieve this end.

First, the client and you should describe desired goals of treatment. Some behavioral goals might include: 1) learn relaxation techniques that can be used in the car on the way home from work, 2) decrease fat consumption to no more than 30 percent of total calories, 3) walk that least five times per week for 20 minutes.

Second, both the client and dietitian should agree on treatment modalities. (4,5) Treatment techniques are described in the next section.

The treatment plan should be signed by both parties and stored in the client's medical record. It provides a forum for the client and you to continually rework the course and context of treatment. Outcomes should be measured or reevaluated to determine the extent to which goals for change have been met.

Treatment Strategies

Self-Monitoring. A technique used both during assessment and treatment, self-monitoring refers to the monitoring, overseeing, observing, or regulating of an aspect of one's behavior. During assessment, it provides the client a forum to identify aspects of eating which are troublesome. For example, a client may not be aware that time of day is a trigger for eating until she or he monitor eating to the extent that all foods and beverages consumed are recorded on paper, for a specified period of time. The information revealed with self-monitoring therefore establishes the context and course of treatment.

With regards to eating behavior, you might monitor a variety of factors, together or separate, as appropriate to the client's needs and problem. Factors which may be monitored with this technique include time of day, type of food, amount of food, place of eating, activity while eating, with whom eating, rate of eating, degree of hunger or fullness, mood (i.e. angry, sad, happy, afraid, lonely), and physical state (i.e. tired, fatigued) (see Appendix 8-B). An adjective list of moods and physical states may assist a client in identifying states of being (see Appendix 8-C,8-D).

In treatment, self-monitoring serves two purposes. First, and perhaps most important, it provides the client a forum to make decisions about that behavior which is monitored, and therefore allows the client to maintain a level of consciousness and intentionality. Focusing on decision making, rather than how well the goal was achieved, reduces the likelihood that such records might only be used to categorize behavior as "good" or "bad." This approach is less shaming and may free the client to accurately record what happened. It is sometimes this "bad" judgment which discourages some clients from keeping such records all together.

A second function of self-monitoring in treatment is to monitor progress. Indeed, it is the basis by which you might judge efficacy. A variety of self-monitoring tools might be used in this endeavor including diaries of food consumed, cigarettes smoked, exercise completed, or records of blood sugar, blood pressure, or pounds lost.

Stimulus Control. Once identified, problematic stimuli can be better managed so that the desired outcome can be achieved. These stimuli are managed through the technique of stimulus control. Stimulus control is used in the phase of treatment where solutions to problems are identified and implemented. The focus should be on managing or coping rather than controlling perfectly. Controlling implies that a stimulus may be extinguished, where in reality the best that may be hoped for is management. Management implies coping differently with a given stimulus.

Before stimuli can be managed in an orderly and coherent way however, goals for treatment should be identified (3-5,18,34). What stimuli is problematic? In what way is it problematic? Under what specific conditions? What outcome does the client and dietitian agree is desirable and achievable? Finally, in what way will the stimuli best be managed? It is upon these, and other questions, the client and dietitian might reflect so that a strategy or strategies for change can be identified and implemented in a sequential manner. The technique of stimulus control has clinical utility with old problems, new problems, and out of control problems. While there are three methods by which this technique may be used, primarily stimulus control modifies food exposure and/or availability and alters food associations. (18) For example, some clients are at risk of eating simply because they saw cookies on the counter top. A stimulus control strategy strives to decrease exposure. Thus, cookies might be stored in the cabinet.

Second, stimulus control may be aimed at changing and/or limiting eating times and places. Thus, one might be encouraged to only snack on fruit between four and six in the evening and only in the kitchen. Such a technique will break food associations between time of day and eating, as well as location and eating.

Finally, stimulus control is aimed at breaking the automaticity of eating. Thus food associations between home from work and cookies, or television and popcorn, might be broken with stimulus control. An example of a stimulus control form is found in Appendix 8-E .

The case of Roger best explains the technique of stimulus control. Roger, a 47-year-old man who sought treatment in a weight loss clinic, complained of excessive eating, usually during the day at fast food restaurants. Because Roger traveled a great deal during his work day, he often stopped at fast food restaurants for snacks and meals. There he often ordered two or three large burgers, fries, and sugared sodas. He was overstimulated with the sight and smell of a fast food restaurant and was unable to change his response. This problematic eating situation was corrected, in part, by changing Roger's driving route. Further, he carried healthy snacks with him and ate these rather than stopping for a "quick" snack. Finally, Roger broke the automaticity of his response near fast food restaurants by finding other ways to cope with triggers which prompted eating such as relieving frustration by stopping on the side of the road and practicing relaxation techniques. Upon doing so, he often found he no longer desired to eat. Over time, Roger lost his desire for fried burgers and fries.

Imagery. Imagery is the process by which a counselor assists the client in recalling or conceiving mentally a hypothetical problematic situation. The manner in which these events are recalled or imagined is predetermined. (41) This technique provides the client a forum to envision problematic situations in the context of healthy coping. Further, problematic situations are categorized on a hierarchy from least difficult to most difficult.

Imagery has clinical utility with all three eating categories; however, it may require one who has an ability to think abstractly. The case of Tom best depicts the utility of this technique. Tom is a 43-year-old man who sought treatment in a weight management clinic. He was sufficiently able to describe his struggles with eating; however, he was less well able to control eating. The dialogue below further describes Tom's eating difficulties and the use of imagery.

Dietitian: "It seems your eating struggles are pretty well-defined. You are able to identify both situations and specific foods which give you trouble. Let's review once more what your struggle is."

Tom: "Well, I just cannot control my eating at buffets, social events where there is a lot of food, and restaurants. I also cannot control my intake of donuts, cookies, and ice cream. If I have them in the house I eat them within a relatively short period of time, within a few hours. Also, a most dangerous time for me is when I am home on a cold winter day. I have nothing to do; so, I eat."

Dietitian: "You really understand your struggle with food well. Let's take a moment now and create a hierarchy of situations and food from least troublesome to most troublesome. 10 will represent the least troublesome food or situation and 100 will represent the most troublesome food or situation. Does this sound okay to you Tom?"

Tom: "Yes, it sounds okay. Let's see, I think 10 is restaurants, 40 is social buffets, 60 is cookies, 70 is ice cream, 80 is an all-you-can-eat buffet, 100 is a donut. I just can't stop with one."

Dietitian: Very good Tom. You completed this without much difficulty. I imagine you have reflected on this quite a bit. You seem to understand your struggle well. Let me see if I understand you correctly. Let's construct your hierarchy together:

100	donuts
90	
80	all you can eat buffet
70	ice cream
60	cookies
50	
40	social buffets (work)
30	
20	
10	restaurants

I see however that you did not list in the house on a winter day. Where would you place this Tom?

Tom: "Let's see, I would put that at 50. Come to think of it, at 30 I would put the teacher's lounge. At 20 I would put the lunch cafeteria at work. Let's see, 90, what is as difficult as donuts for me? I would have to say steak. I guess that's it."

Dietitian: "The next step in our imagery is to begin with the situation which provokes the least amount of worry and anxiety. You described this as restaurants. I imagine then Tom that you could walk into a restaurant and order your chicken meal without too much anxiety or struggle. Is this true for you Tom?"

Tom: "It sure is. It's the easiest one on my list."

Dietitian: "Okay Tom. Try to relax in your chair. Close your eyes. When you are completely relaxed I'd like you to imagine yourself at your favorite restaurant (note: the dietitian would likely spend time training Tom on relaxation techniques before actually trying out the imagery exercise). You walk in the door. The host seats you and your wife at your table. You feel slightly anxious, hungry, and happy to see your wife after a long work day. You sit at your table, review the menu. You feel this is a special time and you want to eat something special. Then you see baked chicken with blackeyed peas, a meal you think would be healthier yet still tasty. I want you to imagine yourself ordering the chicken meal, completely relaxed and without struggle. Imagine yourself able to stop eating when full. You experience no struggle over whether you should finish all of the food on your plate. You simply stop eating when comfortably full, and focus your attention on your conversation with your wife. The waiter comes, removes your plate with some food left on the side, you smile and ask for the check instead of dessert. . . .STOP Okay Tom, let's talk about your experience. (Ask one question at a time.)

What did it feel like? What were your thoughts about the situation? How do you think you might actually feel in that restaurant experience? Suppose you were to eat in a restaurant this evening with your wife, could you act out this imagery experience with her?"

As Tom completed imagery experiences at the lower level, he would slowly move up the hierarchy until achieving success at the level of 100. The focus on treatment would likely be comprehensive in that as Tom successfully imagined eating at each level, he might try out new behaviors with real-life performance-based techniques.

Imagery techniques, combined with other cognitive-behavioral approaches, may be very successful in helping a client move in an ordered fashion through treatment. Imagery, as described here, provides a context and framework for treatment.

Role Playing. Role playing, like imagery, is a treatment technique used in the presence of the counselor. It differs from imagery however in that the counselor takes an active role in the imagery (hypothetical or actual) situation. (17,18,35,41)

Role playing provides the client a forum to practice new behaviors in a safe environment. It is also a place to respond to other's messages. The case of Edith nicely describes this technique.

Edith is a 60-year-old woman who cannot say "no" to others when they offer her food; although she describes being aware of her dilemma and excessive eating. Edith role played this dilemma with her dietitian. This was an important opportunity for Edith, as she was both able to imagine, in an emotive (emotional) and cognitive (mentally clear) manner, her dilemma. At the same time, Edith was able to practice a new ending to her story, in a safe and protected environment. While the dietitian offered some challenge, she did not overly confront Edith and did not demand that Edith behave in a specified manner. With practice, over three role playing exercises, Edith was able to say "no" to the extra, undesired chocolate cake calories that her hostess prepared for dessert—and without feeling guilty. Instead, Edith described feeling that when she did say "no," that she felt empowered, as if she was nurturing herself.

Real-Life Performance-Based Techniques. These techniques are similar to role playing as a treatment; however, in addition, they allow the client to practice new behaviors in vivo. That is, clients are given an opportunity to practice newly learned behaviors in their natural environment, where clients are likely to experience eating dilemmas. With time and practice, the automaticity of new behaviors is enhanced and the likelihood that old, less adaptive, behaviors may surface decreases. (41,42)

This is an important clinical technique for all groups of eating behavior and especially those who feel a sense of control over eating. A simpler term to describe this technique is that of "practical homework." It is an important technique, as it teaches clients they can indeed cope in a new way with problematic eating situations. Real-life performance-based techniques are illustrated with George.

George complained that he just could not enjoy a holiday meal without the "normal" fixings. The dietitian disagreed with him and contracted with George to begin practicing new eating behaviors as early as June. Both George and his dietitian agreed that if he practiced lower calorie and fat habits sufficiently, he would develop coping strategies which allowed him to eat smaller amounts and less fat during the upcoming Thanksgiving Day meal. George practiced moderate eating on three occasions. During each experience he consumed a "typical" holiday meal at a restaurant, while noting both his feelings and the content of his thought during each event. Of particular interest was his attitude that, "it's just not a holiday meal unless I'm full."

With time, both George and his dietitian noticed a transformation in his thinking. After three months of practicing new eating behaviors, exploring triggers to eating, and "trying on" new thoughts and behaviors, George experienced a change in basic attitudes about holiday eating. He no longer felt the need to eat until overfull; instead, George consumed smaller portions of food, feeling both physically and emotionally satisfied.

Self-Reinforcement. Positive reinforcements (operant conditioning) are the methods by which new behaviors are rewarded; therefore, they are the means by which new and more appropriate behaviors increase in frequency. (35,18,42) Perhaps the most basic of self-reinforcers is the positive mood state which occurs with a sense of achievement. Other, more tangible, reinforcers may include smaller sized clothing, a vacation, or a day at the salon.

Self-reinforcement is an important component of behavior change programs. Indeed, self-reinforcement is a predictor of weight loss success. (24,43) A dietitian's task therefore is perhaps to continually focus discussions on *what worked* for the client rather than *what went wrong*. This is empowering for clients. Clients want to feel good about what they are achieving and a dietitian can be instrumental in helping clients achieve this mood state.

While dietitians are important sources of reinforcement, they must not be the only provider of positive reinforcement. It is equally important that a client self-reinforce and that a client receive reinforcement from those in their social network. First, clients should learn to reinforce their own behavior. (3) This is important to increase one's sense of control over the problematic situation and to decrease dependence upon others as continual sources of support. A relationship characterized by merely positives is not necessarily ideal or mutual. Mutual relationships are characterized by those where both members feel a sense of increased zest, empowerment, self- and other knowledge, self-worth, and a desire for more connection. (44)

Not only must a client begin to self-reinforce, others in the client's life may behave in a similar fashion. During a treatment session therefore, the dietitian and client may determine who most often provides the type of support or reinforcement so desired by the client. With such an exploration, clients may learn how they are reinforced by others (through attention, affection, praise, approval, support), and how clients themselves may provide support and reinforcement to another. In effect, what a client may be learning is how to relate mutually and how to develop a level of emotional intimacy with another.

The efficacy of reinforcement is well-documented in research. A weight loss program compared four treatment modalities (20):

1. behavior therapy alone
2. behavior therapy plus post-treatment counseling
3. behavior therapy plus post-treatment counseling plus aerobic exercise
4. behavior therapy plus post-treatment counseling plus social support
5. behavior therapy plus post-treatment counseling plus aerobic exercise plus social support.

The only group to continue losing weight at 18-month follow-up was the treatment group characterized by all four treatment modalities: behavior therapy, post-treatment counseling (26 weeks), aerobic exercise, and social support. Clearly, more comprehensive programs appear more effective than programs which offer fewer components.

Modeling.

Modeling is derived from social learning theory, as first described by Bandura. (45) It is a form of imitation and occurs in a four step process. A client should first *observe* the model's behavior (i.e. eating, speech, thought processes) to a sufficient degree where some of *how* the model performs is remembered. Next, the protege or client may *reproduce* the behavior and/or state of being previously observed. Finally, clients should receive reinforcement and *feedback* for their newly learned behaviors. It is through this process of observation- remembering- reproduction- feedback, that new behaviors are formed and imprinted. Once achieved, new behaviors may become a part of the client's coping repertoire. (Incidently, this is also how dietitians and students learn new counseling skills best—through modeling, refining and practice.)

Clients do not merely model the behavior of strangers however. Clients actively discriminate between persons and select, unconsciously, the most desirable model available. (45) Models share certain similar attributes with their proteges. They are of similar age, sex, race, and attitudes. Further, models are prestigious, competent, and often work in distinguished and important positions. Such research has important implications for dietetic practice.

First, a dietitian may be a model for some and not others. This is normal. The key to a dietitian's experience is to know with *whom* she or he may be an effective model. Perhaps this explains why some dietitians feel completely ineffective with certain clients and yet so successful with others.

Second, dietitians can explain the principles of modeling to clients and assist clients in their journey to find prospective models in their *natural* environment. Once identified, and a trusting relationship is developed between model and protege, the client may seek advice, reinforcement, praise, or coaching from his or her model. (46) Indeed, there is a certain order to the modeling relationship.

The principle of modeling applies to mentoring relationships, and to self-help groups where one selects a sponsor. Models are invaluable sources of methodology, reinforcement, praise, trust, and other positive experiences, and perhaps provide some of the social support many behavioral therapies declare is so important in behavioral change.

Systematic Desensitization.
A technique used to relieve one of the pains associated with phobias (extreme anxiety in relation to objects, animals or people), systematic desensitization may not be appropriate for use by a dietitian (3-5, 39-41). Still, it may be useful information for the dietitian, as in cases of making a referral decision.

The process of systematic desensitization is achieved with three steps. (5) First, a client is taught methods of deep muscle relaxation. Second, a client is instructed on how to construct an anxiety hierarchy (similar to the hierarchy constructed during imagery). Finally, anxiety producing phobias, objects, or animals from the hierarchy are matched with relaxation training. The goal of systematic desensitization is to teach a particular client a new way of coping. Instead of coping by using anxiety, one learns to substitute the relaxed state for the anxiety state, to the degree that the relaxed state becomes automatic. It may be clear to some that the assumptions of this technique are rooted in classical conditioning; thus, it is a technique particularly suitable for one who feels a sense of *loss of control*. Those who suffer with compulsive eating, bulimia, and/or anorexia may benefit from systematic desensitization.

This technique is included, not with the intention that a dietitian may use this technique upon reading, but rather, for the purpose of information. Indeed, many clients dietitians counsel may benefit from such a technique. It is important for dietitians to know therefore, what clients may benefit from referral and when to refer a client to a behaviorally-oriented counselor.

Those who may benefit from systematic desensitization may suffer with a variant of anxiety disorder (6), as well as those who feel *out of control* with eating or eating-related behavior. (35) Symptoms of generalized anxiety disorder include persistent anxiety as manifested by excessive anxiety and worry concerning many life events, an inability to control the worry, and worry which is associated with motor tension, restlessness, apprehension, or vigilance. (6,47)

COGNITIVE RESTRUCTURING TREATMENT STRATEGIES
Men are disturbed not by events, but by the views they take of them.

Epictetus (4)

The actual assumptions of cognitive therapies are perhaps as old as Epictetus, described as a stoic Roman philosopher who lived around the time of 55 AD. He professed that one's problem is rooted in how one perceives one's problem, rather than what the problem may actually be. Indeed, one's problem is a function of one's values, beliefs, ideologies, and philosophies of living. When these beliefs and values are absolute in nature, as opposed to relative, one will likely experience emotional sequelae or responses (anxiety, guilt, shame, depression), as well as behavioral sequelae (eating, punching a wall, drinking alcohol, smoking). Moreover, these responses or sequelae are viewed as maladaptive answers to a mismanaged problem. Basic assumptions of cognitive therapy are further outlined in Table 8-3.

Table 8-3 Basic Assumptions of Cognitive Therapy

1. People are born with powerful aptitudes to think both rationally and irrationally.
2. People have vast resources for growth, and therefore, can indeed change their destiny in personally significant ways.
3. People's tendency for irrational thinking is exacerbated by family and culture.
4. To understand disturbed behavior, the therapist must understand how people perceive, think, emote, and act.
5. When people experience life disturbances, it is because they care too much about what others think.
6. Cognitive-behavioral techniques effectively change behavior and cognitions in a brief period of time.
7. The technique is designed to help people examine and change their most basic values.

In the quest to correct a maladaptive problem, one might first explore one's basic ideologies. These ideologies are often a reflection of early learning in the family and in society. For example, one's family may have taught, "*You must always eat all of the food on your plate; You must never cry; You must never show others when you are vulnerable.*"

The problem of adopting irrational ideologies is further exacerbated when one attends school during middle childhood, and thereafter, as one's exposure to irrational ideologies is expanded. Indeed, irrational ideologies (racist, sexist or other bigoted ideas, use of violence to solve problems, the idea that material goods will lead to happiness and popularity, and so on) are ubiquitous—they emanate from teachers, television, music, media, most any place people are. The problem therefore becomes one of exposing, eluding, and circumventing irrational ideology. Once exposed, irrational ideologies can be replaced with ideologies which are more consistent with one's goals for healthy living. The process by which this occurs is perhaps best described by Albert Ellis in his Rational-Emotive Therapy (RET). (3,5,48)

Albert Ellis developed a cognitive-behavioral counseling technique called Rational-Emotive Therapy (RET) in 1950. (3,5,48) Ellis believed undesired emotional consequences (anxiety, depression, shame, etc.) are created by an individual's faulty belief system. These beliefs can be challenged, however, and replaced with more adaptive beliefs. Doing so may help the client avoid not only the undesired emotional consequence, but the undesired behavior as well (eating, weighing, exercising, smoking, etc.). You may help clients with RET by disputing their irrationally held beliefs and helping them to think more rationally.

Any faulty belief which predisposes the client to aberrant eating, weighing or exercising behavior is an area upon which the dietitian might focus. Clients may abandon treatment because they may think they *cannot* change these undesired behaviors until they understand the origins of their problem. It is a premise of this theory, however, that clients need not understand why they eat as they do to change behaviors. Clients need only to understand the ABCs of their behavior and cognition. Relaying such a message may be freeing for a client. Some do not care to explore to a level deeper than the immediate problem of weight.

Assessment
The cognitive-behavioral theorists will ultimately be interested in knowing how the individual developed ideas or cognitions about reality, how the individual chooses and decides from the many possibilities, and how the individual acts and behaves in relationship to reality.(5)

Like behavioral therapy, a functional analysis is used during cognitive assessment to identify faulty and absolutist attitudes and beliefs. However, the functional analysis used with cognitive techniques differs somewhat from that of behavioral therapy, as thoughts, attitudes, and beliefs are considered a part of the formula (see Appendix 8-F). (3,5,48)

During assessment you might first identify the event which precedes eating. Subsequent to this you assist your client in identifying his or her attitudes, values, or beliefs about the event. It is often one's attitudes which results in both excessive eating and a dysfunctional mood, as these attitudes are often irrational. Irrational attitudes are clearly evident when a client thinks *should, must, ought, always, never*. Irrational beliefs are absolutist. Thus, a client may never feel satisfied because a client cannot achieve his or her goals and may be left feeling badly (shamed, depressed, anxious). Clients may act out this "bad" feeling by eating. The case of Marie illustrates assessment using RET.

Marie complained of overeating and lack of physical activity, especially when anxious. She often ate when feeling as if she could not control a problem in her life. This out of control feeling resulted in significant anxiety. Marie blocked or coped with the anxiety by eating handfuls of jelly beans or chocolates. Her dilemma was further exacerbated by this eating because as she ate she gained more weight and her mobility was further limited. Thus, her goals of weighing less and increasing mobility were yet more distant. Further discussion between the dietitian and Marie reveals the following information.

Figure 8-1   Therapy Discussion Flow Chart

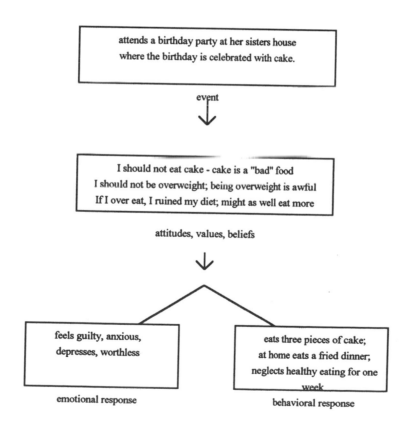

Treatment

Decatastrophizing. This technique was used by Ellis to abate anxiety, which was often an exaggerated negative response to a specific situation. (3,5,48) The technique involves evaluating the client's fear of an identified situation and the *horrible* negative outcome, and helping the client to acknowledge the ridiculousness of the belief and resulting emotion; fear. The case of Adrian illustrates this technique.

Dietitian: "Adrian, you described never eating chocolate because you see it as a horrible food. You further said if you did eat chocolate you would not be able to stop. Can you help me understand more of your experience here?" (The dietitian suspects that chocolate is not the real issue here.)

Adrian: "Well, if I ate chocolate it would be horrible. I would get fat. That's why I can't eat it."

Dietitian: "What is the worst possible outcome you can imagine might occur if you got fat?"

Adrian: "Well, my friends wouldn't like me. I wouldn't fit into my clothes. I just wouldn't fit in with the group. You know, they are all popular, pretty. They have the boyfriends. If I got fat, I wouldn't have that."

Dietitian: "Why would that be horrible?"

Adrian: "Well, then I would be all alone."

Dietitian: "It sounds like being alone carries with it a greater fear than being fat carries. Would you say that's true? What seems more scary to you, being alone or being fat?"

Adrian: "I don't know, being alone I guess. But I still can't get fat."

Dietitian: "So your friends might not want to be with you because fat people are horrible. Suppose you were the fattest person your friends ever met. Why would that make you horrible?"

Adrian: "Well, I shouldn't be fat."

Dietitian: "It might be nicer if you were not fat. You might be able to walk easier. But being fat does not mean that you are horrible. Who told you that you should never be fat? Who told you that you would be horrible if you were fat?";

Adrian: "Well, I guess when I was seven, my Mom did. She put me on these diet pills. I was a chubby little kid. So I lost some weight and it was like everything changed. I got new clothes. My Mom took me places with her. My friends liked me more. I had more friends. I just became a better person. Before that I only got the chubette clothes. My friends made fun of me. I stayed home a lot."

Dietitian: "So being thin means you will not be horrible because you will have more friends, your Mom will give you more attention, and you can buy different clothes. Being fat means you are horrible because you have fewer friends and your Mom won't take you places. It might be nicer to have more and different clothes and friends and your Mom's attention. But being fat does not mean you are horrible. Why is it that you feel it necessary to berate yourself? You seemed to have personalized a sense of badness. Do you see where your logic goes astray? You believe, and you were told by family and friends, that being thin somehow means being more worthy. You might replace this logic with, 'It would be better to weigh less. But being fat does not mean that I am a bad person.' Do you see the difference in what I said and what you are saying?"

Using the client's response, the dietitian can help the client become aware of other possibilities. Further, the dietitian can help the client see the outcome she may imagine as *horrible* is really quite manageable. Thus, the dietitian might use this questioning to move the client to imagining alternative emotional and behavioral reactions, and finally to problem solving.

Challenging the Shoulds, Oughts, and Musts. According to Ellis (48), "shoulds" and "musts" are the foundation of irrational beliefs. Without the dichotomous thinking inherent in these self-imposed rules, irrational thinking would not occur. Perfectionist beliefs upheld by clients always lead to failure because they cannot be achieved; therefore, clients are left feeling even more inadequate than before the rule was imposed. (See Appendix 8-G Irrational Beliefs Daily Log.)

The goal of the dietitian is to help the client dispute irrational beliefs and develop an awareness that such beliefs are absurd or unachieveable. This might be accomplished by comparing facts with fantasies, observing real life phenomenon, trying out behaviors and waiting for the *horrible* event to occur, and then finding that one can indeed cope with the *horrible* event.

Reattribution. Reattribution, a technique where faulty self-perceptions are challenged, is described by Garner and Bemis and used in cognitive therapy with those suffering with anorexia. (32) However, the applicability of this technique may extend beyond that of one with anorexia, as when one experiences distortions in body image.

This technique helps clients perceive an attribute of themselves differently. The nutrition therapist helps the client question the validity of self-perceptions and therefore creates an atmosphere of ambiguity where other cognitions may be considered. Questioning and exploring the evidence of one's beliefs are the primary methods by which this ambiguity is achieved.

Because this technique is confrontative, to be effective it requires a well-formed relationship. That is, there must be a high level of trust, to the degree that the client will not feel criticized or abandoned when irrational thoughts are challenged. Dietitians must therefore attend to the client's affect (emotions), verbal responses, and gestures, searching for gestures of hurt and insult. Should you notice such behavior or feelings, this should be openly discussed.

Decentering. Decentering was first described by Piaget in his theory of cognitive development. (49,50) Piaget asserted that developmentally, one is not able to decenter until middle childhood, between the ages of six to 12 years. In the context of Piaget's theory, decentering means taking into account more than one perspective or explanation, perhaps many, of a particular situation or problem. One who can decenter is able to hold, to understand, to explain that there may indeed be various and very different explanations for one particular problem.

The principle of decentering may be applied to one's self-understanding and to relationships. Relative to one's self-understanding, decentering implies that one may understand an aspect of self from many perspectives. For example, one who decenters sufficiently understands that an overweight condition occurs because one has consumed quantitatively and qualitatively too many calories and has exercised too little. One who does not decenter sufficiently might understand weight gain only and completely in terms of eating a "bad" food. Decentering might also be understood in the context of a relationship. With regard to one's relationships, decentering implies a social situation where both persons in the relationship understand, *I understand you, you understand me, and we both understand a third, more objective perspective.* These are the principles of Selman's social perspective and are very applicable to the dynamic which should exist between a client and a dietitian. (51) For example, a client who does not sufficiently decenter may not understand that you can know his or her experience. Your task, therefore, is to help the client understand that you can indeed feel the experience of the client. It is the experience of the author that clients like and want to know this. It helps them feel understood, significant, and cared for. In fact, conveying to a client that you understand (cognitively) and can feel (emotionally) a client's experience, is being empathic and is a core requirement of a therapeutic relationship. (34)

While decentering is an ability acquired and used in cognitive processing during middle childhood, researchers who studied this phenomenon in years after Piaget have demonstrated that even during adolescence, some individuals maintain a level of egocentricity. In his work with adolescence, Elkind demonstrated that adolescent egocentricity is apparent in behaviors such as fault finding, argumentativeness, self-consciousness, self-centeredness, indecisiveness, and identifying hypocrisy. (52) Many adults behave in a similar fashion. Thus, this issue of decentering, and helping clients to decenter, is seemingly important to many of the clients dietitians' treat.

Garner and Bemis (32) used this technique with those suffering with anorexia. The outcome of this technique is one's ability to acknowledge a perspective different from one's own. For example, a person with anorexia might imagine that others can detect when she or he gains three pounds and everyone notices. Through decentering, this person can begin to understand that others may not notice something so overly important to the client.

Decentering is a technique applicable to clients other than those suffering with anorexia. Actually, it is a very personal technique because it has to do with what you imagine others know about you. It is applicable to a person of any weight and perhaps most applicable with persons who are overly concerned with how others regard them. (46) The case of Jane demonstrates the clinical use of decentering.

Jane sought treatment for weight loss. She understood her struggle with food as eating too many "bad" foods during the week. She further described that she could not bear to be fat. In fact, the reason why she was now separated from her husband was because he could not bear her "fatness" as well. She described her marital relationship as "close" when she was thin and "distant" when she was fat. Thus, using Jane's reasoning, the primary problem in her life was one of being "fat," and not one of perhaps marrying a man who did not love Jane at the level of her vulnerable core. Indeed, Jane's struggle with food is penetrating and likely indicates a more serious struggle with her sense of self, her sense of differentiation, and her sense of worthiness, respect, and esteem.

A dietitian working with Jane might recognize the depth of her pain, actively work toward establishing a trust and rapport not based on "diet," but based on the human contact between Jane and the dietitian. This would help Jane to develop an awareness that people can indeed like her and develop a mutual relationship with her for reasons other than her weight. The dietitian therefore would be educating Jane on her other attributes which are desirable, her strengths. Thus, it may be apparent that techniques are not used in isolation. This last example demonstrates reattribution as well as decentering.

Once rapport is developed, the dietitian might gently begin to explore Jane's ideology of "fat and goodness." Where did it come from? What was the most salient life experience which taught her to believe this? What role model in her life demonstrated this ideology to her? Under what conditions might this ideology not be true? When had this ideology perhaps not held true for Jane in the past? Through gentle, understanding, and empathic confrontation the dietitian can create a level of ambiguity within the client's ideology. Once formed, this ambiguity can be molded and transformed to more rational thinking in terms of oneself, one's relationships, and one's problems.

PSYCHOEDUCATIONAL TREATMENT STRATEGIES

Techniques which involve both a cognitive component and a behavioral component are called psychoeducational techniques. Many dietitians already use psychoeducational techniques in their counseling practices, although they may not name them as such.

This portion of the chapter explores psychoeducational techniques in four ways: first, the word is explored; second, the techniques are differentiated from both behavioral and cognitive techniques; third, clinical utility is discussed; and fourth, sample techniques (distraction, delay, and parroting) are explored and modeled.

Root Words

The root "psycho" generally implies of the mind or mental processing. Freud was the first to describe such processing. (53) Relative to psychoeducational techniques, "psycho" implies physical and mental impulses or urges. Included under this category are states of being (i.e. hunger, fullness, mood) and physical sensations (i.e. bodily feelings).

The suffix "educational" suggests knowledge, which is acquired through a process of teaching and learning. Thus, psychoeducational implies a process of learning about oneself, self understanding (one's physical and mental impulses, instincts, and/or patterns of behavior), gaining new knowledge (i.e. the number of grams of fat in a teaspoon of butter), and learning to regulate one's behavior in accordance with some standard.

Differentiation

Guerney, Stollak, and Guerney (54), initiators of the psychoeducational movement, describe this technique as a method, not focused on "curing," but rather, on "managing" physical and mental impulses appropriately. Thus, through psychoeducational technique a client develops greater self-understanding of impulsivity, temperament, hunger cues and other bodily sensations and learns to regulate behavioral responses in accordance with need, societal ideals, and/or some standard.

It may be apparent to the reader that psychoeducational techniques are indeed different from both behavioral and cognitive techniques. They differ from behavioral ones in that behavior change with psychoeducational techniques occur because of a two-fold process. First, one's level of self awareness and understanding must be increased and second, the client is then trained how to manage his or her temperament and/or impulse.

Psychoeducational techniques differ from cognitive techniques in that the cognitive ones focus primarily on one's system of attitudes and beliefs. Further, cognitive techniques do not employ a procedural component directed at understanding one's impulses, temperament, and/or bodily sensations.

Clinical Use

Psychoeducational techniques are suitable for a variety of dietary problems. They may be used in cases of anxious eating, depressive eating, and unintentional eating. A client who suffers with anxiety might use food to manage this state of being. However, the client may not be aware of the function food serves in this situation. Through a process of exploration the dietitian might help the client identify ways in which food functions in his or her life.

Some clients use food to manage depressive states of being. Often people who are depressed complain of an "empty" feeling. Sometimes this feeling of "emptiness" is framed (described) as hunger. It may be that a person's internal states of hunger and depression become confused. (8) Psychoeducational techniques might help a client become physically and mentally aware that emptiness and hunger are in fact two different states of being and thus, must be treated differently.

Finally, some eat for unknown reasons. These clients are simply not in touch with their physical and mental processes. Both exploration and education is necessary to help this client increase his or her level of self awareness so that eating might be better managed.

Psychoeducational techniques may be helpful therefore, when a client requires both behavioral change, as well as cognitive change. In addition, a client might benefit from "self awareness" training. These techniques are outlined by Garner, Rockert, Olmsted, Johnson, and Coscina in their chapter on *Psychoeducational principles in the treatment of bulimia and anorexia nervosa (30)*; however, they have applicability with other dietary related problems. Their focus is such that one may manage an urge to eat to the degree that the desire to eat might be extinguished. This may be accomplished with three techniques: distraction, delay, and/or parroting.

Three Sample Treatments

The author often uses these techniques with a weight reducing population. One client, Gretchen, who lost from 469 pounds to 350 pounds over a period of seven months, described her success strategies as distraction, delay, and parroting. Below are explanations and examples of each technique. Further, clinical utility of these techniques will be illustrated with the case of Gretchen, a 40-year-old female who sought weight loss to a healthier, undetermined, weight.

Distraction. Distraction may be used as a first line of defense against urges to eat unnecessary calories or to avoid any behavior which seems somehow undesirable. Well before the urge is experienced, the client must first compile a list of alternate behaviors which may help distract the client from the urge. Gretchen used distraction often. She described experiencing cravings to eat usually in the evening. During her work day she experienced few, if any, urges to eat. The list Gretchen compiled to cope with these urges included riding her stationary bike, removing herself from the kitchen to her bedroom to read a book or watch television, calling a friend on the telephone, or writing a letter. Gretchen often found reading in her bedroom quite effective; however, on occasion this was not sufficient to defend against the urge to eat. When the urge outlasted the defense, Gretchen tried delay.

Delay. Many clients complain of intense urges to eat. Moreover, they describe this urge as a state other than hunger. Still, they feel compelled to eat and sometimes do. When eating does occur, clients are at risk of being drawn into such old thinking patterns as, "Oh I blew it; I might as well finish the package. I'll start my diet tomorrow." The single eating episode may result in increased eating for a variety of reasons. Delay, used by itself or in combination with parroting, may prevent this automatic response.

The author has often heard clients remark, "If I wait 10 minutes often the urge to eat goes away." Indeed, this is true for many clients. But how might a dietitian use this technique and with what type of client? Delay might be used as a scheduled homework assignment. The dietitian might assign the client the following task.

Counselor: "When you feel like eating tomorrow you might try to delay eating. It might be helpful to think of this as your homework, and we can talk about your success at our next appointment. Tomorrow when you feel the urge to eat you may try repeating to yourself, "I will not eat for 15 minutes" (a parroting technique). At the end of 15 minutes you might reevaluate your need to eat. Often the urge to eat goes away after 10 or 15 minutes. I feel it is important that you try this technique, if only to learn that you can indeed bear this urge without acting on it. You don't have to eat simply because you feel the urge to eat. How does this sound to you? "

Client: "It sounds reasonable to me. But I never tried to stop eating once the urge came over me. I just ate. But what if I cannot stop my urge to eat?"

Counselor: "What do you imagine it might be like for you to feel this urge to eat and not act on it? (imagery) Can you describe for me what you might think and feel?"

Client: "Well, I might feel anxious. I might begin to think, 'I need to eat this chocolate.' I might not be able to stop myself from eating."

Counselor: "What do you imagine this chocolate might do for you? (imagery) How do you imagine feeling maybe 30 minutes after eating the chocolate? What do you think the chocolate might be doing for you at that moment that another behavior cannot accomplish for you?"

The dietitian and client may continue the conversation using the technique, delay, as a forum to explore the client's experience of eating, while at the same time revealing irrational thinking, and educating the client on more appropriate ways of thinking and eating. The process is an evolutionary one, in that it may occur over a period of weeks, and may require continual reinforcement on behalf of the dietitian and others. A counseling goal for both the dietitian and client might be to substitute the dietitian's role of reinforcing and exploring for another person who regularly communicates with the client. In doing so, reinforcement will be more available. The client will therefore have a forum to more regularly reinforce more appropriate ways of thinking and behaving with regards to food.

Gretchen often found delay to help defend against eating urges. She often combined delay with distraction. She might first defend by reading in her room, then acknowledge that she would wait 10 more minutes, and become engrossed in some activity. At times however, Gretchen found herself still craving to eat after the 10 minute period had elapsed. When this occurred, Gretchen used parroting techniques.

Parroting. As the name implies, parroting is a technique where the client repeats certain phrases to himself or herself in an attempt to dissipate and extinguish eating urges. To be most effective, these statements should be written well in advance of an eating urge. When the urge occurs a client is often too vulnerable to strategize and is more at risk of responding to the urge rather than defending against it. While the ultimate result of parroting is that the irrational urge is disputed and abated, a more profound change may occur within the client's belief system. Parroting provides clients a forum to reprogram previously held, maladaptive beliefs. These beliefs can only be reprogrammed when new, more adaptive statements are practiced and repeated frequently. Gretchen found parroting quite effective, especially when combined with distraction and delay. She regularly used the following statements:

Come on Gretchen, you're not hungry. You just ate dinner.

Go find something else to do Gretchen; you already ate your allotted 400 calories.

This is not hunger you are feeling; it is boredom. Go to sleep.

Don't go in the kitchen right now, that will put you at risk. You're not hungry.

One bite will make a difference. You don't need it. I frequently develop the urge to eat when I feel depressed;
but, this does not mean that my body needs food.
Food will not help me feel less depressed and/or less anxious.
If I always do what I've always done, I will always get what I've always gotten.

Gretchen's parroting statements all focused on eating urges; but, this technique may help to manage other behaviors as well. Some clients complain of excessive urges to exercise, not to exercise, to smoke, or to weigh themselves.

You can be instrumental in helping your clients develop parroting statements. First, explain to your client the purpose and utility of such statements. Second, provide examples from your own life, or another client's, of how parroting was both helpful and effective. Groups may be especially useful in this regard. Group members may model and role play the way in which they use parroting techniques to cope with unwanted eating urges. Finally, provide continued support to clients who feel they cannot control their urge to eat by giving them permission to eat when techniques do not work. Often, merely knowing that one has permission to eat makes the urge somehow less shameful and more manageable.

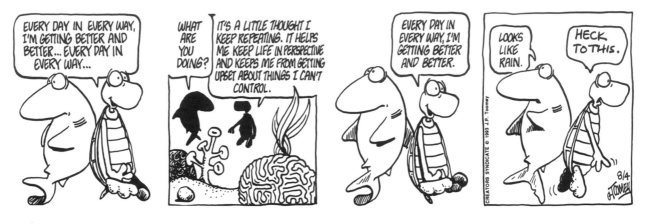

Used with permission of J.P. Toomey and Creators Syndicate.

SHERMAN'S LAGOON   By J.P. Toomey

CLINICAL IMPLICATIONS AND CONCLUSIONS

The cognitive-behavioral model of counseling theory draws on such methods as self-monitoring, stimulus control, imagery, role playing, real-life performance-based, self-reinforcement, modeling, systematic desensitization, disputing, decentering, reattributing, distraction, delay, and parroting. Indeed, these are efficacious methods; in addition, their use is well-supported with empirical research (2-5). Further, research is beginning to focus on identifying *which treatment is most effective with which individual, with what problem, at what time.* Clinicians are not merely slaves to their intuition. (2-5)

While it is well-established that cognitive-behavioral programs help *some* individuals achieve their desired health goals, these methods are not a panacea for changes in weight, eating, cholesterol, blood sugar, hypertension, and/or cigarette smoking. Indeed, some individuals seem to exhibit no improvement.

Many dietitians have worked with clients who spend months at the same weight, with the same eating problems, without significant changes in laboratory values or anthropometric data. Despite your most insightful advice, a most creative diabetic calculation, or a most perfect dietary formula, by clinical standards an individual *may fail* to recover. It may indeed be a discouraging experience to work with such individuals. Should you focus solely on physical recovery as a source of professional reinforcement, you may be left feeling ineffectual. One might look deeper then for evidence of improvement.

Individuals may benefit from other relational factors, which are not overtly apparent to either you or the client. For example, perhaps you created a relationship based on trust where it had not been previously experienced. Perhaps the client experienced a greater degree of mutuality in relationships outside of counseling, because of the mutuality which was modeled and experienced between you and your client. Perhaps the client simply feels a greater sense of significance because of the unconditional respect and warmth given by you. These are factors which may not be accounted for in lost weight, lowered blood pressure, or lowered blood sugar. These are human factors which may be experienced even if you do not *prescribe* a diet, *provide* an educational handout, or *calculate* exchanges. These factors are perhaps less well measured and less well explained; however, these factors exist.

It is the author's contention that a client's emotional condition is equally as important as a change in one's physical condition. Dietitians may indeed be sources of *normative* relational experience. This is indeed important, and sufficiently so, to the degree that a dietitian and client may dedicate an entire session to the discussion of how trust was developed between them. The implications of such trusting situations are profound.

According to Erik Erikson, trust is the basis of one's personality, religious, emotive, and ideological experience. (55, 56) Dietitians may consider their counseling appointments, therefore, in developmental terms.

The challenge for dietitians then is perhaps not method, and not even technique, but rather, staying attuned to the human and relational factors of dietetic counseling. It is the author's contention that these factors are often ignored, that dietitians feel uncomfortable focusing on relationship and the *individual* within. Rather than focusing on *technique* therefore, dietitians might focus on the *relationship* created between dietitian and this person. It is perhaps this relationship which is most therapeutic.

LEARNING ACTIVITIES

1. Observe a nutrition counseling session for either a weight management or anorexia/bulimia. Evaluate the session with the therapist using the questions outlined on pages 135-136 related to ethical counseling.
2. After observing the above counseling session, identify the different cognitive, behavioral or psychoeducational techniques that were used.

REFERENCES

1. Minuchin S, Fishman HC. *Family Therapy Techniques*. Cambridge, Massachusetts: Harvard University Press; 1981.
2. Corey G, Corey MS, Callanan P. *Issues and Ethics in the Helping Professions*. (3rd ed.). Pacific Grove, California: Brooks/Cole Publishing Company; 1988.
3. Corey G. *Theory and Practice of Group Counseling* (2nd ed.). Pacific Grove, California: Brooks/Cole Publishing Company; 1985: 337-374.
4. O'Leary KD, Wilson GT. *Behavior Therapy: Application and Outcome*. (2nd ed.). Englewood Cliffs, New Jersey: Prentice-Hall, Inc.; 1987.
5. Ivey AE, Ivey MB, Simek-Downing L. *Counseling and Psychotherapy: Integrating Skills, Theory, and Practice*. (2nd ed.). Englewood Cliffs, New Jersey: PrenticeHall, Inc.; 1987.
6. American Psychiatric Assocation. *Diagnostic and Statistical Manual of Mental Disorders*. Washington DC;1994.
7. Brownell KD, Foreyt JP, Eds. *Handbook of Eating Disorders: Physiology, Psychology, and Treatment of Obesity, Anorexia, and Bulimia*. New York: Basic Books, Inc., Publishers; 1986.
8. Bruch H. *Eating Disorders: Obesity, Anorexia Nervosa, and the Person Within*. New York: Basic Books, Inc., Publishers; 1973.
9. Reiff DW, Reiff KKL. *Eating Disorders: Nutrition Therapy in the Recovery Process*. Gaithersburg, Maryland: Aspen Publishers; 1992.
10. Wilson GT, Pike KM. Eating disorders. In: Barlow DH, ed. *Clinical Handbook of Psychological Disorders: A Step-by-Step Treatment Manual*. 2nd ed. New York: The Guilford Press; 1993.
11. Glanz K, Snelling A, Payne D, Semenske AR. Strategies for modifying behavior to reduce cardiac risk. In: Kris-Etherton PM, VolzClarke P, Clark K, Dattilo AM, eds. *Cardiovascular Disease: Nutrition for Prevention and Treatment*. The American Dietetic Association. 1990; 224-247.
12. Report of the Expert Panel on Blood Cholesterol Levels in Children and Adolescents. Washington DC, U.S. Department of Health and Human Services, 1990.
13. Report of the Expert Panel on Population Strategies for Blood Cholesterol Reduction. Washington D.C., U.S. Department of Health and Human Services, 1990.
14. Rabb C, Tillotson JL (eds.): Heart to Heart. Washington D.C., U.S. Department of Health and Human Services, 1983.
15. Report of the Expert Panel on Detection, Evaluation, and Treatment of High Blood Cholesterol in Adults. Washington D.C., U.S. Department of Health and Human Services, 1989.
16. Remmell PS, Gorder DD, Hall Y, Tillotson JL. Assessing dietary adherence in the Multiple Risk Factor Intervention Trial (MRFIT). *Journal of the American Dietetic Association*. 1980; 96: 351.
17. Williams AB. Behavior Modification. In: Holli BB, Calabrese RJ. *Communication and Education Skills: The Dietitian's Guide*. Philadelphia: Lea & Febiger; 1986: 81102.
18. Brownell KD, Kramer FM. Behavioral management of obesity. *Medical Clinics of North America*. 1989;73(1): 185-201.
19. Perri MG, Nezu AM, Patti ET, McCann KL. Effect of length of treatment on weight loss. *Journal of Consulting and Clinical Psychology*. 1989; 57(3): 450-452.
20. Perri MG, McAllister DA, Gange JJ, Jordan RC, McAdoo WG, Nezu AM. Effects of four maintenance programs on the long-term management of obesity. *Journal of Consulting and Clinical Psychology*. 1988; 56(4): 529-534.
21. Wadden TA, Stunkard AJ, and Liebschutz J. Three year follow-up of the treatment of obesity by very low calorie diet, behavior therapy, and their combination. *Journal of Clinical and Consulting Psychology*. 1988; 56(6): 925-928.
22. Graham LE, Taylor CB, Hovell MF, and Siegel W. Five year follow-up to a behavioral weight loss program. *Journal of Consulting and Clinical Psychology*. 1983;51(2):322-323.
23. Westover SA, Lanyon RI. The maintenance of weight loss after behavioral treatment. *Behavior Modification*. 1990; 14(2): 123-137.
24. Kayman S, Bruvold W, Stern JS. Maintenance and relapse after weight loss in women: Behavioral aspects. *Am J Clin Nutr*. 1990; 52: 800-807.
25. Wing RR. Behavioral treatment of severe obesity. *Am J Clin Nutr*. 1992; 55: 545S-551S.
26. Brownell KD, Wadden TA. Etiology and treatment of obesity: Understanding a serious, prevalent, and refractory disorder. *Journal of Consulting and Clinical Psychology*. 1992; 60(4): 505-517.
27. McDonald LS, Woolsey M, Murray A. Weight management. In: Kris-Etherton PM, Volz-Clarke P, Clark K, Dattilo AM, eds. *Cardiovascular Disease: Nutrition for Prevention and Treatment*. The American Dietetic Association. 1990; 175-189.
28. Buckmaster L, Brownell KD. Behavior modification: The state of the art. In: Frankle RT, Yang MeiUih, eds. *Obesity and Weight Control: The Health Professional's Guide to Understanding and Treatment*. Rockville, Maryland: Aspen Publishers, Inc.; 1988:205-224.
29. Morton, CJ. Weight loss maintenance and relapse prevention. In: Frankle RT, Yang Mei Uih, eds. *Obesity and Weight Control: The Health Professional's Guide to Understanding and Treatment*. Rockville, Maryland: Aspen Publishers, Inc.; 1988: 315-332.
30. Garner DM, Rockert W, Olmsted MP, Johnson C, and Coscina DV. Psychoeducational principles in the treatment of bulimia and anorexia nervosa. In: Garner DM, and Garfinkel PE, eds. *Handbook of Psychotherapy for Anorexia Nervosa & Bulimia*. New York: The Guilford Press; 1985: 513-572.

31. Fairburn CG. CognitiveBehavioral treatment for bulimia. In: Garner DM, and Garfinkel PE, eds. *Handbook of Psychotherapy for Anorexia Nervosa & Bulimia*. New York: The Guilford Press; 1985: 160-192.

32. Garner DM, Bemis KM. Cognitive therapy for anorexia nervosa. In: Garner DM, and Garfinkel PE, eds. *Handbook of Psychotherapy for Anorexia Nervosa & Bulimia*. New York: The Guilford Press; 1985: 107-146.

33. Fairburn CG, Marcus MD, Wilson GT. Cognitive Behavioral therapy for binge eating and bulimia nervosa: A comprehensive treatment manual. In: Fairburn CG, and Wilson GT. *Binge Eating: Nature, Assessment, and Treatment*. New York: The Guilford Press; 1993: 361-404.

34. Egan G. *The Skilled Helper: A Systematic Approach to Effective Helping*. 3rd ed. Monterey, California: Brooks/Cole Publishing Company; 1986.

35. Williams R, Long J. *Toward a self-managed life style*. (3rd ed.). Boston: Houghton Mifflin; 1983.

36. Linehan M, Bootzin R, Cautela J, London P, PerloffM, Stuart R, Risley T. Guidelines for choosing a behavior therapist. *Behavior Therapist*. 1978; 1(4): 1820.

37. Eysenck HJ. Behavior Therapy. In: Eysenck HJ, Martin I, eds. *Theoretical Foundations of Behavior Therapy*. New York: Plenum Press; 1987; 335.

38. Watson JB. *Behaviorism*. Chicago: University of Chicago Press; 1930.

39. Mineka S. A primate model of phobic fears. In: Eysenck HJ, and Martin I. *Theoretical Foundations of Behavior Therapy*. New York: Plenum Press; 1987; 81-111.

40. Levey AB, Martin I. Evaluative conditioning: A case for Hedonic Transfer. In: Eysenck HJ, and Martin I. *Theoretical Foundations of Behavior Therapy*. New York: Plenum Press; 1987; 113-131.

41. Wilson GT. Behavior therapy. In: Corsini RJ, and contributors. *Current Psychotherapies*. Itasca, Illinois: F.E. Peacock Publishers, Inc.; 1984:239-278.

42. Lowe CF, Horne PJ, Higson PJ. Operant conditioning: The Hiatus between theory and practice in clinical psychology. In: Eysenck HT, and Martin I. *Theoretical Foundations of Behavior Therapy*. New York: Plenum Press; 1987; 153-165.

43. Heiby EM. Assessment of frequency of selfreinforment. *Journal of Personality and Social Psychology*. 1983;44(6): 1304-1307.

44. Miller JB. *What Do We Mean By Relationships*? (Work in Progress No. 22). Wellesley, MA: Stone Center; 1986.

45. Bandura A. *Social Learning Theory*. Englewood Cliffs, New Jersey: Prentice-Hall; 1977.

46. Rose, SD. *Group counseling with children: A behavioral and cognitive approach*. In: Gazda GM, ed. *Basic Approaches to Group Psychotherapy and Group Counseling*. 3rd ed. Springfield, Illinois: Charles C Thomas; 1982.

47. Brown TA, O'Leary TA, Barlow DH. Generalized anxiety disorder. In: Barlow DH, ed. *Clinical Handbook of Psychological Disorders: A Step-by-Step Treatment Manual*. 2nd ed. New York: The Guilford Press; 1993; 137-188.

48. Ellis A. Rational-Emotive therapy. In: Corsini RJ, and contributors. *Current Psychotherapies*. Itasca, Illinois: F.E. Peacock Publishers, Inc.; 1984: 196-238.

49. Piaget J. Piaget's theory. In: Mussen PH. ed. *Manual of child psychology*. 3rd ed. New York: John Wiley & Sons, Inc.; 1970; 703-732.

50. Ginsburg HP, Opper S. Piaget's *Theory of Intellectual Development*. 3rd ed. Englewood Cliffs, New Jersey: Prentice-Hall; 1988.

51. Selman RL. The child as a friendship philosopher. In: Asher SR, Gottman JM. eds. *The Development of Children's Friendships*. Cambridge, Massachusetts: Cambridge University Press; 1981; 242-273.

52. Elkind D. *All Grown Up and No Place to Go*. Reading, MA: AddisonWesley; 1984.

53. Freud S. *A General Introduction to Psychoanalysis*. Garden City, NY: Doubleday; 1943.

54. Guerney B, Stollak L, Guerney L. The practicing psychologist as educator: An alternative to the medical practitioner model. *Professional Psychologist*. 1971; 2: 276-282.

55. Erikson EH. *Childhood and Society*. New York: W.W. Norton & Company; 1963.

56. Erikson EH. *Identity and the Life Cycle*. New York: W.W. Norton & Company; 1980.

Acknowledgments:

The author of this chapter wishes to express acknowledgment and gratitude to Pat Queen Samour, Wanda Shelton, Amy Peterson, and most of all her family, Alex, Phillip and Meredith, for their continued support and guidance, which they so freely provided while this manuscript was written.

Appendix 8-A

NUTRITION COUNSELING TREATMENT PLAN

Patient Name:_____

Date:_____

Objectives of Treatment:

1._____

2._____

3._____

4._____

Problematic Behaviors	*Target Strategy*	*Estimated Date of Meeting Goal*
1._____	_____	_____
_____	_____	_____
2._____	_____	_____
_____	_____	_____
3._____	_____	_____
_____	_____	_____
4._____	_____	_____
_____	_____	_____

_____   _____
Client's Signature   Dietitian's Signature

Appendix 8-B

SELF MONITORING FORM

Time	Food	Amount	With Who	Activity	How Fast?	Mood

Appendix 8-C

MOOD ADJECTIVE LIST

loving - friendly - thankful
adaptable	affectionate
agreeable	amorous
caring	empathic
forgiving	generous
genuine	giving
grateful	longing for
mindful	optimistic
passionate	patient
sensitive	sincere
tender	tolerant
trustful	understanding

happy
accepted
at ease
cheerful
glad
joyous
lighthearted
magnificent
peaceful
poised
refreshed
relaxed

hurt - frustrated
awful	bothered
clumsy	crabby
sore	threatened
harassed	imprisoned
mistreated	perturbed
pressured	restless
rotten	sore
strained	swamped
terrible	threatened
uneasy	unhappy
unsatisfied	wounded

ashamed - guilty - embarrassed
awkward	blamed
cheapened	condemned
degraded	disgraced
dishonored	doomed
exposed	foolish
humiliated	punished
regretful	ridiculous
shamed	silly

confused
baffled
dismayed
disorganized
distracted
forgetful
overwhelmed
puzzled
tricked
uncertain

sad - depressed - gloomy
disappointed	discouraged
falling apart	grief stricken
hopeless	let down
mournful	pained
pessimistic	sad
serious	solemn
sorrowful	tearful
troubled	weary

energetic
active	agile
alert	animated
attentive	busy
daring	diligent
eager	encouraged
enthusiastic	excited
hardworking	interested
lively	resourceful
self-confident	spirited
tireless	vital

worried
alarmed
anxious
concerned
disturbed
fearful
hesitant
nervous
panicky
restless
unsettled

weak - defeated - shy
disenhearted	helpless
impotent	inadequate
incompetent	inferior
intimidated	insecure
needy	neglected
powerless	self-conscious
stifled	timid
troubled	unable
unqualified	unstable
vulnerable	worthless

angry - aggravated
agitated	annoyed
bitter	cranky
enraged	furious
infuriated	resentful

content - comfortable
agreeable	bright
cheerful	easy going
gratified	pleased
secure safe	supported

lonely - forgotten
abandoned	betrayed
empty	ignored
isolated	rejected
stranded	unimportant

Appendix 8-D

PHYSICAL MOOD ADJECTIVE LIST

energetic - alert
active agile	alive
animated	attentive
capable	fresh
lively	peppy
powerful	quick
rested	strong
sturdy	tireless
vivacious	wakeful

lethargic - fatigued - sleepy
dazed	debilitated	disabled
drained	drowsy	exhausted
feeble	fragile	frazzled
inert	inactive	limp
listless	nodding	run down
sleepy	sluggish	tired
weary	worn	yawning
	unstable	

painful - hurt -sore
abrasion	ache
acute	bruised
chronic	crampy
discomfort	distress
inflamed	injured
piercing	stabbing
suffering	swelling
tender	wounded

well - healthy
comfortable	healing
fit	flexible
fresh	hearty
good	invigorated
refreshed	restful
robust	relaxed
stimulated	strong
tranquil	trim

restless - jumpy
agitated	fidgety
jittery	quiver
nervous	shaky
shiver	sleepless
spasmodic	tingling
trembling	twitching
unsettled	unsteady
unstable	wobbly

ill - sick
chills	diarrhea
dizzy	faint
feverish	flushed
infected	lousy
nauseated	queasy
unwell	vomit

hot
boiling
burning
heated
sweating
warm

cold
chilly
frigid
frozen
icy
numb

hungry
devouring
famished
gluttonous
insatiable
ravenous
starved
voracious

full
bloated
bursting
content
comfortable
gorged
satisfied
satiated

slender - thin
bony	emaciated
gaunt	lean
lanky	scrawny
skinny	slim

heavy - fat
chubby	flabby
fleshy	hefty
huge	massive
plump	portly
stout	weighty

Appendix 8-E

STIMULUS CONTROL

Trigger	Strategy
1	a. b. c. d. e.
2	a. b. c. d. e.
3	a. b. c. d. e.
4	a. b. c. d. e.
5	a. b. c. d. e.

Appendix 8-F

IRRATIONAL BELIEFS FORM

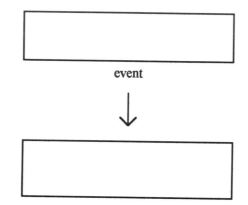

event

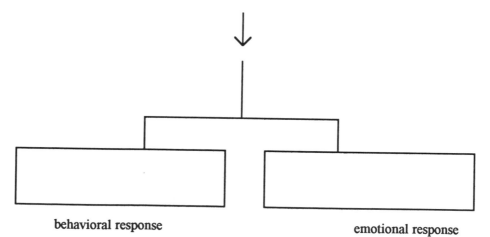

thoughts, beliefs, and/or attitudes about the event

behavioral response   emotional response

Appendix 8-G

IRRATIONAL BELIEFS DAILY LOG

Event	Thoughts about Event	Emotional Response	Behavioral Response

9

Nutritional Diagnostic Codes and Measurable Outcomes

Mary Ann Kight, PhD, RD, Professor of Nutrition, University of Arizona

---

After reading this chapter, the reader will be able to:
- [ ] define dietetic human condition codes
- [ ] correlate D-S NDC's to regulatory standards
- [ ] identify rationale for creating a practice-based NutritionD degree

---

Considering the expected growth of nutrition specialists in such fields as medicine, nursing, and pharmacy, there are at least three areas of clinical practice besides education and counseling that are necessary for our clinical practice to mature to an advanced level. These include:

- training in diagnosing nutritional problems, including deficiencies and writing diet and nutritional prescriptions (both of which take place sporadically now), should evolve as university programs create, and practitioners graduate from, clinical experience-based (like a medical residency instead of PhD-based) NutritionD doctorate programs (see FYI at the end of this chapter);

- using nutrition codes in hospital and outpatient billing and medical records to show the penetrating scope of nutrition's influence in patient focused care (see sample forms in Appendix 9-A and 9-B) and, thereby, penetrate the concept of "reimbursement only for ICD-9 CMs;"

- embracing outcomes (documented client results) as the measure of effectiveness of nutrition intervention—it is not enough to disseminate information; intervention must be diagnosis-directed and of sufficient duration to produce improved outcomes.

Dietetic-Specific Nutritional Diagnostic Codes (D-S NDCs)

The dietetic human condition codes are the first diagnostic human condition codes specific to dietetics and are complementary to medical and nursing codes. (1) As published, they differentiate 74 nutritional problem or disorder states using descriptors, qualifiers, and related defining characteristics. (See Figure 9-1.) The descriptors and qualifiers are labels for disorders such as altered body composition integrity, altered nutrient disposition, nutritional noncompliance, feeding route inadequacy, undesirable interactions between medications and food or nutrients, undesirable metabolic set-point, and other problems relevant to a nutritional diagnostic practice. (2)

The codes and related nutritional diagnostic practices are consistent with new clinical standards of practice (interventions) and care (outcomes) recommended by government agencies, accrediting bodies and professional organizations. (2) The codes can be a guiding force for making decisions about the role of dietitians as advanced-level clinicians because:

- the codes are aimed at delineating a client-centered profession's advanced-expert scope of practice,

- diagnoses provide a distinct focus for establishing interventions and measurable outcomes. (3)

Dietitian as Diagnostician

Additionally, it becomes evident that establishing diagnosis-related measurable outcomes can be a secondary force in directing dietitians who are interested in becoming principal investigators of clinical outcomes research. In this somewhat futuristic, yet emerging role, the dietitian as diagnostician: (4,5,6)

1. observes and assesses the status of clients for signs and symptoms (i.e. evidence) of nutritional problems;
2. recognizes the end point of assessment is the diagnosis of problems and considers possible meanings or diagnostic inferences (deductions) that might be derived from the presenting evidence;
3. uses clinical/ diagnostic (deductive) reasoning to "rule in" (or identify) the most logical and relevant inferences (deductions), to gather additional data as guided by the selected inference (s), and to search pertinent literature as each inference dictates;
4. translates each ruled-in inference into a diagnostic statement, i.e. the most clearly related code (D-S NDC) identified as the most likely etiology manifested by the presenting evidence;
5. decides upon and develops an intervention plan (including education and counseling as necessary) for implementation and testing as directed by the etiology component of each diagnostic statement;
6. implements the developed plan;
7. monitors and documents any observed change in presenting evidence as: a measure of outcome of each diagnosed problem; a measure of impact of the implemented plan; a measure of quality in the service provided;
8. recognizes that tracking of cases can provide valuable insights relevant to research designs for predicting, improving, compressing and preventing unwanted outcomes and for establishing dietitians as principal investigators in the movement toward clinical outcomes research.

Essential to this futuristic role is a "diagnosing mind" which constructs inferences and intellectual maps instead of, or in addition to, obeying pre-determined algorithms or flow diagrams. It assembles bits of information such as signs and symptoms into composite chunks known as diagnostic categories. This then gives explanatory, intervention and testable power to otherwise overlooked pieces of nutritional problem related information. Thus intellectual mapping is commutative (characterized by a combination of elements that are often independent of the order in which the elements are taken) and is expected of expert clinicians. Algorithms and flow diagrams are more ordered and routinized (repetitious in character) and therefore more likely to be used by entry-level clinicians. (7)

1995 JCAHO Standards

Consistent with this new role are the 1995 Joint Commission on Accreditation of Healthcare Organizations (JCAHO) Nutrition Standards. (8) These new JCAHO standards provide startup opportunity to incorporate the dietetic codes and "diagnosing minds" into the healthcare system.

These new standards position dietitians to observe and assess for evidence of Dietetic (D) Coded:

- inadequate nutrient intakes (D 10.001- D 10.011)
- questionable anthropometric measurements (D 2.001)
- undesirable weight status (D 23.004, 23.005 or 23.006)
- questionable laboratory tests and/ or their results (D 2.006)
- manifestations of nutrient deficiency (D 2.001, D 10.001-10.011 or 17.001)
- manifestations of nutrient excess (D 6.001-6.005 or 22.001)
- questionable medication effects (D 23.002)
- conditions affecting ingestion, digestion, absorption or utilization of nutrients (D 2.005)
- food intolerances and allergies (D 12.001 or 12.002)
- questionable food preferences (D 11.002)
- questionable diet prescription or number of days NPO i.e. nothing by mouth (D 14.005)
- evidence of education and /or counseling needs (D 4.001 or D 4.002)

Thus these new standards can be linked to 31 of the possible 74 D-S NDCs, representing a startup "minimum code set" for implementation.

The Future Reality of the Clinical Dietitian

As human nutritional health problems become better known and accepted, dietetic professionals having profession-specific expertise in physical assessment, diagnostics, and diagnosis-related outcomes research will strengthen their hold on nutrition services, academic chairs of human nutrition and dietetics departments, dietetics education and credentialing groups, nutritional science research groups, and professional dietetics and nutrition organizations. (9)

Clearly, client-centered dietitians are intended to move forward in terms of nutritional diagnostics and dietetic educators are intended to re-orient their teaching to nutritional problem, diagnostics-based practice doctorates (10) and mentoring-type instruction. (11)

This would involve a three-tiered approach:

- Tier one would center on the nutrition history, nutrition physical and initial diagnostic impression;

- Tier two would focus on further (deeper) nutritional diagnostic reasoning/ inference making and diagnosis directed interventions, including education and counseling;
- Tier three would address clinical outcomes research.

Dietetic educators and clinicians are now poised to advance from entry-level practice to diagnostics-based doctoral level training and expert clinician privileges respectively.

REFERENCES

1. Kight MA. Start up characterizations/ diagnostic criteria for using dietetic-specific nutritional diagnostic codes. *Diagnostic Nutrition Network.* 1994; 3 (1,2).
2. Thomson C. New beginnings for the RD: The dietetic human condition codes. *RD*, Esential News for Dietitians from Sandoz Nutrition. 1994; 14 (3): 1,16.
3. Waltz CF, Strickland OL, Lenz ER. *Measurement in Nursing Research*. Philadelphia, PA: FA Davis Co.; 1991.
4. Kight MA. Working with diagnosis related groups (DRGs): Diagnosis in the practice of selected health-medical team members. *Nutr Support Services.* 1985; 5 (2): 39-46.
5. Thomson CA, Kight MA, Longstreth M. Influence techniques and activities clinical dietitians use when interacting with physicians. *J Am Diet Assoc.* 1990; 90: 1242-1246.
6. Kight MA. A dietetic-specific diagnostic reasoning approach to communicating in code. *Diagnostic Nutrition Network.* 1993; 2(2): 2-5.
7. Campbell EJM. Point of view: The diagnosing mind. *Lancet.* 1987; 1 (Apr-Jun): 849-851.
8. Joint Commission on Accreditation of Healthcare Organizations. *1995 Comprehensive Accreditation Manual for Hospitals.* Oakbrook Terr., IL: Joint Comm. Pub.; 1994.
9. Kight MA. *Dietetic Voices of the Future Conference*, Jan. 29-30, 1994, Tucson, AZ.
10. Christie BW, Kight MA. Educational empowerment of the clinical dietitian: A proposed practice doctorate curriculum. *J Am Diet Assoc.* 1993; 93 (2): 173-176.
11. Association of American Medical Colleges. *ACME-TRI Report: Educating Medical Students.* Washington, DC: Assoc. of American Medical Colleges Pub.; 1992.

Figure 9-1 Dietetic-Specific Nutritional Diagnostic Codes

Absence of/Limited — D1.000
- □ Nutrition Service/Professional Nutritionist Contact — D1.001
- □ Nutritional Collateral Systems — D1.002

Altered/Alteration In — D2.000
- □ Body Composition Integrity
- □ Bowel Elimination — D2.001
- □ Drug Disposition — D2.002
- □ Metabolism — D2.003
- □ Nutrient Disposition — D2.004
- □ Nutritional Biochemistry Integrity — D2.005
- □ Water, Fluids — D2.006

Conflict in — D3.000
- □ Feeding and Treatment/Diagnostic Schedules — D3.001

Deficit in — D4.000
- □ Nutrition Education — D4.001
- □ Nutrition Knowledge — D4.002

Dependent on — D5.000
- □ Home Enteral/Parenteral Product Assistance — D5.001
- □ Home Food Service Assistance — D5.002
- □ Home Therapeutic Diet/Product Assistance — D5.003

Excessive — D6.000
- □ Caloric Allowance/Intake — D6.001
- □ Fiber Allowance/Intake — D6.002
- □ Protein Allowance/Intake — D6.003
- □ Vitamin/Mineral Allowance/Intake — D6.004
- □ Water/Fluids Allowance/Intake — D6.005

Imbalance — D7.000
- □ Electrolyte — D7.001
- □ Energy — D7.002
- □ Nutrient — D7.003
- □ Water, Fluids — D7.004

Impaired — D8.000
- □ Activity Performance — D8.001
- □ Cognition & Behavior — D8.002
- □ Fecundity/Fertility — D8.003
- □ Growth/Development/Function — D8.004
- □ Home Maintenance of Dietary Needs — D8.005
- □ Lactation Performance — D8.006
- □ Social Performance — D8.007
- □ Work Performance — D8.008

Inactive Role In — D9.000
- □ Maintaining Adequate Nutrition — D9.001

Inadequacy — D10.000
- □ Caloric Allowance/Intake — D10.001
- □ Carbohydrate — D10.002
- □ Fat-Essential Fatty Acid — D10.003
- □ Feeding Route — D10.004
- □ Fiber Allowance/Intake — D10.005
- □ Food-Diet Consistency — D10.006
- □ Mineral — D10.007
- □ Protein-Amino Acid Allowance/Intake — D10.008
- □ Vitamin — D10.009
- □ Water, Fluids/Fluid Balance — D10.010
- □ Treatment Time — D10.011

Inappropriate — D11.000
- □ Caloric Distribution — D11.001
- □ Dietary Habits — D11.002
- □ Feeding Route — D11.003
- □ Food Role Perception/Food Abuse — D11.004
- □ Protein Distribution — D11.005

Intolerance — D12.000
- □ Drug/Chemical Substance in Food — D12.001
- □ Food(s)/Nutrient(s) — D12.002

Misinformation — D13.000
- □ Nutrition — D13.001

Misuse — D14.000
- □ Enteral Product — D14.001
- □ Nutrient Supplement — D14.002
- □ Other Food Substance — D14.003
- □ Parenteral Product — D14.004
- □ Therapeutic Diet/Product — D14.005

Nonacceptance — D15.000
- □ Food Item(s)/Nutritional Product(s) — D15.001

Noncompliance — D16.000
- □ Nutritional — D16.001

Possibility of/Possibility of Developing — D17.000
- □ A Specific Disease Interaction — D17.001
- □ Morbidity, Increased Duration/Severity of Illness — D17.002
- □ Mortality, Increased Risk of — D17.003

Potential — D18.000
- □ Consequences of Altered Nutrient Function(s) — D18.001

Prevention, Decreasing/Eliminating Need for/Use of — D19.000
- □ Drug Therapy — D19.001

Self Assessment Risk Factors — D20.000
- □ Nutritional — D20.001

Suboptimal — D21.000
- □ Pregnancy Outcome — D21.001
- □ Nutritional Resiliency — D21.002

Toxicity — D22.000
- □ Nutrient — D22.001

Undesirable — D23.000
- □ Food-Diagnostic/Treatment Schedule Interaction — D23.001
- □ Medication-Food/Nutrient Interaction — D23.002
- □ Metabolic Setpoint — D23.003
- □ Overweight Status — D23.004
- □ Underweight Status — D23.005
- □ Weight (e.g. loss/gain) — D23.006

Unwellness — D24.000
- □ Nutritional — D24.001

Other

FOR YOUR INFORMATION

Practice-based NutritionD Degree

Mary Ann Kight, PhD, RD

Visualize yourself as a Doctor of Clinical Nutrition working in a hospital with clinical privileges and your own office, or in private practice prescribing and providing the nutrition intervention for a patient from home care to inpatient to your private office. One day that might be a reality. As we learn more about nutrition's affect on genetic markers and predisposition to disease, how to assess and alter a person's nutritional biochemistries, or how to diagnose nutritional deficiencies and toxicities through visual signs, we will need practitioners with advanced clinical and diagnostic skills. Dictitians are the logical professionals to seek this training and recognition, but the opportunity will no doubt be competitive.

Advanced level role delineation for clinical dietitians goes hand in hand with the concept of advanced-level education. The clinical doctorate in nutrition is consistent with national nutrition priorities (disease prevention and wellness). It also falls in line with two of the major missions of most nutritional sciences and dietetics departments: the reduction of morbidity and disease prevention. These nutrition departments can best serve initially as support for the concept. They also may be in a position to refer students, who feel constrained at the thought of a more traditional doctoral program to a practice doctorate.

Academic Development

Practice doctorate options are a growing academic value in university systems, e.g. the Pharmacy D (a residency-type, practice oriented doctorate) is now offered by universities in addition to the dissertation-based PhD (doctor of philosophy) degree in one of the Pharmaceutical Sciences. Students have always valued the availability of options and choices. They value having a choice among classes, instructors, advisors, among colleges, majors and degrees. Students with years of clinical nutrition experience as well as those new to the field will see a clinical doctorate as a career investment that will make them unique and in demand in health care. Thus, optional doctoral degree programs for practitioners need to be developed.

Successful development will require an educational investment that supports growth of a new academic culture with collaborative linkages to nursing, pharmacy, laboratory sciences and medicine. Regional academic centers should be created that address core competencies for advanced practice nutrition research and development. Core competencies would be nutrition history taking, physical examination, diagnostic reasoning/ inference making, advanced care process management, intervention (including education and counseling), theory building and clinical outcomes research. Additionally, this new human nutrition academic culture should foster resourceful, mentoring-type instruction and self-directed lifelong problem-based learning.

Summary

The concept of a practice-based NutritionD degree is relevant to improving the human condition; therefore, the need has been established. The start up academic culture and prototype core topics are in place at the University of Arizona, Tucson with several other institutions in the planning stages. It is time for other academic institutions to initiate planning similar programs including ones that offer classes on site or in part through telecommunication.

Appendix 9-A

D/Dietetic-Specific Nutritional Diagnostic Codes (D-S NDCs)*

Absence of / Limited	**D1.000**	**Excessive**	**D6.000**	**Inadequacy**	**D10.000**	**Misinformation**	**D13.000**	**Prevention, Decreasing/**	
☐ Nutrition Service/Pro-		☐ Caloric Allowance/		☐ Caloric Allowance/		☐ Nutrition	D13.001	**Eliminating Need for/**	
fessional Nutritionist		Intake	D6.001	Intake	D10.001	**Misuse**	**D14.000**	Use of	**D19.000**
Contact	D1.001	☐ Fiber Allowance/Intake	D6.002	☐ Carbohydrate	D10.002	☐ Enteral Product	D14.001	☐ Drug Therapy	D19.001
☐ Nutritional Collateral		☐ Protein Allowance/		☐ Fat-Essential		☐ Nutrient Supplement	D14.002	**Self Assessment**	
Systems	D1.002	Intake	D6.003	Fatty Acid	D10.003	☐ Other Food Substance	D14.003	**Risk Factors**	**D20.000**
Altered/Alteration in	**D2.000**	☐ Vitamin/Mineral		☐ Feeding Route	D10.004	☐ Parenteral Product	D14.004	☐ Nutritional	D20.001
☐ Body Composition		Allowance/Intake	D6.004	☐ Fiber Allowance/		☐ Therapeutic Diet/		**Suboptimal**	**D21.000**
Integrity	D2.001	☐ Water, Fluids		Intake	D10.005	Product	D14.005	☐ Pregnancy Outcome	D21.001
☐ Bowel Elimination	D2.002	Allowance/Intake	D6.005	☐ Food-Diet Consistency	D10.006	**Nonacceptance**	**D15.000**	☐ Nutritional Resiliency	D21.002
☐ Drug Disposition	D2.003	**Imbalance**	**D7.000**	☐ Mineral	D10.007	☐ Food Item(s)/		**Toxicity**	**D22.000**
☐ Metabolism	D2.004	☐ Electrolyte	D7.001	☐ Protein-Amino Acid		Nutritional		☐ Nutrient	D22.001
☐ Nutrient Disposition	D2.005	☐ Energy	D7.002	Allowance/Intake	D10.008	Product(s)	D15.001	**Undesirable**	**D23.000**
☐ Nutritional		☐ Nutrient	D7.003	☐ Vitamin	D10.009	**Noncompliance**	**D16.000**	☐ Food-Diagnostic/	
Biochemistry Integrity	D2.006	☐ Water, Fluids	D7.004	☐ Water, Fluids/Fluid		☐ Nutritional	D16.001	Treatment Schedule	
Conflict in	**D3.000**	**Impaired**	**D8.000**	Balance	D10.010	**Possibility of/Possibility**		Interaction	D23.001
☐ Feeding and		☐ Activity Performance	D8.001	**Inappropriate**	**D11.000**	**of Developing**	**D17.000**	☐ Medication-Food/	
Treatment/Diagnostic		☐ Cognition & Behavior	D8.002	☐ Caloric Distribution	D11.001	☐ A Specific Disease	D17.001	Nutrient Interaction	D23.002
Schedules	D3.001	☐ Fecundity/Fertility	D8.003	☐ Dietary Habits	D11.002	☐ Morbidity, Increased		☐ Metabolic Setpoint	D23.003
Deficit in	**D4.000**	☐ Growth/Development/		☐ Feeding Route	D11.003	Duration/Severity		☐ Overweight Status	D23.004
☐ Nutrition Education	D4.001	Function	D8.004	☐ Food Role		of Illness	D17.002	☐ Underweight Status	D23.005
☐ Nutrition Knowledge	D4.002	☐ Home Maintenance		Perception/Food		☐ Mortality, Increased		☐ Weight	
Dependent on	**D5.000**	of Dietary Needs	D8.005	Abuse	D11.004	Risk of	D17.003	(e.g. loss/gain)	D23.006
☐ Home Enteral/		☐ Lactation Performance	D8.006	☐ Protein Distribution	D11.005	**Potential**		**Unwellness**	**D24.000**
Parenteral Product		☐ Social Performance	D8.007	**Intolerance**	**D12.000**	**Consequences of**	**D18.000**	☐ Nutritional	D24.001
Assistance	D5.001	☐ Work Performance	D8.008	☐ Drug/Chemical		☐ Altered Nutrient		**Other**	
☐ Home Food		**Inactive Role in**	**D9.000**	Substance in Food	D12.001	Function(s)	D18.001		
Service Assistance	D5.002	☐ Maintaining Adequate		☐ Food(s)/Nutrient(s)	D12.002				
☐ Home Therapeutic		Nutrition	D9.001						
Diet/Product									
Assistance	D5.003								

*© 1993 by M.A. Kight and Biodietetic Associates

Problem_____: _____

DATE PROBLEM IDENTIFIED	DATE PROBLEM RESOLVED

Etiology: _____

Signs/Symptoms: _____

Plan: _____

Outcome (Expected/Actual): _____

Problem_____: _____

DATE PROBLEM IDENTIFIED	DATE PROBLEM RESOLVED

Etiology: _____

Signs/Symptoms: _____

Plan: _____

Outcome (Expected/Actual): _____

EL DORADO HOSPITAL AND MEDICAL CENTER
DEPARTMENT OF NUTRITION SUPPORT SERVICES

NUTRITIONAL PROBLEMS

NSS-0512 Rev. 10/93   © CBTV

Reprinted with permission, El Dorado Hospital and Medical Center. M.A. Kight and Biodietetic Associates

Appendix 9-B

NUTRITION   SERVICE

INITIAL CONSULTATION

CODE	X	SERVICE	FEE
999799		Initial-Basic	
999813		Initial-Intermediate	
999835		Initial-Indepth	
		*SR/MC	
999006		Initial-Basic	
999028		Initial-Intermediate	
999040		Initial-Indepth	

D-SNDCs RECORDED, specify:

DRG,ICD-9 CM CODES RECORDED, specify:

FOLLOW-UP CONSULTATION

CODE	X	SERVICE	FEE
999857		Follow-up	
999062		*SR/MC Follow-up	
WRITE-IN CHARGES			
999755		Nutrition Supplies	
999766		Neutraceuticals, specify:	

TOTAL CHARGES _____

PAYMENT RECEIVED _____

BALANCE _____

NAME	DATE
ADDRESS	PHONE
INSURANCE	
REFERRING MD	ATTENDING RD

*SR/MC - Seniority/Medicare

NOTE: The code numbering system is specific for services performed by the Registered Dietitians at El Dorado Hospital.

EL DORADO HOSPITAL and MEDICAL CENTER
P.O. BOX 13070 • TUCSON, ARIZONA 85732
PHONE 886-6361

N. S.   PATIENT CHARGE

© CBTV   EDHMC NSS 0501

10

Quality Inpatient Counseling

Bridget Klawitter, MS, RD, FADA

After reading this chapter, the reader will be able to:
- ☐ **recognize the importance of nutrition screening in today's healthcare environment**
- ☐ **identify accreditation standards applicable to the nutrition counseling process**
- ☐ **utilize criteria for documenting client outcomes**
- ☐ **identify issues for nutrition reimbursement in today's healthcare environment**

BENEFITS OF CLINICAL NUTRITION SERVICES IN ACUTE CARE

We all know that well-nourished individuals are more resistant to disease and infection, are better able to tolerate other therapies, and recover better from acute illness, surgical interventions, and trauma. Inadequate nutritional intake can precipitate disease or increase its severity. Early detection of nutrition-related problems and appropriate nutrition interventions are effective in helping the patient recover more quickly and decrease the number of days requiring hospitalization.

Registered dietitians and registered dietetic technicians are critical members of health care teams. Medical nutrition therapy, coordinated by a registered dietitian, is an integral part of disease prevention, treatment and recovery, and is necessary to maintain quality of care and achieve cost savings. It involves two phases: (a) assessment of the patient's nutritional status, and (b) treatment, which includes diet therapy, counseling, or the use of specialized nutritional support.

Value of Screening in Cost Containment

Clinical dietetic practitioners should use a comprehensive nutrition screening program to zero in on patients who possess co-morbid nutritional conditions so that physicians can formerly diagnose and together we can more adequately treat patients' needs. Computer linking between departments such as nursing stations, the lab, and the clinical dietetic department allows dietetic practitioners to obtain the clinical nutrition data to facilitate the identification of patients at nutritional risk. A nutrition screening program is an inexpensive method to streamline clinical nutrition care and identify those patients at nutritional risk who are most likely to benefit from special nutrition intervention during their hospital stay.

A growing body of evidence in the literature points to protein-energy malnutrition (PEM) as a complication that can potentially increase morbidity, mortality, and mean length of stay. Because PEM cuts across diagnostic and treatment categories, traditional methods of identifying high risk patients may need to be more sensitive in order to detect nutritional risk.

Many third party payments to healthcare providers are based on the average cost of caring for patients classified by diagnostic related groups (DRG's). Classifications of a claim considers a number of factors including: principle diagnosis, other diagnoses (called "complications" or "co-morbid conditions" or "cc's"), surgical procedures, and the patient's age and sex. (3) In some studies, the addition of nutrition diagnoses has contributed as much as $150,000 to $312,000, which more adequately covered the actual costs of care. (4, 5, 6) Nutrition screening results can also provide a basis for communication with physicians. Screening data may also help establish the need for medically appropriate, cost-effective nutrition interventions, including counseling.

The clinical dietetic practitioner can control costs by monitoring the use of high-tech nutrition therapies, including parenteral nutrition. Substantial savings can be realized when enteral feedings are substituted for parenteral nutrition. Clinical dietitians can also play an essential role in ensuring the most cost-effective enteral products are used through their departmental management of the enteral formulary.

Changes in Healthcare Climate and Clinical Practice

At The American Dietetic Association's Future Search Conference in 1994, speakers stated that health care in America in the year 2000 will not look anything like it does today. (1) It will be increasingly affected by regulatory changes, increased market competition for patients, and hospital mergers and affliations. Our jobs will look different too (see Chapter 15). Concerns about escalating costs and limited services in managed care, coupled with consumers' expectations not being met, create a growing concern about the quality of patient care. Hence, quality assessment and cost benefits of nutrition services take on new significance.

The opportunities to provide inpatient nutrition counseling continue to decrease as patients are discharged from acute care settings sooner and sicker. At the time of discharge patients are often not ready for comprehensive nutrition counseling nor is the typical hospital environment conducive to private therapy sessions. The rapid turnover and short lead times limit a clinical dietitian's ability to identify specific counseling needs, provide counseling, and evaluate the patient's knowledge and understanding prior to discharge.

Despite the above circumstances, patients and physicians expect (and accrediting agencies are beginning to require) that appropriate nutrition education take place, if possible, in the hospital setting so the patient and his or her family do not aggravate, but instead encourage; continued improvement of the patient's physical state. In casual conversations, the majority of dietitians seem to agree that it is most appropriate to counsel patients on survival or "need to know" information during brief hospitalizations and to refer the patients to more comprehensive nutrition counseling in the outpatient setting. But the majority of patients still only receive abbreviated nutrition intervention in the hospital setting and seldom are referred to outpatient counselors for more comprehensive instruction or follow-up, except perhaps in the case of diabetes.

CONSIDERATIONS FOR INPATIENT COUNSELING
When Time Is Short

The typical abbreviated, but essential, "need to know" information used in inpatient counseling follows:
- Establish behavioral diagnoses
    1. distinguish between behavioral and nonbehavioral causes (weight gain due to decreased activity versus as a result of taking prednisone)
    2. define behaviors in relation to condition (less physical activity coupled with increased calories leads to weight gain)
    3. rank behaviors in order of importance (increased activity versus decreased calories)
    4. assess behavior changeability (easier to decrease portion sizes than find time for exercise)
    5. prioritize behaviors based upon importance and changeability
- Assess what client wants to learn
    1. may be perceived as immediate need (How many calories do I need? or Why do I need to limit sodium?)
    2. acknowledges independence in decision-making
- Adult patient must acknowledge there is a problem (see Chapter 2)

When time is not a factor, inpatient counseling can follow the guidelines discussed in earlier chapters. See page 31 for information on how to counsel a critically ill patient.

Protocols, CQI and Discharge Plans

By developing and using practice guidelines and protocols (or critical pathways or care maps), which standardize practice in order to produce positive outcomes, you can ensure efficiency and effectiveness in your delivery. (See side bar Nutrition Component of Typical Cardiac Pathway.)

Dietitians should evaluate the outcomes of nutrition interventions so that cost effectiveness and cost benefits can be delineated. (See FYI at the end of this chapter, Clinical Dietitians Use Case Studies to Document Cost-Benefit.) On-going Continuous Quality Improvement (CQI) should be an integral part of inpatient as well as outpatient services with the focus on outcomes as a result of counseling interventions.

Many patients in the acute care setting require comprehensive nutrition plans of care when they are discharged to promote continuity of care and prevent early rehospitalizations. Discharge planning should start the day of admission and be designed to provide continuity of care and allow for a smooth transition for the patient from one care setting to another. This means systems must be set up to facilitate the transition to outpatient nutrition services in the clinic, community, or in other institutions. Discharge planning is a transdisciplinary process and should be considered a priority by dietetic professionals.

Locations For Counseling Will Be Changing

As hospital stays become shorter, clinical dietitians need to plan to change *where* they counsel patients. Several other factors also contribute to shifts from inpatient acute care to outpatient ambulatory care and consequently a need for expanded nutrition services in those settings: the aging population, advances in medical technology, increased health care costs, increased focus on prevention and wellness, the AIDS epidemic, and the coexistence of malnutrition with chronic diseases. (1,2)

QUALITY IMPROVEMENT

Three terms are important to understand:

- *Quality assessment* measures the level of quality care at some point in time but does not connote any effort to change or improve that level of care. (3)
- *Quality improvement* emphasizes coordinating and integrating various health care professionals in the assessment of processes that affect patient outcomes. (4)
- *Continuous Quality Improvement* (CQI) is an all encompassing concept, which includes the measurement of the on-going level of care provided, and when indicated, the attempt to continually improve it.

Quality improvement can be determined from either *structure, process, or outcomes*: (5)

Structure consists of tangible or organizational components involved in patient care (i.e. facilities, equipment, personnel, or organizational structure). The program review process may include reviewing current nutrition counseling programs and assessing the need for other programs like group diabetes or breast feeding classes. Structure indicators (an indicator is an index used to monitor the stability or change in a designated process) may also review the policies that guide patient education and counseling or review the accuracy and appropriateness of nutrition educational materials.

Process denotes what actions are carried out in the provision of care (i.e., interventions, counseling, or treatment). In patient education, process indicators target the delivery of patient teaching and may include counselor effectiveness, documentation, and the flow of the counseling process.

Outcomes are the effects on the health status of the patient. Outcome indicators evaluate behavioral changes in the patient by measuring knowledge and skills at the time of the counseling and often after discharge. The process of CQI is dependent upon linkages between structure and process, and between process and outcomes. For example, the availability of adequate clinical dietetic staff to conduct nutritional counseling and decrease the number of readmissions for uncontrolled blood sugars in a child with diabetes.

REGULATORY REQUIREMENTS IN INPATIENT AND LONG-TERM CARE

The basic functions of external controls (by government or private agencies) in health care are to offer formal standards, to survey providers (hospitals, drug rehabilitation centers, etc.), to assess the degree of compliance with those standards, and to impose sanctions or incentives in response to reported deviations from the standards. (5)

OBRA and Long-Term Care

The 1987 Omnibus Budget Reconciliation Act (OBRA) requires the inspection of nursing homes and other skilled nursing facilities receiving Medicare and/or Medicaid funds from the federal Health Care Financing Administration (HCFA). Each state also has long-term care licensure requirements, which are usually similar to the federal guidelines but may be more rigorous. OBRA requires states to conduct inspections with a focus on the needs of individual residents and the quality of services being offered to them. (6)

Residents' needs may range from denture problems and multiple medications to too much gas and brittle bones. Many have keen interest in food and nutrition. It is important to document any discussions with the resident in regards

---

Nutrition Component of Typical Cardiac Pathway

Susan DeHoog, RD, Dir., Clinical Nutrition, Univ. of Washington Medical Center, Seattle, WA

Goals: to improve patient outcomes, promote recovery, and promote healthy eating behaviors
Nutrition concerns are:
- maintenance of lean body mass (LBM)
- anorexia
- meeting 50% of nutritional needs prior to discharge
- infection
- effects of drugs
- anemia
- protein-calorie malnutrition (PCM)
- initiation of oral intake
- fluid imbalance/ hydration status

Nutrition Interventions:
Post Op Day #1 (POD #1)
- NPO
- nutritional assessment
POD #2
- active bowel sounds in all four quadrants
- tolerating solid food without nausea and/or vomiting
- 4 gram sodium, heart healthy diet
POD #3
- evaluate adequacy of oral intake via nutrient intake analysis
- assess for constipation
- supplements to supply additional Kcal, if necessary
- initiate tube feeding if patient is still intubated
POD #4
- instruct on nutritional requirements for wound healing (first 6 weeks post op)
- instruct patient/ family on a heart healthy diet
POD #5
- eating 50-75% of nutritional needs without nausea and /or vomiting
- patient and family will describe the benefits of the heart healthy diet and how they will meet the requirements
- if patient is assessed to have inadequate knowledge, a discharge summary/ plan for continuum of care is initiated (refer to the outpatient clinic dietitian or referring health care provider).
POD #6
- patient is discharged

Bibliography
DeHoog SJ. *Re-engineering Clinical Nutrition Processes.* Redmond, WA: In Press; 1995. Food and Nutrition Department: *Diagnostic Related Nutritional Care Plans:* UWMC, Seattle, WA, 1994.

to the prescribed diet, choices regarding meals, snacks, and activities, and care or treatment. Surveyors will also look for a comprehensive transdisciplinary care plan with measurable objectives and a timeline to meet identified needs.

JCAHO and Health Care

The "Joint Commission" or JCAHO uses accreditation as a tool to motivate health care organizations to improve systems and processes that most influence client care and outcomes. (5) An accreditation survey assesses the level of an organization's compliance with applicable JCAHO standards. The survey includes written and verbal evidence of compliance and on-site observations by the survey team. The JCAHO also serves to assist organizations in education and consultation regarding compliance to standards.

In its 1995 Accreditation Manual for Hospitals (AMH), JCAHO reiterates that its new approach will require hospitals to shift their thinking away from a checklist of "things to do" towards a more thoughtful "did it work" approach. (6) It is basing accreditation on measured outcomes and actual improvements in patient care, a direction it feels all health care organizations must take. American businesses came around to this realization of accountability many years ago and health care has been just catching up.

Standards Related to the Care of the Patient

Processes in the nutrition care standards are similar to those of other disciplines (see Figure 10-1 Care of Patients Function). (2)

Figure 10-1   Care of Patients Function

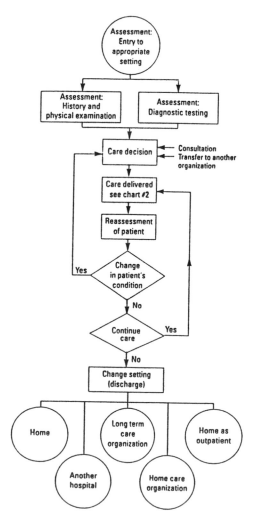

Used with permission Copyright 1995 Joint Commission of Accreditation of Healthcare Organization. In Accreditation manual for hospitals. Chicago: The Commission; 1995.

Originally, the implementation of the standard regarding nutrient-drug counseling was the responsibility of dietetic services, but it was recognized that a transdisciplinary approach is needed.(9) Much controversy has centered around this standard and it has been rated less effective than other standards in its ability to improve patient care. (12) There is a lack of agreement over which drug-food interactions are clinically important, but monoamine oxidase (MAO) inhibitors are most frequently mentioned followed by anticoagulants, tetracycline, and diuretics. (10) Ideally, each patient should be counseled on all clinically relevant drug-nutrient interactions. However, limitations in time, resources, and personnel do not make this possible and those patients at greatest risk for substantial interactions should be targeted for counseling. Other patients should at least receive written materials (i.e. computer print-out with the pertinent information). Eventually, as hospitals go to paperless charting and dietitians carry portable handheld computers, it will not be difficult to have drug-nutrient information available at bedside.

Surveyors encourage transdisciplinary collaboration in the care of patients. This includes such disciplines as physicians, dietitians, nurses, pharmacists, physical therapists, and social workers. Collaborative care teams and critical pathways are more commonly found now in response to this area of emphasis by surveyors. Dietetic practitioners in the acute care setting need to become involved in clinical nutrition and education committees whenever possible to represent the nutritional aspects of total patient care and facilitate these transdisciplinary approaches for the provision of nutritional care.

Organizations must provide the resources to systematically assess and meet the educational needs of the patient and family in a coordinated, multidisciplinary way. The education standards themselves are essentially unchanged from prior standards except for an added emphasis on patient and family responsibility for the patient's ongoing care needs, including the recognition that active participation in one's treatment is an important factor in a patient's outcome. This includes the use of medications and medical equipment, potential nutrient-drug interactions, counseling on modified diets, and how/when to obtain further treatment if indicated. Health care organizations do have flexibility on how they comply with the education standards; the standards for example do not dictate which profession(s) will be responsible for an educational process. *This could mean however, that nutritionists are not used for diabetes, breastfeeding or other nutrition-related educational consults.*

The flowchart for the education function illustrates the three areas that impact the patient: the organization's focus on education; the direct impact of education on the patient and his or her family; and the program evaluation in relation to patient outcomes (see Figure 10-2 Education Function). (2)

Figure 10-2   Education Function

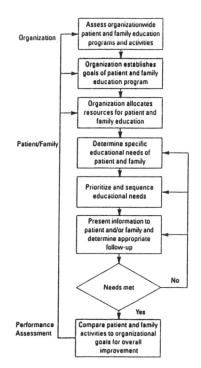

The primary goal of the standards for education is to provide the client with knowledge of their condition/illness and their treatment so that they may learn behavior and skills that will promote recovery and improve function. Client education/counseling is to be specific to the needs, abilities, and readiness of the individual patient as appropriate to the length of stay. This includes counseling on potential nutrient-drug interactions, nutrition interventions and/or modified diets as appropriate.

The standards also compel providers to share discharge instructions with the organization or individual(s) responsible for the continuation of care (2). This includes the assessment of patient needs, ensuring that they are smoothly transitioned from one care setting to another, and the provision of information to patients, family or other providers of care who are receiving the patient. These standards are often referred to as the framework for case management. The flowchart for the continuum of care function (see Figure 10-3 Continuum of Care Function) demonstrates that, based on the initial assessment of the patient, the most appropriate plan of care is to be developed. (2)

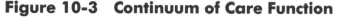

Figure 10-3 Continuum of Care Function

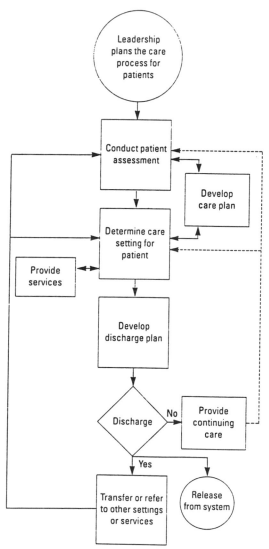

Used with permission. Copyright 1995 Joint Commission of Accreditation of Healthcare Organization. In Accreditation manual for hospitals. Chicago: The Commission; 1995.

Components of the standards related to continuity of care require a process or system to ensure clinical continuity and communication between providers of care as patients move from one care setting to another. The ultimate goal is continuous, appropriate and well coordinated care—a "seamless" provision of services.

DOCUMENTATION OF PATIENT CARE (13)

Institutions, as well as various departments within institutions, use a variety of forms and formats to document clinical care provided to patients. The primary purpose of documentation is to direct the care of the client, especially when multiple disciplines are involved, and to record the client's status or response to the interventions. Routine interventions are generally formulated into standards of care while client-specific interventions are formulated into a plan of care. The documentation process is also crucial to the review and evaluation function of total quality management (TQM is the process of ensuring high quality output to enhance customer service and improve customer satisfaction) (14) as well as justification for reimbursement in some situations. Continuous Quality Improvement (CQI) is the process of continual information feedback, evaluation and improvement of delivery systems and outcomes based on objectivitely measured quality parameter. (15) A third term, PI or Performance Improvement, is just emerging in some locales and differs very little from both earlier terms but uses the most successful components of each.

Traditionally, those institutions governed by such regulatory agencies as JCAHO or the Department of Health and Human Services do not have specific charting formats for documentation delineated in the regulatory standards however the standards do identify documentation requirements. Institutions can define their own documentation formats as long as they are in compliance with all legal, accreditation and professional standards. The focus of the new JCAHO standards has been progressively shifting toward outcome evaluation, which may necessitate changes in the way some institutions chart.

Historically, notes have been narrative, however, many institutions have implemented charting formats to encourage an efficient retrieval of information in regards to specific problems or situations. Such formats in the literature include focus and SOAPIER charting. (See examples in FYI "Documentation Format Examples" at the end of this chapter.) Too often progress notes document only repetitive routine interventions and assessments while significant information regarding the client and/or significant others and their interaction with the healthcare provider is lost. (PIE [problem, intervention, evaluation] charting is more of a nursing process in most institutions unless they are fortunate enough to have multidisciplinary charting formats using PIE for all disciplines.)

Nutrition Plan of Care

The nutritional plan of care for a client should identify a priority set of problems for that individual as well as communicate what to observe, teach or implement in order to achieve certain outcome criteria. The plan of care also serves to identify specific interventions for the client, family or specified disciplines to implement. The typical components of the plan of care include:

- problem statements
- outcome criteria/goals
- interventions
- evaluation.

Many facilities integrate multiple disciplines into the care of each individual client. A primary responsibility of these transdisciplinary groups is to continually assess and improve patient care through the development of clinical care pathways and/or protocols. (See FYI "Nutrition Education in a Typical Pathway", page 184.)

The nutrition *problem statement* is a statement of concern (other than the medical diagnosis) for which the nutrition staff provides intervention that can be evaluated. Problem statements can often be prefaced with the statement, "Alteration in. . . as related to. . . ," as is often seen in the nursing documentation process. For example, "alteration in oral intake related to poor dentition" or "alteration in bowel elimination R/T low fiber intake."

Outcome criteria (or goals) should be statements describing a measurable indice or behavior of the client/family denoting a favorable response (changed or maintained) after implementing the plan of care. In effect, the outcome criteria serve as standards for measuring the effectiveness of the plan of care. If outcome criteria are not being achieved, the diagnosis should be reevaluated and the plan of care and/or goals revised. Collaboration among disciplines is instrumental in designing an effective nutrition plan of care. *Interventions* are autonomous actions by each discipline involved in the client's care, based on scientific rationale, and executed to benefit the client in an anticipated way related to their diagnosis and outcome criteria. Interventions may either be independent (i.e. a discipline-specific prescribed treatment) like a dietitian prescribed diet order or delegated (i.e. physician prescribed diet order with monitoring by another discipline to determine compliance or effectiveness). Interventions may be either activities that are performed for or with the client like monitoring oral intake or assisting with daily menu completion using exchanges, or may be activities such as assessments to identify new problems or determine the status of existing problems. Whenever possible, interventions should provide for active participation by the client with a goal of maximizing their health capabilities.

Evaluation of the client's status compares it to the outcome criteria anticipated from the plan of care. Continuous evaluation allows each discipline, either individually or collaboratively, to determine if the client is progressing as planned. *Summary evaluation statements* for each anticipated outcome should specifically address what the client has accomplished or is able to do, verbalize or perform. The evaluation phase should be continual from the time the plan of care is implemented to the termination of care and any referrals made. *Progress notes*, regardless of where in the medical record they may be located, serve to document significant data or events in the care of the client.

Discharge planning is an important component of the plan of care. As mentioned previously, the discharge planning process should begin at the time of admission. Discharge planning may include:

- written nutrition instruction materials
- follow-up outpatient visits
- referrals to other homecare or community resources.

At times, referrals outside the immediate area may be indicated and early discharge planning allows time for the appropriate arrangements to be made and all discharge summary documentation to be completed.

WHY CHARGE FOR INPATIENT CLINICAL SERVICES?

Diagnosis-specific coding for reimbursement is vital to documenting alterations in nutritional status. Although dietetic specific codes have been proposed (16) (see Chapter 9 for dietetic procedural/diagnostic billing/medical records codes), current systems in the majority of acute care settings dictate that documentation by dietetic practitioners use medical-specific coding.

Dietetic practitioners must be prepared to answer some tough questions from hospital administrators. (17) The lack of specific nutrition billing codes often makes it difficult to track the fruits of dietetic services specifically. Often, administrators consider clinical dietetic services as "insignificant" revenue sources. This makes it all the more important that you market what you provide like:

- improved patient outcomes and satisfaction,
- reduced number of readmissions through effective nutrition counseling and outpatient follow-up,
- increased DRG nutrition-related revenue,
- growing revenues from inpatient and outpatient counseling and other clinical services.

The increase in capitated plans makes the issue of revenue generation a difficult discussion to support, but the benefits of disease prevention and health promotion are even stronger. However, an analysis of 1601 nutrition intervention case studies compiled by the American Dietetic Association revealed that the average annual cost savings for patients could equal thousands of dollars, i.e. $10,538 for gestational diabetes; $6,556 for a tube/IV feeding; $2,496 for hypercholesterolemia; $2,178 for Type II diabetes. (18)

In the past many dietetic practitioners have been hesitant to charge for inpatient and/or outpatient nutrition services such as assessments and nutrition counseling. Changes in third party payer mixes as well as reimbursement policies have had a dramatic effect on acute care billing for clinical nutrition care. Clinical nutrition departments now must differentiate routine services from nonroutine services. Nonroutine services are generally physician-ordered and provided to selected at risk patients. Basic nutrition care usually includes:

- Screening of patients identified at nutritional risk
- Obtaining food preferences or allergies
- Menu distribution process
- Quality control: meal rounds, tray assessments, surveys
- 3 meals per day and nonpharmaceutical nourishments and snacks
- Phone consultations
- Resolution of patient satisfaction issues

All other services are considered specialized and billable. If you charge for services, charge fair fees and promote the value of your services, not just the revenue potential. Following are the reasons many hospitals charge for nonroutine nutrition services:

- Provides financial accountability for dietetic services
- Promotes fair distribution of clinical staffing by prioritizing clinical nutrition services
- Provides cost benefits in relation to decreased LOS (length of stay) when nutrition intervention involved
- Improves quality of patient care through early intervention and preventive nutrition
- Assigns value to clinical nutrition care
- Enhances professional image

Reimbursement

Respondents to the 1993 American Dietetic Association membership database survey indicated that outpatient dietitians are more likely to bill for their services (46%) than inpatient dietitians (35%) and dietitians in private practice bill clients or third party payers most frequently (65%). (18) A recent fee for service national survey of inpatient clinical nutrition services indicated that only 24% of those surveyed billed for diet instruction (counseling). (19)

A nine step process has been suggested for establishing a system to promote reimbursement for nutrition services: (20)
1. assess the environment
2. establish a rationale and implementation plan for charging
3. evaluate services currently being provided
4. identify, define, and describe billable and nonbillable services
5. establish fees or charges
6. process charges and bill appropriate parties
7. document services rendered
8. monitor reimbursement
9. educate users and market nutrition services

An understanding of procedure codes is valuable when trying to pursue reimbursement for nutrition services. Procedure codes represent services and products on health insurance claim forms and are many times, in conjunction with diagnosis codes, the basis for decisions regarding coverage and reimbursement. Factors that may affect reimbursement for services include: (21)

- Physician driven
- Reasonable and medically necessary
- Use of procedure codes
- Thorough documentation
- Diagnosis (counseling for obesity is usually not covered unless there are complications)
- Payer source(s)
    Discount from charges (a predetermined amount e.g. 10% off all/selected services)
    Reimbursement per diem (a set payment per day regardless of service)
    Reimbursement per case (set payment based on diagnosis e.g. DRG's)
    Capitated payment (set payment based on so much per covered life per year regardless of services provided)
- Location (hospital-based vs. clinic-based vs. private practice may determine contracts available and/ or billing codes utilized)

Inadequate staffing is often heard as the reason some nutrition services are lacking. More than 25% of the hospitals polled by Modern Healthcare (22) have trimmed their workforces, some as much as 24%. In a study reported by Compher and Colaizzo (23), registered dietitian staffing in hospitals decreased by 11% from 1986 to 1989 at a time when total hospital staffing increased by 2.9%. Charging for inpatient services in hospitals experiencing tough financial situations may facilitate justification of current staffing levels. The survival of hospital-based clinical dietitians may be dependent on establishing their value in both practice areas and in the institution's financial circles as well as documenting the cost-effectiveness of medical nutrition therapies, including nutritional counseling, such as decreased readmissions due to diet noncompliance and the reduction of health risk factors related to nutrition.

SUMMARY

Sweeping changes in health care are changing the ways clinical dietetics and inpatient counseling are practiced. In some areas of the country many jobs are in jeoparady while a short distance away another hospital may be adding clinical dietetic staff because they are aggressively seeking opportunities and changing with the times. Patients expect to be fed tasty, healthy food while in the hospital and to be adequately instructed on what they should eat to recover from illness, injury or surgery, or prevent disease. That's not too much to ask.

LEARNING ACTIVITIES
1. Write a chart note for a client nutrition counseling session you have observed in both formats: FOCUS and SOAPIER.
2. Contact nutrition therapists and interview them in regards to their techniques and success in obtaining reimbursement for services. What techniques could you use?
3. With a colleague, write a sample nutrition component for a critical pathway. What is your goal? What are your concerns? Interventions? How do you measure success?

REFERENCES
1. Brook RH, Williams KH, DaviesAvery A. *Quality assurance in the 20th century: will it lead to improved health in the 21st?* 1975; Santa Monica: Rand Corporation, p.5530.

2. Joint Commission of Accreditation of Healthcare Organizations. 1995; *Accreditation manual for hospitals*. Chicago: The Commission.

3. Donabedian A. The quality of care: how can it be assessed? (Chapter 2). In Graham NO. ed. 1990; *Quality assurance in hospitals: strategies for assessment and implementation*. Rockville: Aspen Publishers, p. 1430.

4. Vladeck BC. Quality assurance through external controls. In Graham NO. ed. 1990; *Quality assurance in hospitals: strategies for assessment and implementation*. Rockville: Aspen Publishers.

5. Herbelin K, McElroy D, McGee T. A blueprint for success with OBRA inspections of nursing facilities. 1994; *Dietetic Currents*.21:1 4.

6. *Quality watch: Joint commission introduces three new areas of survey concentration*. 1992; Hospitals. 62:64,66.

7. Joint Commission on Accreditation of Healthcare Organizations. Summary analysis 1995 JCAHO standards. 1994; *Briefings on JCAHO*. :124.

8. Sweeting S. Total quality management. 1994; *DGCP Newsletter*. 12:910.

9. Huyck NI. Patient education: implementing a food and drug interaction program. 1991; *Topics in Clinical Nutrition*. 6:3441.

10. Jones CM, Reddick JE. Drugnutrient interaction counseling programs in upper midwestern hospitals: 1986 survey results. 1989; *J Am Diet Assoc*. 89:243245.

11. Lasswell AB, Loreck ES. Development of a program in accord with JCAHO standards for counseling on potential drugfood interactions. 1992; *J Am Diet Assoc*. 92:11241125.

12. Wix AR, Doering PL, Nalton RC. Drugfood interaction counseling programs in teaching hospitals. 1992; *American Journal of Health Promotion*. 49:855860.

13. Adapted from Klawitter BM. Documentation for nutritional care: overview of concepts and standards. 1995; *The Connector*. (In press).

14. McDonald SC. Total quality management (TQM) in healthcare. *J of Canadian Diet Assoc*. 1994; 55:12-14.

15. Cameron AM (ed.) *Incorporating nutrition care into critical pathways for improved outcomes*. Houston: Ross Products Div./ St. Luke's Episcopal Hospital. 1994: pg.3.

16. Kight MA, Gammon M. Startup characterizations/diagnostic criteria for using dieteticspecific nutritional diagnostic codes (DS NDC's) in adult care situations. 1994; *Diagnostic Nutrition Network*. 3:26.

17. *Business success in dietetics: generating revenue and saving costs*. Columbus, OH: Ross Laboratories; 1990.

18. Holmes V. ed. How you can promote the value of your services. *ADA Courier*. 1994; 33:2.

19. Chima CS. Fee for service survey for inpatient clinical nutrition services. *CNM Newsletter*. 1994; 13: 7-9.

20. Smith KG, Konkle DR, Semen M. Charging for hospital-based nutrition services. In NSPS Committee, eds. *Reimbursement and insurance coverage for nutrition services*. Chicago: American Dietetic Assoc; 1991:35-50.

21. Savage NK. Procedure codes for nutrition services. *DGCP Newsletter*. 1994; 12:7-8.

22. Burda D. Cutting down: hospitals' labor costs are top target, annual human resources survey shows. *Modern Healthcare*. 1993; 23: 49-58.

23. Compher C, Colaizzo T. Staffing patterns in hospital clinical dietetics and nutrition services: a survey conducted by the DNS practice group. *J Am Diet Assoc*. 1992; 92: 807-812.

FOR YOUR INFORMATION

Clinical Dietitians Use Case Studies to Document Cost-Benefit

Barbara Williams, MS, RD, ARA Health Services

Inquisitiveness, intuition, as well as a passion to develop resolutions to practical problems you see every day in practice keeps you viable and up-to-date. One of the most important problems facing clinical dietitians today is the proof that nutrition intervention produces improved health in clients that will far out-weigh and cost less than other forms of intervention like medications, surgery, hospital stays, physician consultations, or no intervention. Too many practitioners assume that collecting and analyzing cost-benefit data is difficult and beyond their skill or knowledge, when in fact it is not, especially if you use case studies and the following simple forms.

The following three forms can be used to organize your case study information and present it to employers, managed care purveyors, referring physicians, insurers, and so on:

- Figure FYI 10-1 Outcome Documentation
- Figure FYI 10-2 Case study format for documentation
- Figure FYI 10-3 Medical Nutrition Therapy Saves Health Care Dollars (summary of four case studies)

FYI Figure 10-1   Outcome Documentation

The case study technique is an easily learned type of research frequently used in clinical and counseling settings. Case study research is "a descriptive technique in which you report on a single case or a few cases. The term 'case' refers to the object of the study. A case study can be just about anything." (1) Another important term is "outcome" which means the result. In nutrition intervention that would mean as a result of your consultations with the client what does he or she do or think differently? What does the client know now that he or she didn't know before? Have any blood chemistries improved? Are there any good emotional changes or maturing developmental skills? If nothing changes for the better for the client as a result of seeing you, then why should that client or any other come to see you?

FYI Figure 10-2   Case study format for documentation

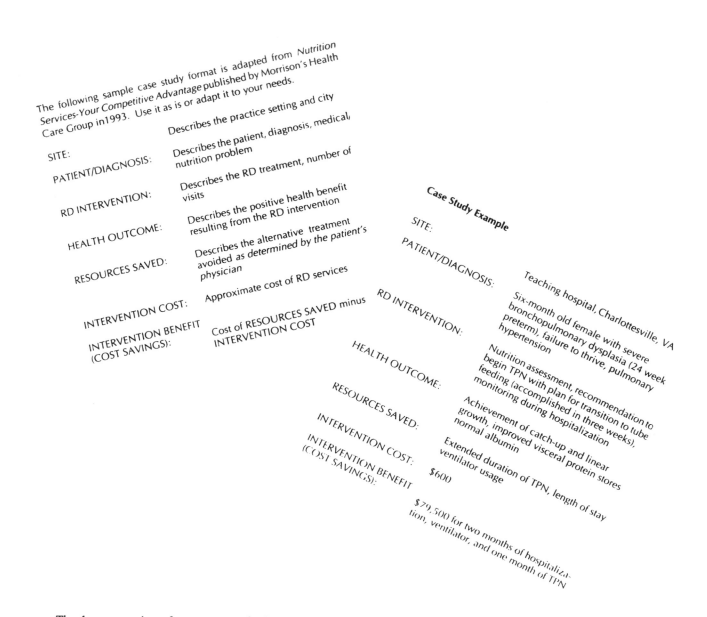

The following sample case study format is adapted from *Nutrition Services-Your Competitive Advantage* published by Morrison's Health Care Group in 1993. Use it as is or adapt it to your needs.

SITE: Describes the practice setting and city

PATIENT/DIAGNOSIS: Describes the patient, diagnosis, medical, nutrition problem

RD INTERVENTION: Describes the RD treatment, number of visits

HEALTH OUTCOME: Describes the positive health benefit resulting from the RD intervention

RESOURCES SAVED: Describes the alternative treatment avoided as determined by the patient's physician

INTERVENTION COST: Approximate cost of RD services

INTERVENTION BENEFIT (COST SAVINGS): Cost of RESOURCES SAVED minus INTERVENTION COST

Case Study Example

SITE:

PATIENT/DIAGNOSIS: Teaching hospital, Charlottesville, VA Six-month old female with severe bronchopulmonary dysplasia (24 week preterm), failure to thrive, pulmonary hypertension

RD INTERVENTION: Nutrition assessment, recommendation to begin TPN with plan for transition to tube feeding (accomplished in three weeks), monitoring during hospitalization

HEALTH OUTCOME: Achievement of catch-up and linear growth, improved visceral protein stores normal albumin

RESOURCES SAVED: Extended duration of TPN, length of stay ventilator usage

INTERVENTION COST: $600

INTERVENTION BENEFIT (COST SAVINGS): $79,500 for two months of hospitalization, ventilator, and one month of TPN

The documentation of your case study data should provide details on the patient's condition, the nutrition therapy, and the resulting benefits and cost savings. A failure to calculate costs makes the tools incomplete. Calculation of cost must be accurate, consistent, and not inflated. The list of complications and their prices and alternative therapy must be reasonable and fair, along with the exact dose and cost of any medication saved. Summarize the information from FYI Figure 10-1 onto FYI Figure 10-2. As seen on FYI Figure 10-3, several case studies can be summarized on one form to be used to show that various clients benefitted from nutrition intervention and considerable money was saved.

FYI Figure 10-3   Medical Nutrition Therapy Saves Health Care Dollars

	Case Study 1	Case Study 2	Case Study 3	Case Study 4
Site:	Community Hospital, Pennsylvania Inpatient Nutrition Services	Community Hospital, Pennsylvania Outpatient Nutrition Services	Nursing Home, Washington	Hospital, Washington Inpatient Nutrition Services
Patient/Problem:	37 year-old female with hyperemesis and weight loss of 9 lbs. in 11 1/2 weeks of pregnancy.	41 year-old female with morbid obesity, high blood pressure, heart disease; unable to do cardiac cath because of obesity.	80 year-old male with dementia and dysphagia from a stroke, lost 14 lbs. in 90 days and developed pneumonia. Receiving chloral hydrate, making patient too sleepy to eat.	54 year-old male with abdominal wound cellulitis and fistula, insulin dependent diabetes and obesity. Patient had fistula for 2 years.
RD Intervention:	1 consult and 1 follow up over 9 days. Total of 90 minutes.	Individual counseling consisting of 8 visits over 11 weeks. Total of 4 1/2 hours.	8 hours of consultation time. Changed diet, had patient eat in dining room, inserviced nursing staff on feeding, recommended discontinuing medication.	Individual counseling consisting of 8 visits over 1 month. Total of 8 hours.
Health Outcome:	Placed on NG tube feeding, within 12 hours nausea stopped; within 24 hours consuming 90% of meal without nausea or vomiting. Discharged on oral diet with NG tube in place.	Weight loss of 21 lbs. after 4 weeks of counseling, able to do cardia cath, blood pressure decreased.	Pneumonia resolved, patient no longer choked on food, improved food intake, gained weight, became more alert.	Patient placed on TPN, fistula closed. Lost 18 lbs. in 1 month.
Resources Saved:	3 days of TPN with 500 ml lipids = $690 plus 3 additional hospital days for continued nutrition and education on home TPN = $2,250.	Blood pressure medication cut in half, saving $1,080 per year. Cholesterol lowering medication eliminated, saving $1,080 per year. Avoided 2 day hospital stay for exploratory procedures to determine extent of heart disease, saving $1,500.	Prevented hospitalization - $4,000	Prevented surgical intervention - 4 days at $1,000/day = $4,000. Prevented further use of TPN - $4,000 for placement, TPN for 30 days = $12,000
Intervention Cost:	$80 RD time plus $9.54 for 3 days of NG tube feeding.	$260	$300	$480
Intervention Benefit:	$2,850	$3,400	$3,700	$19,520

After collecting the data, market it. It is extremely important that you compile the data in such a way that it is useful when making presentations to others who can support you. Never assume that others know and understand the importance of what you do, show them the proof!

REFERENCE

1. Borden KS, Abbott BB. *Research Design and Methods: A Process Approach.* Mountain View, CA: Mayfield Publishing Co.; 1988.

Thank you to the following persons for contributing the Attachments, which can be duplicated and used by readers.
Diane Friedman, MS, RD, Consultant Dietitian to ARAMARK Healthcare Support Services
Lynn Jenkins, RD, Asst. Dir. of Patient Services, The Cheshire Medical Center, Keene, NH
Terry Crossan, RD, Outpatient Dietitian, Chester Co. Hospital, West Chester, PA
The Washington State Dietetic Association

FOR YOUR INFORMATION

Nutrition Education in a Typical Pathway

Susan DeHoog, RD, Dir., Clinical Nutrition, Univ. of Washington Medical Center, Seattle, WA

When patients are admitted to the hospital our role and responsibility is to provide medical nutrition therapy and education to the patients, along with providing nutritional expertise and education to the interdisciplinary health care team. In accordance with the changes of the Joint Commission on Accreditation of Hospitals Organization (JCAHO), the emphasis has shifted to interdisciplinary patient care. This includes an interdisciplinary approach to the education and continuum of care provided to patients. We must demonstrate, verbally and in writing, that we have conferred with the other health care professionals regarding the education of the patient and/or significant other.

Therefore, we need a functioning mechanism designed to standardize and communicate nutrition care approaches and processes. This includes both inpatient and outpatient areas. One element of this mechanism is to be part of the clinical pathways developed by the facility. Clinical pathways track a patient's interventions and outcomes throughout their hospital stay. They are established to ensure processes are standardized and result in a defined positive outcome. Each day of hospitalization has identified interventions and outcomes. Clinical pathways can start in the outpatient department; be implemented inpatient and conclude back in the outpatient area.

All assessments are based on the average length of stay for the disease state. For example, nutritional status hospital day one (HD #1) with intravenous cisplatin, the outcome is for the patient to maintain 50% of nutritional needs with or without antimetics. By HD #4, patient/family education needs to be completed. (Average length of stay is six days). Discharge planning usually begins when the patient enters the hospital.

All hospital clinical dietitians need to be active in your hospital's education and nutrition committees. The nutrition committee, whose members usually include medicine, surgery, nutrition, pharmacy and nursing, promotes the optimal use of nutrition resources for patient care. The education committee, which can include the same disciplines, oversees all educational mechanisms.

This could include all nutritional instructions and all potential food/drug interactions. The process should include follow up care either to a nutrition clinic, private practice dietitian, or a dietitian at the referring facility. Diseases such as heart disease, kidney disease, cancer, diabetes, hypertension, and other leading causes of death where lifestyle impacts the disease process all need education intervention.

Your process of education can be as follows:

1. The dietitian assesses the patient's learning ability and readiness for learning, comprehension and ability to implement changes. Consideration is given to literacy, cognitive limitations, religious food-related practices, family beliefs, values and culture. When indicated, an interpreter will be used.
2. The patient and/or significant other receive education specific to the patient's diagnosis, assessed needs and abilities.
3. The dietitian assesses the patient's and/or significant other's comprehension and ability to implement changes. Learning needs may need to be prioritized.

Discharge

JCAHO standards require that any discharge instructions given to the patient are also provided to the facility or individual responsible for the patient's continuing care. A copy of the discharge summary and instructions need to be forwarded to the patient's primary care provider. The discharge summary should contain the following information: (see form that follows)

  1. Pertinent information on weights, labs, food intake, calculated needs, medications
  2. Summary of nutritional problems and therapies
  3. Outcome of nutritional therapies
  4. Statement of patient education to include:
     • patient and/or significant other has been instructed on prescribed needs
     • expected adherence to prescribed diet
     • comprehension of nutrition information and self-care
     • drug/nutrient interaction education, if appropriate
  5. Statement on expected "progress"
  6. Recommendations for follow up

7. Continuum of care plans
8. Statement that indicates other members of the health care team have been advised of the education provided to the patient and/or significant other.

BIBLIOGRAPHY

Hospital healthcare standards manual. Oakbrook Terrace, Ill: Joint Commission on Accreditation of Health Care Organizations;1995.

Grant TA, DeHoog SJ. *Nutrition Support Planning: Nutritional Assessment and Support*, 4th ed. Seattle, WA: 1991; 205-228.

FOR YOUR INFORMATION

Documentation Format Examples

FOCUS CHARTING

Focus: Altered knowledge: diabetic diet

D (data): "I don't understand my diet. It's much too complicated for me. My wife will have to take care of it." 32-year old male admit with newly diagnosed diabetes, to receive oral hypoglycemic agent coupled with diet for control of blood glucose. Admission labs: glucose 255, cholesterol 245. Height: 72" Weight: 215# Order received for instruction on 1800 calorie low-fat low-cholesterol diet for discharge. Diet history reveals erratic meal patterns, frequent soda and alcohol intake (had 4 beers night before admission). Eats out frequently, usually fast foods or convenience store items. Wife working and not available for counseling before discharge. Strong family history of heart disease and diabetes.

A (action): Assist client in identifying diet changes he can make. Suggest use of diet soda and provide suggestions for lower fat lower cholesterol options when eating out. Monitor menu selections and intake while hospitalized. Provided qualitative diabetic guidelines and started counseling on lifestyle changes (diet and activity) that client can consider. Instructed on use of exchanges for menu completion. Continue with diet counseling inpatient with followup as outpatient (including wife) recommended.

R (response): Client expresses willingness to make some changes, i.e. drink diet soda and decrease alcohol intake. Client able to state importance of controlling blood sugars and cholesterol levels. Able to complete menu with assistance using exchanges.

SOAPIER CHARTING

S (Subjective data): "I don't understand my diet. It's much too complicated for me. My wife will have to take care of it."

O (objective data): 32-year old male admit with newly diagnosed diabetes, to receive oral hypoglycemic agent coupled with diet for control of blood glucose. Admission labs: glucose 255, cholesterol 245. Height: 72" Weight 215# Order received for instruction on 1800 calorie low-fat low-cholesterol diet for discharge. Diet history reveals erratic meal patterns, Wife working and not available for counseling before discharge. Strong family history of heart disease and diabetes.

A (analysis/assessment): Lack of knowledge regarding diabetic and low-fat low-cholesterol diet principles. Client appears resistant to participating in diet counseling.

P (plan): Assist client in identifying diet changes he can make. Suggest use of diet soda and provide suggestions for lower fat lower cholesterol options when eating out. Monitor menu selections and intake while hospitalized.

I (interventions): Provided qualitative diabetic guidelines and started counseling on lifestyle changes (diet and activity) that client can consider. Instructed on use of exchanges for menu completion.

E (evaluation): Client expresses willingness to make some changes, Client able to state importance of controlling blodd sugars and cholesterol levels.

R (revisions): Maintain current diet as ordered and monitor menu completion. Continue wth diet counseling inpatient with followup as outpatient (including wife) recommended.

Appendix 10-A

Counseling a Person with Diabetes

Melinda Downie Maryniuk, MEd, RD, CDE, Joslin Diabetes Center, Boston, MA

Medical Nutrition Therapy for the person with diabetes is a lifelong process. This is perhaps the most important message that the dietitian should convey to a client at the first encounter. Ideally, the person with diabetes should have their meal plan reviewed by a Registered Dietitian once a year.

The American Diabetes Association's 1994 Nutrition Recommendations do not define the composition of a "diabetic diet." In fact, diabetes dietitians are fond of saying, "there is no such thing as a diabetic diet" meaning that there are as many different kinds of meal plans as there are people with diabetes! By not defining a recommended meal plan, the ADA has endorsed the use of the Registered Dietitian as the person who should determine the approach to meal planning, which will be most well accepted by the client, as well as encourage optimal metabolic control. Exchange lists are only one of many different tools and meal planning methods which may be evaluated for use with the client.

Counseling Steps

Counseling should follow a four step sequence: assessment, goal setting, intervention and evaluation.

During the assessment phase, the dietitian gathers and evaluates data regarding the clients clinical status, their nutrition history, an assessment of their usual intake and an analysis of factors which may support or inhibit the person's ability to make changes. In order to effectively review the clinical data, the dietitian needs to have a good understanding of diabetes as well as the referring physician's goals, such as the target blood glucoses and a target glycohemoglobin. Diabetes specific information that the dietitian should evaluate includes: current level of metabolic control, including glucose and lipids, effectiveness of current diabetes medication regimen and the impact of the dosages and timing on food intake and blood glucoses, frequency and treatment of hypo and hyperglycemia, risk factors and/or presence of diabetes complications.

Goal-directed therapy describes medical nutrition therapy for diabetes. During this second step of counseling, goal setting, it is important to involve the client in the discussion to assess his understanding, willingness and interest in making the necessary eating pattern and behavior changes. Diabetes educators place an emphasis on empowering the patient to take responsibility for their own diabetes management and selfcare. Questions which should be asked include: What do you expect from nutrition counseling? What is the most important goal for you in managing your diabetes and the way you eat? What are some changes you could make to your present plan of eating to follow more closely the diabetes nutrition goals we discussed? The dietitian helps the client set short term and long term goals which are realistic and achievable.

During intervention, the third step of counseling, the dietitian provides information about nutrition and diabetes geared to the appropriate stage or level of the client's needs. Also, a meal planning approach for achieving the goals is selected. There are four basic categories of meal planning approaches: general guidelines, menu approaches, exchange approaches and counting systems. A general guidelines approach may be as simple as teaching the food guide pyramid to the patient or determining a set of specific changes to make in the client's usual eating plan, such as switch from whole milk to 2% milk, consume only 4 ounces of fruit juice at breakfast, and eat meals at the following times: 8am, 12 noon, 6 pm and 9pm (snack). A client who quickly grasps nutrition principles, keeps detailed blood glucose records and is trying to tighten his metabolic control may want to use a counting system approach such as carbohydrate or fat gram counting.

Although the 1994 ADA Guidelines stated that scientific evidence has shown that the use of sucrose as part of the meal plan does not impair blood glucose control in Type I or Type II diabetes, it still needs to be counted as part of the overall carbohydrate allowance. It is misleading for dietitians to teach patients about "fast acting" sugars and "slower acting" starches as both sugars and starches are digested and absorbed at about the same rate. We do need to counsel patients about portion sizes and controlling amounts of high sugar foods and making selections of sugar containing foods which are also lower in fat.

The fourth step in the counseling process, evaluation, is critical to determine the effectiveness of the selfcare plan. Depending on the goals of the therapy, the dietitian may be reviewing the fasting blood glucoses, the glycohemoglobin, lipid levels, body weight, medication levels or other outcomes to assess the effectiveness of the meal plan. Although this is the fourth step, it is not the final step as the process is cyclical returning to the assessment, setting new goals and designing new interventions as needed.

How to Become a Certified Diabetes Educator

It is an exciting time to be a dietitian in diabetes care. Dietitians who see a majority of clients with diabetes are encouraged to become a Certified Diabetes Educator (CDE). In order to qualify to take the CDE written exam, the dietitian must demonstrate having a minimum of 2,000 hours in direct diabetes patient education. For more information on the National Certification Examination for Diabetes Educators, contact the Professional Testing Corporation in New York City, (212) 790-9283, or contact the American Association of Diabetes Educators. Most CDE dietitians find themselves taking on expanded roles as they teach a broad array of diabetes topics including self blood glucose monitoring, hypoglycemia prevention and treatment, exercise guidelines and insulin adjustment guidelines.

CASE STUDIES

The following brief vignettes show the variety of types of counseling encounters dietitians may have with clients:

Craig is an active, 10-year-old boy with Type I diabetes. Craig's brothers, ages 8 and 12, still love to eat the family favorite, sugared flakes cereal, for breakfast. The mother does not know what to do. As the dietitian, you've calculated Craig's breakfast meal plan to include 2 breads, 1 milk and 1 fruit serving. This can also be looked at as 4 carbohydrate (carb) servings or about 60 grams of carb (we typically round the 12 grams of carb in milk up to 15). Whether Craig eats his carb as 2/3 cup sugared flakes (30 grams carb) or 1 1/2 cup unsweetened flakes (also 30 grams carb) should not change the effect on the postprandial blood glucose.

Martha is a 55-year-old woman with a two year history of Type II diabetes controlled with Glyburide. She has been struggling to keep her weight down and her blood glucose in target ranges. Her doctor is considering moving her to insulin unless improvements in control are seen. After meeting with the dietitian, Martha has set the following goals: begin a walking program, 10 minutes every other day for the first week, increasing by 5 minutes each week; begin a fat gram counting meal plan and limit total fat intake to 50 grams each day (about 10 grams at breakfast, 15 at lunch, 20 at supper and 5 at bedtime snack). Fat will be counted using labels and by counting meat, fat and highfat bread exchanges.

John is a 68-year-old man with newly diagnosed Type II diabetes. He has always eaten well balanced meals and he usually eats at about the same time every day. He rarely eats away from home and his weight is normal. Based on your assessment, John may only need to make some changes to reduce the saturated fat in his diet. He doesn't need a new meal plan, but he may just need to learn why he needs to maintain the consistency in the amounts and timing of his meals and the importance of a diet that is lower in fat. John can state what he is willing and able to do to reduce the fat in his meals.

ADDITIONAL RESOURCES:

Franz MJ, Horton EG, Bantle JP, Beebe CA, Brunzell JD, Coulston AM, Henry RR, Hoogwerf BJ, Stacpoole PW. Technical review: nutrition principles for the management of diabetes and related complications. *Diabetes Care*. 1994;17: 490-518.

Maryniuk MD. Diabetes Education: A Dietitian's Role. In: Powers MA, eds. *Handbook of Diabetes Nutritional Management*, 2nd ed., Gaithersburg, MD: Aspen Publishers, 1995.

Pastors JG, Holler HJ. *Meal Planning Approaches for Diabetes Management*. 2nd ed. Chicago, IL: American Dietetic Association, 1994.

Tinker LF, Heins JM, Holler HJ. Commentary and Translation: 1994 nutrition recommendations for diabetes. *Journal Am Diet Assoc*. 1994; 94: 507511.

Appendix 10-B

Counseling a Person with AIDS

Jean E. Schreiner, MS, RD, Owner, Carrot Top Nutrition Resources, Aurora, CO

Counseling a person with AIDS (referred to as PWA in medical settings) about nutrition is an essential component for overall management of the disease. Also, early intervention allows time to establish a relationship and develop rapport with the patient.

By delaying the wasting and malnutrition commonly seen in AIDS patients, dietitians can presumably improve a patient's prognosis. The degree of body cell mass depletion may be a better predictor of survival (1) than any analysis of any specific underlying infection or a CD4 count. Supportive nutrition and dietary measures may significantly improve symptomatic relief and contribute to a higher quality of life. It is the 1994 position of both the American Dietetic Association and the Canadian Dietetic Association that nutrition intervention and medical nutrition therapy along with education should be components of the total health care provided to persons infected with the human immunodeficiency virus (HIV). (2)

Preparing for the Counseling Session

A nutrition therapist must be concerned about all the factors that affect the patient's current nutrition status and his or her ability to buy, prepare and eat food as the disease progresses. Prepare for the counseling session by first evaluating the patient's current symptoms, individual abilities and needs. Use all data available including any recent interview information, charts, nutritional assessments and information from any others involved in his/her care. Consider psychosocial conditions, economic factors, and support systems to develop a workable and realistic plan. Enlist the aid of Social Services, local AIDS information and support groups, and meal delivery services, especially if friends, family or funds are limited. Check the patient's existing insurance coverage and options since nutritional supplements may be reimbursable. Develop a flexible plan with prioritized goals that will improve the patient's quality of life and nutritional status.

The following is a brief review of nutrition related concerns along with other possible complications to consider as you create the individualized plan. Detailed discussions of nutritional concerns and interventions can be found in the resources listed at the end of this article.

Weight Status: If nutritional support is delayed until after significant weight loss, it may be more difficult to change the patient's malnutrition status. Deliberate weight gain may help improve his or her chances of surviving longer with HIV. (3,4) Check weight status and weight history. Use nutritional assessment data to determine which body compartments are depleted. Determine the energy, protein and nutrient goals.

Anorexia: Determine the cause by checking for depression, mouth sores, dementia, anxiety, medications and fear of increased diarrhea. Focus on a calorically-dense diet and supplements.

Nausea/Vomiting: Identify cause(s) and counsel patients regarding appropriate food/liquid choices and timing of meals. If needed, recommend anti-nausea medications to physician.

Dyspnea/Fatigue/Pain: Check patient's ability to eat and evaluate actual intake. Make meal suggestions that include easy food preparation techniques, possibility of meal delivery and helpers to assist at mealtimes. Consider alternative food routes to achieve adequate intake and counsel patient on these options.

Infection/Fever: Check for presence of fluid and nutrient losses and assume increased tissue breakdown. Adjust patient's calorie/protein/nutrient goals and counsel accordingly.

Mouth and Esophageal Sores: Counsel regarding food consistency, types and temperature.

Diarrhea and Malabsorption: Discuss fluid and electrolye replacement and counsel to avoid caffeine, and increasing soluble fiber. Consider possible lactose and fat restriction. Add appropriate supplements specifically for PWAs.

Food Safety: PWAs have an increased vulnerability to food borne illness. They should be counseled concerning food safety at home and eating out, as well as safety of their water sources.

Nutritional Supplements: Check into supplements used, whether traditional or unorthodox and counsel regarding potential harm/concerns in a nonjudgmental way for any unorthodox supplements. Prevent and correct any deficiencies in diet (goal = approximately 200% RDI).

Enteral and Parenteral Feedings: Check into physical facilities and adequacy of feeding equipment. Counsel caregivers and patient (perhaps along with the home health nurse) on the formula and how to administer the feeding. (See resource list for detailed information.)

Drug/Food and Nutrient Interactions: Note all medications used including over-the-counter and their potential influence on nutrient needs, absorption, and side effects. Counsel and educate accordingly.

Counseling Considerations for the Person with AIDS

After considering your client's needs and appropriate interventions, you can prioritize your recommendations, ie. what is an essential intervention and what can be delayed.

Plan the session so that it will be in tune with the patient's condition. Is morning nausea the rule? Will talking during the meal distract the patient from eating a needed high calorie intake? Make sure any home visit or outpatient appointments are planned in the best interest and convenience of the patient's and caregiver's schedule to avoid conflicts with meal delivery times, visits from home health aids, or any other events related to management of his or her care and well-being.

Be aware and sympathetic to the frequent depression that can occur whether it is related to the stress of dealing with a life threatening illness, from medications, or the underlying disease itself. AIDS patients may at times feel too depressed to shop, plan meals or eat nourishing foods. For this and other reasons it is important to include any friends, family, or caregivers in any counseling sessions.

One study revealed the most prominent feelings of PWAs are uncertainty, anxiety and anger over the treatment of their illness by caregivers. (5) Demonstrate your concern and willingness to listen. A positive and nonjudgmental attitude is important. It helps to encourage a patient to be involved in his or her care as much as possible. Making decisions regarding food choices, type of service, and the diet plan can help promote feelings of self-control and esteem. One client once remarked he felt like he was being experimented on because of the many unopened cans of different supplements being sent to his hospital room. An on-site tour of the nourishment area of the hospital kitchen complete with a "taste test" of various supplements got him involved in his care in a positive way.

Information for the client can be provided in an endless number of creative ways. Depending on the patient's needs, the following resources can be useful: verbal plans, written plans with grocery lists, menu ideas, shake recipes, resource lists, eating hints and the address of the nearest food bank. Individual instruction is most common, but a group session with two or more PWAs is useful for discussions regarding food safety, nutritional supplements, or high calorie/protein diet suggestions. Your client should always have your department or office phone number as well as several numbers of other team members, nurses or social workers, where he or she can get fast and reliable answers to questions.

Monitor a patient initially with phone calls and home visits, if your institution allows, or refer the patient to a private practice, managed care, or community dietitian. If this is not possible, continue to provide at home follow-up by calling the client's home caregiver or support services in addition to your calls to the patient. Home health care, particularly nutrition, is not being fully used even though the majority of clients feel they could benefit from home health services. (6)

In summary, early nutrition intervention, with a realistic and flexible nutrition care plan created with the patient's involvement are essential components to overall management of AIDS.

ADDITIONAL RESOURCES

Hickey M S. *Handbook of Enteral, Parenteral, and ARC/AIDS Nutritional Therapy.* St.Louis, MO: Mosby; 1992. For health care profesionals.

National AIDS Clearing House 1-800-458-5231. For consumers and professionals.

Salomont SB, Davis M, Newman CF. *Living Well with HIV and AIDS: A Guide to Healthy Eating.* Chicago, IL: American Dietetic Association; 1993. Twenty-eight pages for consumers and professionals.

Schreiner JE. *Nutrition Handbook for AIDS,* 2nd ed., 1990 and Update Packet 1992. Carrot Top Nutrition Resources, PO Box 460172, Aurora, CO 80046-0172, (303) 690-3650. For health care professionals.

REFERENCES

1. Kotler DP, Tierney AR, Wang J, Pierson RN. Magnitude of body cell mass depletion and the timing of death from wasting in AIDS. *Am J Clin Nutr.* 1989; 50:444-447.
2. The American Dietetic Association and The Canadian Dietetic Association.: Position of The ADA and The CDA: Nutrition intervention in the care of persons with human immunodeficiency virus infection. *J Am Diet Assoc.* 1994; 94:1042-1044.
3. Smith J, Birmingham CL. HIV seropositivity and deliberate weight gain. *N Eng J Med.* 1990:322:1089.
4. Schreiner JE. *Nutrition Handbook for AIDS,* 2nd ed. Aurora, CO: Carrot Top Nutrition Resources; 1990.
5. Dilley JW, Ochitill HN, Peril M, Volberding PA. Findings in psychiatric consultations with patients with acquired immune deficiency syndrome. *Am J Psych.* 1985:142:82.
6. Udine LM, Rothkopf MM. Utilization of home health care services in HIV infection: a pilot study in Ohio. *J Am Diet Assoc.*1994; 94:83-85.

11
Exercise Resistance, Obsession, and Recommendations

Karin M. Kratina, MA, RD

After reading this chapter, the reader will be able to:
- ☐ identify factors that can precipitate exercise resistance
- ☐ distinguish between daily physical activity and exercise promotion
- ☐ identify characteristics of exercise dependence
- ☐ list strategies to counsel the exercise dependent client

Most dietitians recommend physical activity to their clients at some time during a consult. We know that physical activity can improve health. But, as with nutrition counseling, individuals come to see us with a myriad of issues that can interfere with a sound program of physical activity. Exercise is actually a subcategory of physical activity and exercise is not always the goal (see side bar). Since dietitians encounter many clients who are unable or unwilling to follow a moderate exercise program, it is crucial to understand and have solutions for exercise resistance and dependence or obsession. This chapter will also cover the specifics of exercise prescription.

PHYSICAL FITNESS

Characteristics that contribute to physical fitness include cardiovascular-respiratory fitness, muscular strength and endurance, body composition and flexibility. The quantity and quality of exercise needed to attain health-related benefits is significantly lower than that which is recommended for fitness benefits. (1)

OVERCOMING EXERCISE RESISTANCE

"I know I would feel better if I just got some exercise, but I can't seem to get motivated. If I could just lose a little weight first, it would be easier. . .besides, I don't want this fat turning into muscle because I would be just as heavy.

"I don't like to sweat, it makes me feel gross. Three years ago I exercised for six months and it felt good, I'm not sure why, but I did lose 24# then. If only I could get motivated, but I get angry sometimes when I think about exercise. . . I just don't want to. . . .Forget it, I don't even have the time to do it."

Many people know that more activity would be good for them, but they can't seem to get motivated. Even when aware they will feel better with an exercise program, the excuse list is extensive, "I am just too heavy, too old, too uncoordinated, too self-conscious," etc. These individuals often start exercise programs but quit soon after initiating them, even when they report enjoying the exercise. Many say they hate to exercise. Others are interested, but resist moving their bodies with the assumption they'll "get to it some day."

Resistance to exercise must be approached carefully as it can arise for a variety of reasons. An individual may not understand how to do the exercises or may feel intimidated by equipment and/or fancy moves in aerobics. Others may be so overwhelmed by the demands of life that making time for exercise seems an impossibility. Still others are resistant to exercise on a much deeper level. While the excuse list is similar, the true resistance arises from a much different place. Presenting an exercise prescription may motivate these individuals initially, but invariably unless the exercise

Physical Activity and Exercise

Bridget Klawitter, MS, RD, FADA

"Physical activity" and "exercise" are terms that describe different concepts. However, they are often confused with one another and the terms are sometimes used interchangeably in the literature. Physical activity is defined as any body movement produced by skeletal muscles that results in energy expenditure. (1) There are undoubtedly many methods of categorizing daily physical activity, however, Casperson and colleagues (1) have suggested the five categories of occupational, sports, conditioning, household, and other activities. Exercise is a subset of physical activity that is planned, structured, and repetitive and has as a final or an intermediate objective the improvement or maintenance of physical fitness by requiring a relatively high percentage of maximal aerobic capacity over a prolonged period of time.

1. Casperson C, Powell KE, Christensen GM. Physical activity, exercise, and physical exercise: definitions and distinctions for health-related research. Public Health Reports. 1985; 100 (2): 126-130.

resistance is dealt with, the prescription is useless. Counseling needs to focus on determining the source of the resistance and overcoming that resistance.

According to Glasser (2), exercise resistance can develop when:

1) exercise is associated with dieting. Exercise is often connected with dieting which has a 95% failure rate. Most people will fail on their diet and quit their exercise program with a resultant negative attitude towards exercise. They often will see exercise as a necessary evil.

2) exercise is used to change the body into a culturally accepted shape. "For many women, quitting exercise is connected with a despair over societal sex role stereotyping which encourages women to get in shape as a means of increasing their personal value by becoming more sexually attractive. Men and women who try to change their body with exercise are often disappointed in themselves as well as with the exercise when they don't become that ideal shape." (2)

3) exercise is used as an external measure of self-worth. In our culture, "exercise is revered as something that supposedly reflects on an individual's inner character, a testimony to their strength and inner worth." (2) Rebellion is common when exercise is used this way. "If there has been a history of sexual abuse, especially if the perpetrator was male, the rebellion is even stronger. It can reflect a refusal to participate in a sexist or demeaning system." (2)

4) exercise is used as punishment. Exercise can be used to punish oneself when goals such as a limit on food intake or weight loss are not accomplished. They view their bodies as bad and self-indulgent.

5) sexual abuse has occurred. Moving the body can "bring up body memories of the abuse. Exercise can trigger flashbacks of repressed abuse while exercising. It can be restimulating due to the movement of the body, being warm or sweating, or simply because the abuse took place in the body and in some way, the trauma is stored there." (2) Exercising is often curtailed after abuse begins, at puberty or at some point when experiencing being sexually objectified.

Any exercise with the goal of weight loss, competition or perfection will need to be explored. A move must be made to exercise with a focus on pleasure, nurturance, self- fulfillment, movement, social and psychological benefits, energy boosts and a sense of self-mastery in order to help clients move away from exercise resistance.

The decision to exercise needs to come from deep within. False starts with exercise occur because individuals begin for externalized reasons, such as "I should do it for my health," "I need to lose this weight," "My partner really wants me to." The decision to exercise is about reconnecting with the body. Making a commitment to becoming more physical "will have a deep impact on the individual's internal experience. Effective motivation will need to speak to the inner life of the individual and promise an improved experience of living. Emphasis needs to be placed on the way exercise makes one feel in one's body emotionally and spiritually. The changes in external body shape are a side effect and, if viewed as the main goal, will sabotage the healing mind/body connection." (3)

Treating Exercise Resistance

Treating exercise resistance must be accomplished individually. Initially, I often ask clients to commit to no activity at all. Some are pleased by this, some upset wondering how they will lose weight...all are surprised. When they ask why they shouldn't start/increase exercise, I explain I don't believe they are ready to change physical activity patterns and that it will be counter- productive if they attempt to do so.

I usually will not address exercise again for the initial 6 to 8 weeks of nutritional counseling or until the client broaches the topic. At this point, the client is given assignments related to exercise attitudes, but is still asked for a commitment to no prescribed exercise. Assignments are limited only by the imagination. Some ideas are to ask the client to:

1) interview 10 people to determine why they like to exercise;

2) interview 10 people to find out if their exercise focus is to move the body or to change the body and which group seems to enjoy exercise more;

3) watch children play for 30 minutes and record in a journal their observations;

4) play with a child where the child has freedom to move around.

While ideas are endless, *the goal is to bring the client to an awareness of the joy of movement.* Many have never experienced as an adult the joyful pleasure and sense of self-mastery that can come with moving. Reconnecting with this experience is at the core of overcoming exercise resistance. Process these assignments in a counseling session. Help the client form a vision for their relationship with physical activity.

Differentiate between exercise used to change the body and that used to move the body. Exercise resistance is typically fueled when changing the body is a goal. (This motivation also fuels eating disorders.) Ask your client to select two physical activities, one with a goal of exercise, the second with a goal of movement and joy. What is their attitude towards them? Ask that they do these activities and record their experience. In another assignment, the client makes two lists: one of exercises they believe would change the body, the other activities that focus on movement. Again, process in a counseling session.

During this time, challenge cognitive distortions concerning health, fitness and exercise. Most don't realize how little physical activity is needed to be healthy, that it doesn't have to involve an exercise prescription or routine, and that it can be a part of day-to-day life. Fitness should be pleasurable and, unfortunately, popular health advice often ignores less intense, more enjoyable forms of physical activity. "Because of the hype, many people feel discouraged; they can't achieve the ideal prescription of vigorous exercise sessions, and the sleek look of the sinewy models glowing out of magazines covers some how evades them. So they do nothing." (4)

One long-term study found that health benefits began for those who burned up as few as 500 calories a week. This could be accomplished with a 15 minute walk each day or 2 hours of bowling. Death rates declined by 20% even with this small amount of activity. (Death rates dropped another 10 to 20% when using 2000 calories for activities each week.) (5) Just getting moving is enough to give substantial benefit to a "couch potato."

Exercise should be undertaken in a non-competitive environment with activities that will nurture self-esteem. The biggest mistake is to push too hard too soon, so a slow and gentle start is important. Initially, it is best not to concentrate on goals or fitness. Help clients think of pleasurable activities that can be done in the course of the day, as part of life, and preferably without structure. "For example, gardening-hoeing, digging, pulling weeds, and pushing a lawn mower—can increase heart rates by 20 to 25%; for a sedentary person, this may be enough of a boost to improve health." (3) An occasional swim, bouncing up and down in a swimming pool, a wild dance, batting a tennis ball back and forth with a friend, hitting a racket ball against a backboard, bowling, playing catch or Frisbee with a friend. Walk the dog. Take an extra spin around the mall when shopping. Carry all the groceries from the car rather than asking for help. Take a dance class. Play with the children or dog. Rake leaves, shovel snow, push a lawn mower. Make love. Garden. . ." Gardening gets you outside and, instead of running nowhere, you end up growing something new, something alive." (4) Walk with a goal that has nothing to do with exercise. For instance, pick flowers along the way and plan to come home with a little bouquet of flowers for your dining room table. Plan some new landscaping by looking for ideas along the way. Be the judge of a contest to pick the house in the neighborhood with the best grass, cleanest windows or prettiest walkway.

Our clients need to know that every bit of activity counts and adds up to better health, especially in the beginning.

"Encourage your client not to expect improvement overnight. In fact, don't expect anything." (6) Have them compare, and possibly journal about, "their mind and body state before and after exercise. Pay attention to the sensations in the body. Hot, sweaty, breathless—these are all natural results of physical activity. With time they can learn to tolerate and even enjoy these feelings." (6)

Work with the client to adjust activity so that it meets their needs. Talk them through the specifics of their activity to visualize what they will be doing. For instance, if walking has been selected. . .where will they walk, with whom, what will they wear, what will they do when it rains, can they incorporate a walk when they shop at the mall, etc.? If playing ball with a child is the activity planned. . .when, where, with what ball, what time of day?

Encourage the use of affirmations such as, "I feel my strength when I move," "I like myself and feel easy in my body" during exercise. *Do not compliment a weight loss client based on physical size or shape. When congratulated for weight loss, what does that mean when weight is regained? Most inevitably do gain and feel worse about themselves as a result. When somebody says, "I lost weight" a response could be, "How do you feel about that?" Rather than telling someone that they are shaping up, you might say, "You look more content since you have been exercising."*

Avoid talking about fat, burning calories, losing weight or about appearance. Also, avoid talking about exercise:

1) as punishment. "Walk an extra mile to help burn off that brownie."
2) as cure: "Some extra sit-ups will help get rid of that pudge," or "If you exercise, you can have the body you want."

"Remember that fatness does not preclude fitness. Thin people aren't always fit, nor heavy people necessarily unfit. The great dancer Isadora Duncan was a 'big woman' and 200 pound Virginia Zucci, of the Russian Ballet, was famous for her pirouettes." (4) Lynne Cox, who swam the English Channel broke the women's record by three hours, the men's record by one hour, is 5'6" and 180# (and 33% body fat). The winner of the 1994 Nike Fitness Leader of the Year Award was a large women named De Dast-Hakala who teaches step aerobics and champions the cause of large women. Heavy women need to and can move as much as anyone else.

EXERCISE OBSESSION/ DEPENDENCE

You may know her. She arises each morning at 5:30, hitting the pavement before most people are even awake. She doesn't feel ready to face her day unless she does her brisk three miles. She does it, rain or shine. At work she looks forward to her lunch time trip to the fitness center, where they have a special 45-minute workout for people on their lunch break. She's glad that she can get that workout in and be back to work in just a little over an hour. After work she goes to another health club, this one closer to home. She completes one hour aerobics, a half hour on the Stairmaster and also a half hour on the Lifecycle. If, for any reason, she wasn't able to get her lunch time workout in, she'll take another aerobics class. She knows everyone at the gym and she engages in conversations during her workouts. From the outside, she appears to be a motivated, fit and happy person. Actually, she's too exhausted to go out with her friends and is increasingly alone and lonely. Her legs ache constantly, but she continues to work out despite her shin splints. Her doctor is confused by her refusal to slow down; she's usually a very compliant patient. At one point, her doctor forced her to stop exercising for a week. Her depression and anxiety were so overwhelming that she was virtually immobilized until she could get back to her workout.

Men and women such as this are presenting to counseling in increasing numbers. They tend to present not because they want to stop the compulsive activity, but because *they cannot continue*. If these exercisers were willing to take a look at what they are doing, they would find that their activity is not about performance or reshaping their bodies, but about dealing with life. They would find exercise is essential to them to provide a feeling of mental well-being, to release their tension and anger, and even relieve anxiety and depression. They also would find they have few other strategies to cope with these feelings.

While there are many terms in the literature used interchangeably with compulsive exercise, "exercise dependence" is the authors preferred term as it does not refer to a particular sport (dependence can occur to any sport), and because it classifies this behavior with other compulsive behaviors. In 1987, de Coverly Veale proposed diagnostic criteria for exercise dependence using the core features of a dependence syndrome: (7)

1) A narrowing of repartee, leading to a stereotyped pattern of exercise with a regular schedule, once or more daily;
2) Salience with the individual; giving increased priority over other activities to maintain the pattern of exercise, obviously giving up other things in life so that they can maintain their exercise;
3) Increased tolerance to the amount of exercise performed over the years;
4) Withdrawal symptoms related to a disorder of mood, following a cessation of the exercise schedule;
5) Relief or avoidance of withdrawal symptoms by further exercise;
6) Subjective awareness of a compulsion to exercise;
7) Rapid reinstatement of the previous pattern of exercise and withdrawal after a period of abstinence.

Associated features:

1) Either the individual continues to exercise despite a serious physical disorder known to be caused, aggravated, or prolonged by exercise and is advised as such by a health professional;
2) The individual has argumentative difficulties with his partner, family, friends or occupation;
3) The self-inflicted loss of weight by dieting is as a means towards improving performance.

According to de Coverly Veale, "primary exercise dependence" occurs when an individual meets all of the proposed criteria and anorexia nervosa and bulimia nervosa are ruled out. (7) Pure exercise dependence is found most often in middle-aged men in their 40's and 50's. Weight loss by dieting is seen in primary exercise dependence as a means to improve performance; however, if weight loss is too drastic, performance would be impaired, so typically weight is not allowed to drop too low.

Excessive exercise directed towards weight loss or balancing caloric intake is regarded as "secondary exercise dependence." Most often, this kind of activity involves individuals who have a primary diagnoses of an eating disorder.

The prevalence of exercise dependence is not known. Some researchers believe a relatively small percentage of men and women have a severe dependence; others feel that as many as 7% of committed exercisers are dependent on exercise. The author postulates that at least 50% of people with anorexia and bulimia deal with some form of exercise dependence.

A core feature of any dependency is the experience of negative affect when the object of dependence is removed. Glasser described the negative effect that runners experience when they are forced to forego running. Symptoms he found were: depressed mood, irritability, fatigue, anxiety, impaired concentration, sleep disturbance, guilt, tension, vague sense of discomfort. These symptoms were relieved when running was resumed. (2)

There are no conclusive studies as to why these affective withdrawal symptoms occur. Some believe these exercisers are addicted to endorphins, the morphine-like hormones secreted by the body under stress, and that withdrawal from endorphins creates the symptoms. It is the endorphin release that is thought to cause what is commonly referred to as "runner's high."

Another theory regarding exercise dependence is that exercise has become a means of coping. A person may exercise to deal with feelings (tension, stress, anger, guilt, anxiety, loneliness, etc.). Often unaware of the feelings, the dependent person simply acknowledges the drive to exercise which pushes down these feelings. Without exercise, the thoughts and feelings which have been avoided and denied flood back. Essentially, the dependent exercisers have been working out their bodies rather than their problems. Without effective coping mechanisms, they become overwhelmed and are compelled to exercise again to control unwanted feelings. What began as the pursuit of pleasure had become the avoidance of pain.

Treating the Exercise Dependent Client

Typically, compulsive activities are a source of shame and embarrassment. Not so with exercise dependence. This is not a shame-based activity. The exercisers like what they are doing. Exercise dependent clients typically present to treatment because they no longer are able to continue the exercise. Possibly their doctor requires therapy due to injury, or their partner or spouse threatens to leave if therapy is not initiated. These clients tend to be extremely resistant to exploring issues around their exercise.

If the purpose of exercise dependence is to avoid and deny the underlying feelings, anxiety and/or depression, the recovery involves identifying and dealing effectively with these feelings. Without effective coping skills, it is difficult to endure the uncomfortable feelings that arise when exercise is curtailed. An understanding friend, a skilled dietitian, exercise physiologist, or therapist may aid in the process.

Some may be ready to make changes in their exercise patterns, while others may need to stay at their current level of exercise while therapy is initiated. Their relationship with exercise will need to be challenged. An option is to ask them to make changes in their exercise program. I asked one client to wear sandals rather than walking shoes when she power walked. She returned with a very different perspective of her walking and thereafter used her ability to "chose sandals for her walk" (and go for a more relaxing walk) as an indication of the intensity of her feelings. The possibilities are endless for the creative dietitian, especially one who understands that most dependent exercisers have repetitive exercise patterns. For example, ask the client to:

1) Go the opposite direction. Run clockwise instead of counter-clockwise.
2) Change the order of the activities. Do weights first rather than last.
3) Switch activities. Swim instead of run, use a free weight for biceps rather than a machine.
4) Take a different aerobics class.
5) Wear different gear. Run in torn gym shorts rather than sleek running shorts.
6) Quit counting. How do they know when to stop?
7) Express feelings during exercise. Instead of pushing a feeling down, stay present to it while exercising. Move in such a way that the feeling is expressed. A form of aerobic dance, NIA (Non-Impact Aerobics) uses feelings expression. (1)

Frequently, the intensity, frequency or duration of exercise must be reduced. This reduction can occur over time, or can be "cold turkey." Since withdrawal symptoms are usually most intense 36 to 48 hours after ceasing exercise, I challenge clients to omit exercise for three days. I explain what they most likely will experience and help them set up a support system. This intervention often allows the client to see the impact exercise has on their lives and creates openness to pursue these issues.

Exercise dependent individuals will need to examine their belief system around exercise, health, and fitness in order to unravel cognitive distortions. The client will need to understand and accept that training daily is counterproductive, that a low percent of body fat does not necessarily make them healthier, that they will not get out of shape if they take off a day or two, that muscles need days without exercise to recover and refuel, that calories eaten will replace depleted glycogen stores which will help them perform better, or even that minimal movement can contribute to health and be considered exercise.

For instance, in a group I facilitated, a client, "Debbie," was expressing difficulty getting in touch with her feelings. A group member challenged her saying, "Well, you exercise all the time anyway" (inferring that it is difficult to get in touch with feeling when exercising frequently). Debbie disagreed with her stating she exercised "20 minutes a day." I said, "I'm confused because you come to my aerobics class, and that's a 45 minute class. Do you leave before we're finished?" "No," she said "20 minutes. The other stuff, the sit-ups, push-ups and other stuff is not really exercise." I asked her, "What is exercise?" She said, "Exercise is when you get your heart rate up." Someone else said, "You walk all the time, you walk to the store and everywhere." Debbie said, "Walking is not really exercise, because I don't get my heart rate up." We explored her beliefs, but she steadfastly maintained that she exercised only 20 minutes a day. Later, she described another group member as a person who "exercised all the time." I said, "Why is walking exercise for her, but not for you?" She laughed at this inconsistency in her thinking and was willing to discuss it. Thereafter she began to open up and explore her own relationship with exercise.

Alternative coping methods must be strengthened. Clients will need to explore a variety of coping strategies to find those with which he or she is comfortable. A consultation with an exercise physiologist familiar with exercise dependence may be helpful to outline a sound exercise program. Relaxation tapes and writing in a journal can help with feelings and anxiety that may arise. Help clients learn to enjoy movement (see section on exercise resistance).

As exercise is decreased, a client will have more time on their hands. Help your client plan activities that are nurturing and relaxing (movies or dinner with a friend, adopt and train a pet, maintain an aquarium, garden, take a slow walk on the beach, sit and watch the sunset, read a good book) to take the place of goal directed exercise.

Recovery involves learning to trust relationships, to vent feelings, to be assertive, to take risks, and to meet personal needs. Underlying conflict, previously avoided and denied, will need to be confronted and worked through. Self-image and self-esteem will need to be built in areas other than exercise. Ultimately, clients will need to learn to trust and depend on other people in their lives in order to move beyond exercise dependence.

PRINCIPALS OF EXERCISE PRESCRIPTION

An exercise prescription is a "recommended regimen of physical activity designed in a systematic and individualized manner." (8) The prescription includes frequency, intensity and duration of training, the mode of activity and the initial level of fitness. Optimally, fitness level would be determined with an exercise test in which heart rate, electrocardiogram (ECG), arterial blood pressure, and functional capacity are objectively evaluated. However, as will be discussed, in most people, an exercise test is usually not required before starting an exercise program. In any case, careful consideration should be given to the individual's health history and risk factor profile. As a nutrition therapist, if you have not taken a course in fitness evaluation or exercise physiology, consider referring your clients to an exercise physiologist or hire one to work with your clients. (See FYI on a typical client interview in sports nutrition.)

Cardio-Respiratory Fitness

Improvement in cardio-respiratory function is dependent on the intensity, duration, and frequency of the training program. The American College of Sports Medicine (ACSM) recommends the following for the enhancement of health and cardio-respiratory fitness (8):

1) Mode of activity: Any activity that uses large muscle groups that can be maintained for a prolonged period and is rhythmic and aerobic in nature, e.g., running, jogging, walking, hiking, swimming, skating, bicycling, rowing, cross-country skiing, rope skipping or various endurance games.

2) Intensity of exercise: Physical activities corresponding to 40 to 85 percent VO2 max or 55 to 90 percent of maximal heart rate. It should be noted that exercise of low-end intensity may provide important health benefits and may result in increased fitness in some persons (e.g., those who were previously sedentary and had a low fitness level).

3) Duration of exercise: 50 to 60 minutes of continuous or discontinuous aerobic activity.

4) Frequency of exercise: Three to five days per week.

5) Rate of progression: In most cases the conditioning effect allows individuals to increase the total work done per session. In continuous exercise this occurs by an increase in intensity, duration or by some combination of the two. The most significant conditioning effects may be observed during the first 6 to 8 weeks of the exercise program. The exercise prescription may be adjusted as these conditioning effects occur with the adjustment depending on participant characteristics, the exercise test results and/or exercise performance during exercise sessions.

Intensity of Exercise

Exercise intensity should be low enough to be tolerated by the participant during 20 to 60 minutes of activity, yet sufficient to induce a training effect. Various techniques can be used to prescribe and monitor exercise intensity, but for the purposes of this discussion, exercise intensity will be prescribed by heart rate.

Target heart rate range is determined by taking 60 to 80% of the difference between a maximal and a resting heart rate (HR). People in lower fitness levels should exercise closer to 60% HR max. Since determining HR max is not always possible, Katch and McArdle recommend the use of "age-adjusted maximum heart rates" (9) (See Table 11-1), by subtracting the person's age from 220.

Table 11-1   Age Adjusted Target Heart Rates

Target Heart Rate Range	Lower Limit	Upper Limit
Age of individual		
(for example, age 40)	220	220
	- 40	- 40
Age-adjusted maximal heart rate	180	180
Individual's Resting heart rate	- 60	- 60
Heart rate reserve	120	120
Conditioning intensity (60-80% HR range)	x.60	x.80
	72	96
Resting heart rate	+60	+60
Target heart rate range	132	156 beats per minute

The target heart rate range is only a guideline to follow in prescribing exercise. An individual's response to the exercise must be evaluated and the intensity altered to provide for the participant's comfort and safety while achieving a training effect. Counting the pulse for 10 seconds immediately after exercising and multiplying by six gives a good estimate of the exercise heart rate.

Increased intensity of exercise is associated with increased cardiovascular risk, orthopedic injury and decreased compliance. Therefore, programs with low to moderate intensity with longer duration are recommended. Heart rate fluctuates during exercise so intensity is prescribed in a range as in the example. Signs and symptoms of coronary artery disease (CAD) or other diseases may require exercise intensity being maintained at levels below those calculated.

Duration of Exercise Sessions

The conditioning period may vary from 20 to 60 minutes, excluding warm-up and cool down. The conditioning response is a result of the product of the intensity and the duration of the exercise. Significant cardiovascular improvements have been realized with 5 to 10 minutes of exercise that is at 90 percent of functional capacity. However, since high intensity, short duration sessions are not desirable for most participants. Better results are obtained with low intensities and longer duration. Such programs may also have a lower risk of orthopedic injury and have a higher caloric expenditure.

Frequency of Exercise Sessions

"The recommended frequency varies from several daily sessions to 3 to 5 periods per week according to the needs, interests and functional capacity of the participants." (1) For some individuals, sessions of 5 minutes duration several times a day may be desirable. Typically however, participants should exercise at least 3 times a week on alternate days. "The amount of improvement in VO2 max tends to plateau when frequency of training is increased above 3 days per week. The value of the added improvement found with training more than 5 days a week, is small to not apparent in regard to improvement in VO2 max. Training of less than 2 days a week does not generally show meaningful change in VO2 max." (1)

Rate of Progression

How quickly an individual progresses in the exercise program depends on their functional capacity, health status or age preferences, and needs or goals. Initially, exercise should include light calisthenics and low level aerobic activities, where there will be a minimum of muscle soreness and avoidance of injuries or discomfort. Initially, the aerobic conditioning phase should be at least 10 to 15 minutes. This initial stage usually lasts from 4 to 6 weeks, depending on the rate of adaptation of the participant. Somebody with a low fitness level may take as many as 10 weeks in this initial phase.

Over the next 4 to 5 months, intensity is typically increased to the target level with the duration increased every 2 to 3 weeks. Cardiac patients and less fit individuals should have more time to adapt at each stage. They may initially use discontinuous aerobic exercise and progress to more continuous aerobic exercise. The duration of exercise for these participants should be increased to 20 to 30 minutes before an increase in the intensity. After the first six months of training, the participant usually reaches a satisfactory level of cardio-respiratory fitness. Continuing the same work-out schedule will enable them to maintain fitness, although further improvement is minimal. At this point, the program can be reviewed and goals altered.

Body Composition

We know that excess body fat is harmful to health, but there are many misconceptions about the assessment and interpretation of body composition. Thinness has become a national obsession with dieting and exercise used to meet this cultural ideal. Some believe that professionals may contribute to the extreme concern with thinness by encouraging the "thinness = health" equation and by allowing those that will never be thin to believe they can become thin by following "the formula." This ignores research that indicates that people come in all shapes and sizes and that some people are genetically loaded to be larger than "normal."

Unfortunately, "professionals have frequently established targets for body composition that are unrealistically low, in terms of health benefits. Thinner is not necessarily healthier, evidenced by similar mortality risk across a wide range of body composition values. Health risk increases significantly only at the upper end of the body composition distribution." (9)

The American College of Sports Medicine states that "we should tolerate a broad range of body composition values as normal" and recommends that "intensive intervention of weight loss should be implemented in persons at the upper end of the distribution." (8) Additionally, they recommend that clinicians "should be aware of the wide range of normal values, and not encourage all participants to achieve a particular value." (8) In light of this information, we need to interpret each persons body composition individually, taking into account their clinical status and other risk factors. We may need to become more comfortable aiding our clients to health at larger weights. (See Appendix 11-A Weight Loss at Cooper Clinic.)

HERMAN

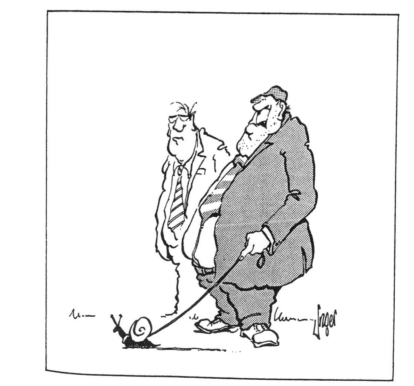

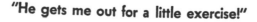

"He gets me out for a little exercise!"

Muscular Strength and Endurance

The goal of muscular strength and endurance training is to increase the strength and endurance of the muscles so that they become more efficient in dealing with every day demands placed on them, such as mowing the grass, carrying groceries and moving luggage. Strength is defined as the amount of force exerted by a muscle group for one movement. Endurance is the ability of the muscle group to maintain continuous repetitions over time. The American College of Sports Medicine recommends strength training two times a week, consisting of 8 to 10 exercises with the major muscle groups, a minimum of one set of 8 to 12 repetitions.

Muscular strength and endurance are developed by the overload principle. Muscular strength is best developed by using heavy weights (that require maximum or nearly maximum tension development) with few repetitions and muscular endurance is best developed by using lighter weights with a greater number of repetitions.

While increased frequency of training and additional sets and/or repetitions "elicit larger strength gain, the magnitude of the differences is usually small." (9) One study compared training two-days-a-week with three days a week for an 18 week time period. (10) The subjects performed one set of 7 to 10 repetitions to fatigue. The two-day-a-week group showed a 21 percent increase in strength compared to a 28 percent increase in the three-day-a-week group. In other words, 75 percent of what could be attained in a three-day-a-week program was attained in a two-day-a-week program.

Flexibility
Any exercise program should include activities that promote maintenance of good flexibility, particularly at the lower back. Stretching exercises are designed to improve and maintain range of motion in a joint or series of joints. These exercises should be performed slowly with a gradual progression to greater ranges of motion. The participant should move into the stretch slowly, hold for 10 to 30 seconds and repeat 3 to 5 times. They should not stretch to a point of significant pain. Stretching exercises should be performed at least three times a week and can be included in the warm-up and cool-down periods around the aerobic conditioning phase.

Warm-Up and Cool-Down
Each exercise session should include a warm-up of 5 to 10 minutes and a cool-down of 5 to 10 minutes. The warm-up period gradually increases the metabolic rate from the resting level to that level required for conditioning and may include walking or slow jogging, light stretching exercises and calisthenics or other types of muscle conditioning exercises. The cool-down includes exercises of diminished intensity, such as slower walking or jogging, stretching and in some cases, relaxation activities.

EVALUATION OF PARTICIPANTS PRIOR TO EXERCISE PARTICIPATION
It is important to evaluate individuals prior to exercise testing or exercise participation. Individuals are divided into three risk classifications (1):
1. Apparently healthy - those who are asymptomatic and apparently healthy with no more than one major coronary risk factor (Table 11-1).
2. Individuals at higher risk—those who have symptoms suggestive of possible cardiopulmonary or metabolic disease (Table 11-2) and/or two or more major coronary risk factors (Table 11-1).
3. Individuals with disease—those with known cardiac, pulmonary, or metabolic disease.

Table 11-1   Major Risk Factors (1)

1. Diagnosed hypertension or systolic blood pressure greater than 160 or diastolic blood pressure greater than 90 mmHg on at least two separate occasions, or on antihypertensive medication

2. Serum cholesterol greater than 6.20 mmol/L (greater than 240 mg/d)

3. Cigarette smoking

4. Diabetes mellitus*

5. Family history of coronary or other atherosclerotic disease in parents or siblings prior to age 55

---

* Persons with insulin dependent diabetes mellitus (IDDM) who are over 30 years of age, or have had IDDM for more than 15 years, and persons with non-insulin dependent diabetes mellitus who are over 35 years of age should be classified as patients with disease and treated according to the guidelines for those people who fit in Table 2.

Table 11-2   Major Symptoms or Signs Suggestive of Cardiopulmonary or Metabolic Disease.** (1)

1. Pain or discomfort in the chest or surrounding areas that appears to be ischemic in nature

2. Unaccustomed shortness of breath or shortness of breath with mild exertion

3. Dizziness or syncope

4. Orthopnea/paroxysmal nocturnal dyspnea

5. Ankle edema

6. Palpitations or tachycardia

7. Claudication

8. Known heart murmur

**These symptoms must be interpreted in the clinical context in which they appear, since they are not all specific for cardiopulmonary or metabolic disease.

Recommendations

"No set of guidelines on exercise testing and participation can cover every conceivable situation." (8) The American College of Sports Medicine provides the following recommendation in an attempt to provide some general guidance: (8)

Apparently Healthy Individuals   Apparently healthy individuals can begin moderate (intensities of 40 to 60 percent VO2 max) exercise programs (such as walking or increasing usual daily activities) without the need of exercise testing or medical examination, as long as the exercise program begins and proceeds gradually and as long as the individual is alert to the development of unusual signs and symptoms. (9) To classify moderate exercise, it must be within the individual's current capacity and be able to be sustained comfortably for a prolonged period, for example, 60 minutes.

Prior to beginning a vigorous exercise program, men over 40 and women over 50 should have a medical examination and a maximal exercise test. Vigorous exercise (intensity greater than 60 percent VO2 max) is defined as exercise intense enough to represent a substantial challenge and results in significant increases in heart rate and respiration. It usually can not be sustained by untrained individuals for more than 15 to 20 minutes.

Individuals at Higher Risk   An exercise stress test prior to beginning a vigorous exercise program is desirable for higher risk individuals of any age. Individuals at higher risk are those with two or more major coronary risk factors (Table 11-1) and/or symptoms suggestive of cardiopulmonary or metabolic disease or who fit the diabetes guidelines. For those without symptoms, an exercise test or medical examination may not be necessary if moderate exercise is undertaken gradually with appropriate guidance and no competitive participation. Maximal exercise tests in patients at high risks should be physician supervised.

Individuals with Disease   Persons of any age with symptoms suggestive of coronary, pulmonary or metabolic disease should have a medical examination and a physician supervised maximal exercise test prior to beginning an exercise program.

Summary

Recommendations should be made in the context of participant's needs, goals and initial abilities. In this regard, a sliding scale as to the amount of time allotted and intensity of effort should be carefully gauged for both the cardio-respiratory and muscular strength and endurance components of the program. An appropriate warm-up and cool-down, which would include flexible exercises, is also recommended. The important factor is to design a program for the individual, to provide the proper amount of physical activity and to attain maximal benefit at the lowest risk. Emphasis should be placed on factors that result in permanent lifestyle change and encourage a lifetime of physical activity.

"Exercise should be done neither as a punishment for looking bad nor as a necessary evil for looking good. It's a gift you give yourself because you need and deserve it. So start playing to play, instead of to win, and you'll find yourself in a no-lose situation. Dinah Shore once said, 'I've never thought of participating in sports just for the sake of exercise, or as a means to lose weight . . . or because it was a social fad. I really enjoy playing. It's a vital part of my life.' " (4)

REFERENCES

1. American College of Sports Medicine. *The Recommended Quantity and Quality of Exercise for Developing and Maintaining Cardiorespiratory and Muscular Fitness in Healthy Adults.* Position Stand. Indianapolis: 1990.
2. Glasser W. *Positive Addiction.* New York: Harper & Row; 1976.
3. White F, White T. *Treating Overweight and Emotional Overeating Disorders.* Santa Barbara, CA: Handouts from workshop; Sept. 1994.
4. Ornstein R, Sobel D. *Healthy Pleasures.* New York: Addison-Wesley Publishing Company; 1989.
5. Leon AS, Connett J, Jacobs DR, et al, Leaisure time physical activity levels and risk of coronary heart disease and death. *J of Amer Medical Assoc.* 1987; 258: 2388-2395.
6. Freedman R. *BodyLove: Learning to Like Our Looks and Ourselves.* New York: Harper & Row; 1989.
7. de Coverley Veale DM. *Exercise Dependence.* British Journal of Addiction. 1987; 82(7):735-740.
8. American College of Sports Medicine. *Guidelines for Exercise Testing and Prescription.* Philadelphia: Lea & Febiger; 1992.
9. McArdle WD, Katch FI, Katch VL. *Exercise Physiology: Energy, Nutrition, and Human Performance.* Philadelphia: Lea & Febiger; 1992.
10. Braith RW, Graves JE, Pollock ML, Leggett SL, Carpenter DM, Colvin AB. Comparison of two versus three days per week of variable resistance training during 10 and 18 week programs. Int. *J Sports Med.* 1989;10: 450-454.

ADDITIONAL READING

Benyo R. *The Exercise Fix.* Champaign, IL: Leisure Press; 1990.
Gavin J. *The Exercise Habit.* Champaign, IL: Leasure Press; 1992.
Prussin R, Harvey P, DiGeronimo T. *Hooked on Exercise.* New York: Fireside/Parkside—Simon & Schuster; 1992.
Yates A. *Compulsive Exercise and the Eating Disorders.* New York: Brunner/Mazel, Inc.; 1992.

FOR YOUR INFORMATION

Typical Sports Nutrition Consultation

Kathy King Helm, RD, LD

The client is a 17-year-old female named Mandy. She is a senior at Central High School and the best player on the Girl's Basketball Team. Last year she blew out both knees and has spent the remainder of the time in rehabilitation under the supervision of a personal trainer. Mandy has the ability to get a college scholarship in basketball if this year goes well for her. Her mother called for an appointment because Mandy gained about 30 pounds this past year and needs to get it off without jeopardizing her basketball season which opens in four weeks.

Mandy is 5'5" at 174 # and 27% body fat. She appears stocky and solid in build. She is an only child and her father was a good athlete and professional football player. He has been her coach since she was four years old, but now they argue too much for him to coach her. Her mother is overweight, but very conscious about what to buy and prepare for meals. She wants to support Mandy and yet put the responsibility to eat well on Mandy's shoulders. Mandy is an honor student.

Mandy has a personal trainer who has helped her regain her strength and agility since her injuries. She works out six days per week, usually for 2-4 hours total in a variety of aerobic, flexibility, and strength routines.

Mandy goes to basketball practice an hour before school starts and can't practice with breakfast in her stomach. School lunch is either the hot meal, which she seldom eats, or a salad bar with 3/4 cup of dressing and four crackers. Afternoon snacks are usually with team members at a fast food restaurant and consists of burritos, hamburgers or pizza, fries, malts or colas. The evening meal is lighter because she works out three nights per week for two hours with her trainer and works out on her own or with team members the other two evenings. Weekends are "pig-outs" with her friends.

Therapist: "Mandy, I am really proud of you and what you have accomplished. By working together we can help you lose weight and still stay strong for basketball. Are you willing to change how you eat if we make it reasonable?"

Mandy: "Sure. I've had a really hard year mentally and physically. This time last year the doctor said I'd never play again and I knew I'd prove him wrong. But I went through hell last spring when my second knee went out. I didn't know if I could handle the pain again, but I did. I ate too much when I couldn't exercise and I've only lost 6# since starting with my trainer."

Mandy's Mom: "We really pulled back and let her make up her own mind about everything. She wants to play basketball again and her doctor and trainer say she's stronger than before. I think I buy the right foods at home, but she doesn't always eat at home."

Therapist: "I agree. Her food records show she eats well at home. Mandy, it's common for athletes to gain weight when they stop exercising. Later when you started rehab and working with your trainer, weight from increased muscle mass could cover up weight loss from burned off fat. Tell me, have you ever had to lose weight in the past?"

Mandy: "The people in our family are not petite. I've always been a jock, so I never had to worry about gaining weight. So this is my first official 'diet.' "

Therapist: "Instead of calling it a 'diet,' think of it as learning how to eat again. You have to eat enough calories to support the training you do each day, but you will be eating less than you used to, so you will be losing weight. Let's start with breakfast. What are you willing to eat after practice but before school starts?"

Mandy: "I don't have time then, but I have study hall first hour and I can eat there."

Therapist: "Are you willing to try a granola bar, dry cereal, fruit, or little box of juice? You need more liquids and carbohydrates after practice."

Mandy: "I can do that."

Therapist: "Lunch is a really good time to get more food and liquids stored for afternoon practice. It's no wonder that you are starved later on and over eat with just a salad for lunch—and a very high fat one at that. What kind of lunch are you willing to bring from home?"

Mandy: "I will eat a peanut butter sandwich or ham. That's about it."

Therapist: "What about fresh fruit? (Nothing I have to peel.) You mentioned yogurt on your food record. Will you take yogurt or drink low fat milk?"

Mandy: "I can buy milk there or I can take yogurt with a sandwich."

The discussion continued until Mandy had identified what she would eat on school days. During basketball season Mandy often skipped meals on the weekend and slept in or ate out. She was willing to eat more regularly at home in order to better maintain her energy and fluid intake while she loses weight.

Therapist: "Mandy, your mom seems to know what to buy and how to prepare lower fat meals. That's what an athlete needs: a diet high in fruits, vegetables, grains, and fluids; lower in fat; and moderate amounts of protein. Your diet has been very high in fat. I will give you this sheet where I've written down what we've agreed upon for meal ideas, but can you give me an idea of what you plan to eat each day?"

Mandy remembered what to eat and even added a few new selections.

Therapist: "That's great! I want you to keep a written record for me and bring it next week along with your training schedule. We'll talk about how to eat on the day of competition next week. Please call me if either of you have any questions before we meet again."

Mandy: "My basketball coach has some muscle building powder he wants me to take, but mom wants you to see it first."

Therapist: "No problem. Either drop the product information by this week or bring it next time. This week I want you to do the best you can. You will be getting yourself ready for this year's basketball season through your efforts. Time is short right now, but I don't want you to be too rigid with yourself. I want you to enjoy eating, but just change some of what you eat. How does that sound?"

Mandy: "I can live with that. My dad just took a job out of town, so I think it will be easier to do this now. He won't be back until Thanksgiving."

Therapist: "Is your dad concerned about your weight?"

Mandy: "He makes fun of overweight women. He always yells at me when I come off the court when I play a game because he wants me to play better. I'm already the best player on the team."

Mandy's Mom: "Her dad is getting better. I tell him that if he loves me and Mandy, he will love us no matter what size we are, and he agrees. In fact he is getting a stomach himself."

Therapist: "You said earlier that your dad was an athlete and professional ball player. That could make him overly concerned about looking fit. By the time he sees you in several months, your season should be in full swing and your weight will be coming down. You appear to be relaxed and confident. Is that true?"

Mandy: "I feel a lot older than I did last year. Kids are coming to me for advice. The quarterback had to go through a similar operation to mine a month ago and I called him up to tell him what to expect. We're sort of friends now."

Therapist: "You never know how life works, but it sounds like you have really grown from your knee experience. You sound like you will be OK whether basketball is your whole life or not."

Mandy: "I didn't believe I was important without basketball but now I do."

Mandy's Mom: "We've become much closer after this year. . . .Thank you for seeing us."

Therapist: "I have thoroughly enjoyed myself and I look forward to seeing you next week."

Appendix 11-A

Weight Loss Program at Cooper Clinic

Georgia Kostas, MPH, RD, LD, Director of Nutrition, Cooper Clinic, Dallas, TX

For 16 years weight loss counseling at the Cooper Clinic has involved individual and group counseling with a registered dietitian and often a team approach with a physician, exercise physiologist and psychologist. The mainstay of the Kostas/ Cooper weight loss philosophy is that each client receives an individualized eating program that is livable, workable, practical, flexible, and based upon the needs, goals, lifestyle and personality of that client.

Weight loss clients meet with a registered dietitian on a regular basis either weekly or bi-weekly for six or 12 weeks, or whatever length of time is needed to accomplish the goals. During this time the dietitian may refer the client to another team member for more specific assistance. It is absolutely critical that the client feels involved, feels accepted, and does not feel criticized or deprived. Therefore, if the client wants to include specific foods such as chocolate, ice cream or hamburgers, those foods are part of the eating plan.

When the guilt of eating is removed, the emotional release and positive response a patient enjoys empowers him or her to move forward to achieve positive results in losing and managing weight. To achieve any permanent lifestyle changes, the client must feel his or her particular needs are met, problems are addressed and solutions found. Also, the client must feel the barriers to change have been identified along with solutions on how to remove those barriers. With workable strategies, attainable goals, and multiple options the involved patient takes charge and stays motivated. Getting the client involved in the solutions to his problems has lifetime rewards, including learning to problem-solve in other areas of his or her life.

Typical Program

A consult begins with a nutrition assessment and evaluation, which includes a diet/weight loss questionnaire, medical questionnaire, lab work, body composition measurements, and analysis of a three-day food record mailed in before the appointment. In most instances the client is at the Clinic for a day-long, medical physical, and that is why so much information is available for the initial consultation, which lasts just 45 minutes because of the large number of clients that must be seen each day.

Rather than cover the myriad of nutrition issues that may apply, the dietitian "zeros in" on three or four key factors that will make the greatest impact on the client's ability to lose weight successfully. The concept clients find most enlightening and encouraging is "little things add up to make a big difference." One of our most effective teaching tools is our Eating Out brochure that describes a typical meal at a restaurant (Italian, Mexican, Steak House, and so on) versus healthier selections. The client learns that most restaurant meals contain 1500-2000 kilocalories, but with new choices the meal can be as satisfying at half the calories.

Although the dietitian does not provide individualized exercise prescriptions, each client is given the Cooper Clinic recommendations for exercising aerobically 30-45 minutes, 3-5 days a week, and strength training 20-30 minutes, 2-3 times per week. It is emphasized that exercise lowers body fat, increases lean body mass, increases metabolic rate and reduces inches, which can be powerful motives for adding exercise.

The next step is to develop the specific eating plan using the five different approaches described in *The Balancing Act Nutrition and Weight Guide* workbook used by weight loss clients, if needed. The five approaches include:

1. KISS or Keep It Simple System, based on low-fat, high-fiber eating and using the new USDA Pyramid Guide
2. Fat gram plan
3. Food Group (Exchanges) plan
4. Two-week set of fixed menus using exchanges for those people who don't want to think about what to do
5. Mix and Match Meal Plan, for busy people who want to eat-on-the-run and select meals at a glance; there are 20 menus for each of the three meals a day, which combine to approximately 1000-1500 kcal per day and 20-30 grams of fat.

As success is based upon the long-term, not quick-fix philosophy, we encourage clients to commit to permanent changes by signing up for a six or 12-week follow up series. At each of these 30 minute sessions, we discuss activities and problems of the previous week, expected new or stressful situations that will occur or any other item of special concern. Also at this time, one of 10 educational units on behavioral habit changes that are imperative to long term weight loss are presented and discussed.

Measures of Success

Our clients' most successful tools for weight loss are:

- written food records (reviewed with the dietitian at each session)
- regular exercise
- accountability to a health professional who provides support and encouragement

What ultimately helps a person become successful is the friendly, caring, personalized service received by the client from the dietitian and also from all the support staff, e.g. the receptionist, the personal greeting at the door, and the person taking payment. Positive interactions and encouragement are essential for the patient's sense of acceptance and enthusiasm to proceed with a very challenging course.

Case Study

Ted was a distraught businessman who had gained 25 pounds in the last year while he exercised consistently and counted calories. After intense questioning, he stated that he traveled a lot by air for his company. He didn't eat the meals on the plane and only drank water! On further investigation, he casually revealed, "If I have anything at all, it's just a bag of peanuts." My eyes lit up.

"How many bags?"

"Just three bags per flight."

"How many flights per week?"

"Just six."

"How many weeks?"

"Fifty."

"300 calories per flight x six flights per week x 50 weeks per year = 90,000 calories or 25 pounds!!"

Give clients encouragement, hope and simple, practical tools to achieve their goals.

RESOURCE

Kostas G. *The Balancing Act Nutrition & Weight Guide*. Dallas, TX: Georgia Kostas; 1994.

12
Group Process
Kathy King Helm, RD, LD

After reading this chapter, the reader will be able to:
- [ ] list the six components of the group process
- [ ] describe the steps (dimensions) of the group process
- [ ] identify at least two advantages of group counseling
- [ ] identify at least two disadvantages of group counseling
- [ ] define the roles and responsibilities of the facilitator

---

Working with clients in groups can be challenging as well as rewarding. Traditionally, nutritionist have used groups when teaching multiple clients about a nutrition topic like diabetes, sports nutrition, breast feeding, or weight loss. Group instruction to learn new skills, such as menu planning, low fat meal preparation and stress management, can be as effective as individual instruction if careful attention is given to classroom plans or workshop designs and *sufficient practice in the skill* being taught is provided. (1,2,3) Group instruction can also be a useful preface to individual counseling. This allows the general information to be given to a group followed by more focus and implementation in individual therapy. Counseling a group of clients is different than teaching a group or counseling one-on-one.

When teaching a nutrition topic, interchange of information between the leader and participants usually is limited and traveling in one direction—from the leader to the group. The information usually is the same for all group members with only abbreviated comments to members with different needs.

Counseling in a group setting is time saving when compared to individual counseling. You can see 10 patients in little more time than it takes to counsel one person. It is cost effective in that you can generate more revenue in a shorter period of time and your patients usually save money because they pay less for a group meeting than for individual counseling. Group settings are more social with more opportunity to have various viewpoints and problem-solving opportunities.

In case it sounds easy to make more money by seeing patients in groups, counselors will tell you it's not. Acting as a group facilitator is not a job that should be taken lightly. The facilitator's effectiveness depends on adequate and frequently, extensive preparation, careful diagnosis, planning, knowledge, and always, consideration of alternatives. (4)

Group members often arrive with very different expectations, different behavioral and psychological needs, and different communication styles. Instead of having one person to help and one personality and family problem to deal with, you may have 10. One member may feel, as facilitator, you pay too much attention to other members. Another may feel your questions or the discussion are too personal. One person in the group may refer all his or her friends to your program and another in the same group may drop out after the second session due to disappointment.

Brownell reported in 1984 that group therapy (in behavioral weight loss programs) (5) was more successful than individual counseling in helping patients achieve their goals. Some people and problems, such as those that need social acceptance and peer support, respond well in groups if the group is a good match. However, other people need and respond to the individual support and close rapport established with their personal therapist. Human dynamics make it difficult to generalize about something so complex.

Group Therapy
Group therapy is where individuals with similar nutrition-related problems come together to work through those problems. Instead of the therapist working with only one client at a time while the others look on, the group becomes a means for testing reality, a taste of the real society, an accumulation of the personalities and problems that occur on the outside. (4) Of course,

many of the components used in nutrition education lectures like basic physiology, diet therapy, food changes and taste testing may be incorporated in therapy sessions, but they do not constitute the majority of the program.

Group therapy members discover that the group has the capacity to support and love and to provide a release for anger. Group therapy usually attracts a population less severely disturbed or at less nutritional risk than those that require intense, individualized care. As a therapist, you may decide that for some patients, joining a nutrition support group may be an important part of their therapy, especially for patients with eating disorders who have pulled away from interaction with other people. For some patients, the group involvement may come after seeing a nutrition therapist individually or it may be suggested as the first mode of treatment.

A confrontation group is a type of group therapy used to confront group members with honest views about themselves, which can be disconcerting and even traumatic for some individuals. This approach began as an alternative with hard-core drug addicts and alcoholics where, unless change occurred immediately, a self-destructive cycle of events would continue. The confrontation approach is based on the assumption that a person needs to be shaken out of previous patterns, awakened from his lethargy, and made to face his own self-created realities. (4) Taken to an extreme this type of therapy can be terrorizing. Once a person recognizes his misperceptions, there must be follow-up to make sure new, more positive behaviors are internalized. Using this type of therapy exclusively is highly controversial, but if one works in drug and alcohol rehabilitation centers, you may see patients who have recently gone through a similar experience.

Group Process

Good group process is the series of actions or operations that lead toward growth (or success) in a group therapy setting. It is aided by humor, as well as sensitivity, participation, experience, risk and openness. (3,6)

* Humor breaks the tension and helps people share common pleasurable moments. Clients remember things more easily that occur in humorous settings. (3)
* Each member of the group must be sensitive to the needs and feelings of others in the group. While it is part of the group process to challenge and to probe, this must be done in a nonthreatening , nonderogatory manner.
* Active participation by every member of the group is the backbone of good group process.
* Experience is the key to learning in the small group setting. It does not refer to the experience that each person brings to the groups but instead what each person learns and practices.
* A successful group experience means that the group members feel support as they try new, potentially uncomfortable ways of thinking and acting. They may risk changing relationships, comfortable habits and familiar ways of eating.
* Group members must be willing to be open with each other, to admit their deficiencies, to share their ideas, and to let the group profit from their knowledge and experience.

Group therapy involves the same basic dimensions as the one-on-one approach including the following dimensions of group process: (1, 7)

Step 1: Establish a productive counselor/ participant relationship.

This includes establishing rapport with warmth, empathy, and an atmosphere of genuineness. There must be a feeling of trust in order to promote openness and interpersonal communication. Sessions might start with humor, an open-ended question, or an interesting shared experience. Initially, the facilitator should plan some "get acquainted" exercises to help group members get to know each other.

It is important to establish the "ground rules" for the group in the first session. Some facilitators prefer to come up with the rules as a group, others informally offer suggestions, and others pass out a written list that they ask members to commit to and sign. Rules usually consist of such things as: effort will be made to attend every class, all group conversation and sharing will be kept confidential, members agree to participate in discussions, and so on.

Step 2: Balance the facilitator generated and group generated information.

This step includes balancing the didactic nutrition information offered by the facilitator with problem-identification and real-life challenges identified through collaboration and interaction with group members. The facilitator helps members explore the causes and contributing factors to problem behaviors and thoughts. Together, group members and the facilitator may help another member confront irrational beliefs.

Step 3: Design problem-solving strategies.

The facilitator must limit use of directive statements (telling members what to do to solve their problems) and use more nondirective statements (facilitating members to decide for themselves what to do). Group members should be encouraged to become sources of problem-solving ideas. Use role playing, solving typical scenarios, personal experiences, and exploration to come up with ways to take care of old problems.

Step 4: Provide the opportunity for group members to practice new skills.

In Step 3 the person develops a cognitive understanding of the new skills or behaviors. Real learning occurs during the practice sessions. Practice should first take place in the group setting to assure that everyone understands what to do (for example, what to say or do the next time his favorite high calorie snack is offered). The facilitator can ask members to pair off or divide into whatever size group is most appropriate in order to practice the new skill. As each person practices what to say, the other group members offer suggestions, and learn along with him. At subsequent meetings, group members report back on their successes and new challenges encountered while using the skill in "real life."

Step 5: Use positive role models and good pacing to keep the group motivated.

Because the purpose of the group session is to help people overcome their problem thoughts and behaviors, the facilitator should sufficiently acknowledge the positive changes that all members are making. It is not unusual, however, to have someone in a group who reports trying hard but still can't succeed (at losing weight, controlling blood sugar level, or whatever). The facilitator should acknowledge the problem and spend approximately the same time with that person as with anyone. If the person is in denial or obviously needs more time, the facilitator should ask the person to stay later for more personal attention (so the class can continue for the benefit of the majority). This suggestion will usually satisfy the person and keep the rest of the group from getting frustrated.

Step 6: Ask for evaluation and feedback.

This step should be an on-going process whenever the facilitator tries a new strategy or technique with a group. He or she might ask, "Did it work for you to role play today?" or, "What have you learned since we started that has helped you the most (or least)?"

Advantages of Groups

Clients usually rank peer support as the most helpful aspect of groups. A group can help its members feel accepted, loved, and "not alone" in facing whatever common nutrition-related concerns they have. The shared experiences and problem-solving may help a member cope or change thoughts and behaviors more than didactic information does. Groups provide an economical way for clients to afford long-term therapy.

From the therapist's point of view, groups are often dynamic and stimulating, which can add challenge and professional satisfaction. They are a good way to reach a larger number of clients in a shorter time and to generate good revenue for the time invested.

Disadvantages of Groups

Group therapy is not for everyone and group process is not always effective. Group members are sometimes uncomfortable disclosing personal information in a group setting. It's easier to "get lost" in a group and never really deal with your problems because the facilitator's time is limited. While trying to help one or more members, a lot of time can be spent on topics and problems unrelated to the needs of others in the group.

In an individual consultation, the patient and therapist only have one other person to establish rapport with in order to progress into the therapy process. Group members have the opportunity to develop multiple alliances, which can be positive or stressful, depending upon who is in the group. In the group setting even one very negative or overbearing member can make the group sessions trying for everyone.

ROLE OF FACILITATOR

Facilitating a nutrition therapy group is often challenging and it sometimes tests your inner strength. It may call upon your best counseling and interpersonal skills. The person in this position is expected to serve several well defined roles like meeting organizer, contact person, interactive facilitator, and at times, nutrition authority, but most importantly the person is expected to exercise good judgment.

The facilitator is responsible for the following: (6,7)
- organizing the group and establishing a comfortable atmosphere;
- keeping the group focused and productive;
- monitoring the discussion and keeping any records;
- stimulating exploration and self-discovery by group members;

- offering strategies for cognitive and behavioral change;
- acting as a nutrition resource for food choices, menu planning, new food products, and diet therapy questions;
- maintaining control of the therapy situation, which may include keeping interaction between participants nonthreatening, emotionally or physically, or making sure participants act and speak civil to one another, or removal of a disruptive participant.

Although some facilitators demand food records and perfect attendance as requirements for adult group participation, this philosophy is not consistent with adult learning principles because it treats the adult as a child. Keeping food records and regular attendance are considered very effective behavior change tools, but establishing and maintaining rapport and respect are far more important. By showing concern for a client and his or her needs, the facilitator reinforces that the person is more important than his or her weight or other problem. Through mutual problem-solving and breaking tasks into smaller steps the person feels supported, empowered and, in return, often commits to the process and the group effort.

A facilitator should not take it personally if a group member uses the group as a social outlet, as long as he or she isn't disruptive to the progress of the group. It may be that the group serves other needs for that person.

Group members often look to the facilitator as a role model. Therefore, the group will watch closely how the facilitator handles stress, how he or she sets boundaries, how situations that demand assertiveness or flexibility are handled, and whether the facilitator practices what he or she preaches.

ROLE OF GROUP MEMBERS

The members have the responsibility to participate actively in the discussions of the group. However, a member may say at anytime, "I don't have anything to add," or, "I want to listen longer before I comment." Members must be willing to both give and accept constructive criticism, and be willing to practice new skills outside of class time.

Members assume many roles in a group therapy setting. Three types of roles surface as the group handles different problems: task roles, group maintenance roles and individual roles. (4)

Task roles help a group achieve its explicit goals for action:
- the "initiator" discusses what could be done or how to approach a problem;
- the "information source" may add what others have tried or what he has tried;
- the "opinion" person may agree or disagree with what is being offered;
- the "elaborator" will take what has been said and add new insights;
- the "coordinator" will clarify the various suggestions and prioritize them;
- the "critic" or "evaluator" will question facts as presented and assess whether the task is feasible;
- the "energizer" will prod the group to action;
- the "procedural technician" knows where and how to find resources to complete the task.

As a group member at times yourself, it may be easy to recognize yourself in many of these roles. As mentioned earlier, these roles are used to complete a group task.

Group maintenance roles focus on the personal relations among members in a group. They help a group to work together.
- the "encourager" may ask for additional examples or ask if others have similar opinions;
- the "supporter" may agree with others and offer commendations;
- the "harmonizer" may attempt to mediate differences between members or points of view or relieve tension with a joke;
- a "gatekeeper" may ask someone who has not spoken in a while if he or she has anything to add.

Individual roles meet only that person's needs, which are irrelevant to any group task or in helping the group work as a unit. Individual-centered behavior may be aside jokes, personal attacks, bragging about something not related to what the group is working on, and so on. This behavior often induces similar behavior from other group members, which may disrupt the group process.

Some strategies for dealing with disruptive members include: (7)
- use of reflective listening skills: you might say, "Jim, something about the topic of eating meals at home as a child seems to make you uncomfortable and want to change the subject;"
- use of assertiveness skills by the facilitator: you might say, "Terry, I want to hear about your trip too, but please hold it until after group session," or, "Marie, before you take the discussion in another direction, it's only fair that other group members have a chance to speak about their experiences;"
- encouraging all group members to return to the discussion at hand: you might say, "OK, OK, that was a great joke, but I want us all to return to our topic of how you handle stress without eating;"
- removal of the disruptive participant from the group (a very last resort—do this privately if possible).

Why People Join or Leave Groups
Some of the factors that increase the attractiveness of a group: (4)

- Cooperation. A cooperative relationship is more attractive than a competitive one.
- Interaction. Increased interaction among members may increase the attractiveness of the group. People usually want to make friends and hear other points of view, not just sit in a group listening to a lecture.
- Size. Smaller groups are usually more attractive than very large ones. In a smaller group that is still large enough to function well, people become closer, support the cause better, and have a sense of being a significant participant. Six to 12 people is usually the range for more effective group participation.
- Success. Members are more inclined to join groups or continue in groups that are successful or prestigious. The more prestige a person has within the group, or may attain while in the group, the more attractive the group.

It stands to reason that the factors people often cite for leaving a group are the opposite of those listed above. Also, the member's needs or his perception of the group may change or a close friend in the group may stop coming. Usually as long as there is more attraction for the group than negative force against it, the person will stay.

SETTING THE STAGE FOR SUCCESS
It is very important when you plan a therapy group you take into consideration a number of factors:

- *Choose a location that is convenient for the members.* Consider going to a community center with ample parking if your hospital's meeting room is down a maze of hallways in a basement or parking is expensive. In private practice, ask to use a conference room or waiting room after hours when no one else is there if your office is too small.
- *Consider the target group's characteristics when determining the time for the class.* If most of the members will be retired, a daytime class may be more convenient. If the class will be mostly working people, an evening class or maybe early Saturday morning might work. If you don't know which time or day is best, ask the people who call to sign up for the class. If everyone wants Tuesday night and you don't want 25 people in the group, consider offering an early group from 5:30-6:30 PM and another from 7:00-8:00 PM on Tuesday.
- *Consider asking for the class fee by the first session.* This practice will ensure better attendance on the part of the members and better attendance is often equated with better compliance and outcomes. A deposit may be paid in advance to secure the place in the group with the balance paid at the first session. If the therapist takes credit cards, debit slips may be signed in advance to pay for the group in three equal payments. For on-going groups, practitioners usually ask for a monthly payment in advance and some offer a discount if the person pays for three months or so in advance.
- *Don't allow your classes to be too large.* In an informal survey of dietitians who work with groups, six to 12 people is the maximum number they usually allow in a therapy group. Nutrition instruction groups to teach new skills and a body of information with limited interaction may have 15 to 100 people.
- *Consider assessing and/or instructing each member on an individualized regime before the group begins in order to better meet each member's needs.*
- *Don't allow new members to join a week or two late*, or, if you do, or if the group is on-going, take the time to nurture them and bring them into the group so they feel comfortable.
- *Dietitians are not interchangeable.* Each has different skills and abilities. Do not let whoever is working late on Tuesday run the groups. Choose the best person for the job. Group members do not like rotating facilitators. Market the person for the job and let that person be known for her or his skill.
- *It is a misconception to believe that your one hour class gives you rights to a member's whole evening or afternoon.* Start the groups on time (within five minutes of the scheduled time) and end the sessions within 10 minutes of the scheduled time unless you ask for permission to continue some important issue. Members appreciate facilitators who are organized and on time.
- *Make sure the environment is as conducive to good group process as if you were counseling one-on-one.* There should be sufficient sturdy, comfortable chairs usually placed in a circle (children are used to classroom style, but adults want it more informal); good temperature control; adequate lighting; and beverage service, especially if an exercise component is offered before or after therapy.
- *Always prepare for the group sessions and be responsive.* If you offered to look something up for a member at the last session, follow through on your word. If you offered to speak to members in between sessions if they call your office, return the phone calls.

Interactive Techniques to Try

There are a number of techniques to try that will increase member involvement or learning. It often helps to ask members to break into smaller groups to give time to problem-solve or practice a new behavior or skill.

Posting on a flip chart or blackboard is a good way to show the results of small group interaction or group brainstorming. A large number of options can be prioritized by having each member number his or her top five choices. It can help increase idea visibility, stimulate discussion, and focus attention. This method can be overused, however, and it will never save a poorly prepared or unskilled facilitator. (4)

Role playing is most effective in helping participants experience reality instead of just talking about it. They use scripts, so time must be allowed for becoming familiar with the words, getting into character, and practicing with the other actors. Because scripts are used, roles can be replayed with different interpretations. Observers are asked to take notes and gather details to be used in later discussion. After the scene is played, the discussion enlarges from individual player's reactions to implications or alternatives for that situation. (4) Then observers are asked to comment.

Sociodrama or psychodramas are acted out without formal written scripts. In a sociodrama, group members will be asked to act as people in a social situation, i.e., a working mother, a father, and a teenage daughter discussing how each can contribute to making meals more nutritious and less time-consuming. In a psychodrama, group members volunteer problems they want to work on such as how to better handle a spouse's temper at mealtime or food that is always being offered in the lounge at work. The member who suggested the problem may play a part or he or she may choose just to observe. Members who observe may offer suggestions or act out alternative solutions. Both techniques can help members see new alternatives to handling old or anticipated problems.

Replay drama is like to those above, but it differs in that group members replay a real situation or incident that did not go well in order to explore what could have been said or done instead.

Role reversal is used to illustrate how well one person perceives and understands another. Group members may be asked to assume the mannerisms and point of view of the person across the table, or on the other side of an argument. It is ideal for opening stalled communication and/ or when two people see each other as being totally wrong on an issue.

POTENTIAL PROBLEMS WITH GROUPS

Although many problems and their solutions have already been discussed, here are a few others: (6)

The sluggish group. Sometimes groups just don't know where to begin or how to work together. As the facilitator, resist stepping in and carrying the whole conversation. Try asking more open-ended questions to stimulate conversation or use more "get acquainted" exercises like interviewing a partner and reporting interesting information back to the group about that person.

The hostile group. Sometimes individuals in a group blow up at each other or more subtly, allow distrust or anger to fester, which may show up as one or more members withdrawing from group participation. When hostilities occur, the air must be cleared either in front of the group if that is appropriate or in private with the involved parties. *Don't proceed with business as usual because it won't happen. Deal with the problem in a nonjudgmental way. Don't take sides or become personally involved.*

The timid member. A more timid or submissive member may have the most to contribute to the discussion, but be unwilling to fight for equal time. The facilitator should be alert to members and how often they contribute to the discussion. A simple statement like, "Jane, do you have anything to add from your experience?" will provide the member a chance to speak.

The domineering member. A certain amount of dominance by one or more members is common in any group, but if the person assumes the authority role for the group, the group process fails. A facilitator may encourage challenges by other members to what is being said, or ask other members if they have had similar experiences or other solutions in an effort to draw them back into the discussion.

Silence serves a purpose. Don't jump in and break each period of silence. Sometimes everyone needs time to reflect upon what they have just heard or to formulate new thoughts. Stay patient and relaxed. Periods of silence do not reflect poorly on the facilitator. You are not there to keep the troops entertained!

SUMMARY

If a group that comes together actively supports its members while they seek new behaviors and answers, the group process is considered successful. Group therapy can be challenging, stimulating, and productive. It takes practice, supervised training, and experience to act as a facilitator and do it well. If you want to conduct groups, join other therapy groups and see how other facilitators handle the group dynamics and process. If you have a lot of individual counseling skill, consider co-conducting a therapy group with another therapist with group experience (psychologist, psychiatrist, psychiatric social worker, nurse specialist, health behaviorist, etc.). When considering all of the components of successful group process, don't lose sight of the ultimate goal: to help group members achieve outcomes that improve their health and quality of life. (See FYI on page 214 on Residential/Group Centers for Weight and Health Management.)

LEARNING ACTIVITIES

1. Observe a group nutrition counseling/ education session with at least 10 participants.
   a. What roles/responsibilities did the facilitator exhibit?
   b. Identify the "group maintenance roles" you observed.
   c. What interactive techniques were observed?
   d. How would you improve this particular group session?
2. Interview a group nutrition counselor/facilitator.
   a. What/how are the ground rules established?
   b. What are his/her expectations for group member participation?
   c. What do they perceive as their role in the group process?
   d. How are groups planned?
   e. How are groups evaluated?

REFERENCES

1. Ivey A, Authier J. *Microcounseling*. Springfield, IL: Charles C. Thomas; 1978.
2. Hearn M. Three modes of training counselors: A comparative study. Unpublished dissertation. London, Ontario: Univ. of Western Ontario; 1976.
3. Curry J. Facilitating Small Group Learning in Problem Based Learning, in *The Facilitator's Guide to the Small Group Process*, Ohio State University College of Medicine.
4. Napier R, Gershenfeld M. *Groups: Theory and Experience*. Boston: Houghton Mifflin Company; 1973.
5. Brownell K. The psychology and physiology of obesity: Implications for screening and treatment. *J Am Diet Assoc*. 1984; 4:406-413.
6. Snetselaar L. *Nutrition Counseling Skills*. (2nd ed.). Gaithersburg, MD: Aspen Publishing; 1989.
7. Raczynski J. *The Latest in Nutrition Counseling*. Presentation at ADA Annual Meeting, Orlando, FL October 20, 1994.

FOR YOUR INFORMATION

Residential/Group Centers for Weight and Health Management

Marsha Hudnall, MS, RD, Nutrition Director, Green Mountain at Fox Run, Ludlow, VT

Residential centers for health management have been popular since the Roman Empire days when people visited hot mineral spring baths. Today, these places are called spas, or fitness, health or wellness retreats. Some cater to overworked executives or overweight individuals while others cater to individuals looking for new lifestyle philosophies and behaviors.

In the past, most centers' programs concentrated on lots of exercise and healthy cuisine. Today, many programs also offer counseling and programs for the mind so that changes learned during a week or two at the center are better maintained when the person returns home to "real" life. One residential group program for weight and health management is unique in that it was started 22 years ago by a Registered Dietitian, and it's philosophies and programs are now more timely than ever before. The market has finally caught with what Thelma Wayler, MS, RD knew all along.

Green Mountain at Fox Run

The diet boom had just begun in 1973 when Ms.Wayler started a weight management center based on a revolutionary concept—diets don't work. Two decades ago, when Thelma told women that one brownie never made anyone fat and encouraged women to start exercising, she made waves with both her nutrition colleagues and the public. Waves that got her national attention, including a full-page feature in the *New York Times* and appearances on programs such as *The Donahue Show*. Now, 22 years later, her message is embraced by most practitioners in the weight management field.

Today, Thelma's education-based program, Green Mountain at Fox Run in Ludlow, Vermont (now directed by her son Alan H. Wayler, PhD, a nutritional biochemist) continues to offer cutting-edge information and a practical, take-home experience to women from all over the world. They come because they're tired of dieting. Rather than give up on health altogether, they seek a lifestyle approach to weight and health management that offers a livable means by which to feel well, look good, and stay that way.

Program

Participants attend either one, two, four or more week sessions beginning on specific starting dates. This ensures a sequential and structured format for imparting information in a consistent fashion. The program day is comprised of a mix of workshops, behavior groups, physical activity, and stress management classes. Along with the professional staff of Registered Dietitians, exercise physiologists and behavioral specialists, Green Mountain employs massage therapists, most of whom are registered nurses.

Sessions are limited to 42 women to ensure a highly personalized experience. A group-based approach is used for workshops and behavior sessions to take advantage of the powerful educational dynamic it offers. Additionally, participants can meet one-on-one with professional staff in private counseling sessions.

Case Study

At the suggestion of a registered dietitian, Joanne came to Green Mountain. At 42-years-old, she was watching her weight steadily climb, no matter how much she dieted, and her blood cholesterol level was over 300. She was a compulsive eater and was increasingly discouraged about ever taking charge of her weight and health. She was ready to give up.

At Green Mountain, along with about 40 other women aged 18 to 80, who were feeling similarly about their weight and health, Joanne began a journey that resulted in a new way of thinking and acting about food, her weight and herself. The team of registered dietitians, exercise physiologists and behavioral specialists taught her that at the core of healthy living lay the principle of feeling good, enjoying her life, and getting pleasure from the food she eats. She learned about eating smart (which, again, included foods she enjoyed even if they were rich in fat and calories). She learned that if she truly wanted to take charge of food instead of having it rule her, she would need to begin eating according to her individual needs and realistic desires. She would be in charge of making decisions about food and eating and taking responsibility for those decisions. Joanne began to develop and adopt a new approach to eating with the help of registered dietitians, who helped her take the lead in deciding her goals and approach and gently guided her when she encountered obstacles.

Joanne also learned about sensible exercise, how to do it, enjoy it, and stay with it. She explored her attitudes about physical activity and how she dealt with stress and developed plans for coping with high-risk situations under the guidance of behavioral experts. Several of the women at Green Mountain with Joanne weren't even there for weight issues, but to learn how to better cope with stress.

Perhaps most importantly, however, she had a chance to put her new knowledge and plans into action while living in a "safe" environment. That's the beauty of a residential setting. Removed from the daily stresses of life, in a peaceful, relaxed setting among the rolling mountains of Vermont, Joanne was able to take chances with her eating. She enjoyed the meals, which occasionally included ice cream or cheesecake for dessert, and saw she could eat such foods without gaining weight. She ventured to dinners at local restaurants and put the strategies she had developed to work.

Joanne spent about two-thirds of every day engaged in some type of physical activity. She started out slowly, but was soon walking steep hills daily. She tried all kinds of activity, from step aerobics, to free weights, to stretch classes, to recumbent biking, to the NordicTrak. She found what she liked and planned a reasonable program to continue at home that she could fit into her busy life.

Joanne's weight dropped (along with her blood cholesterol levels). It wasn't because she was starving herself (indeed, she was eating at least 1800 calories a day on average), or because she was exercising strenuously. It was because she had adopted a sensible, healthy approach that allowed her to enjoy life without obsessing about food, exercise or weight. She had changed her focus from weight to health, from a specific figure on the scale to how she felt.

Today, five years later, Joanne has kept off the weight she lost. Never down to her previous "ideal" weight, but she had learned that goal was not realistic nor necessary. She has returned to Green Mountain three times over the five years, for "recharging." She periodically faces stresses that challenge her new-found abilities, so she occasionally makes use of Green Mountain's telephone counseling program, to speak with one of the staff who help her work through specific problems she is facing.

Summary

Dietitians, physicians, psychological therapists, nurses and other health specialists refer clients and use Green Mountain as an adjunct to their ongoing treatment program. Residents receive a broad and intensive treatment experience away from the distractions of everyday life to permit focus on establishing priorities for weight and health goals. The resident begins or reinforces the process, but returns home to the support of a professional where the ongoing work of reeducation and counseling continues. Our message is that successful weight and health management is an ongoing process that requires periodic reinforcement.

13

The Challenge of Maintaining Change

Idamarie Laquatra, PhD, RD, Vice President of Scientific
Affairs and Training, Diet Center Worldwide, Inc.

After reading this chapter, the reader will be able to:
- ☐ **identify four motivational processes that may enhance maintenance of a skill**
- ☐ **describe at least two external situational variables that may decrease skill maintenance**
- ☐ **identify maintenance skills that clients can utilize to minimize long-term relapse**

Maintaining lifestyle and eating changes has been an area of intense interest and concern to practitioners. Why do many clients have such a difficult time maintaining dietary changes in their lives? Although problems with maintenance seem to be publicized more frequently in the area of weight control, the truth remains that any dietary change faces maintenance challenges. For example, most individuals who suffer from myocardial infarction have little problem altering their behaviors to accommodate a low saturated fat and low cholesterol eating pattern. As health returns, however, their priorities often change, causing them to lose their focus and backslide to old behaviors.

Maintenance of change once treatment is discontinued does not occur naturally. (1) The skills needed to change behavior differ from those required to maintain the change. Individuals who do extremely well during the treatment phase may or may not have success at maintaining new behaviors. In fact, some therapists feel more concerned about those clients who have no problems of adherence during treatment, because the clients may not have been confronted with situations to "test" their coping strategies.

Maintenance of any skill involves an interaction of motivational processes within the client with situational variables in the posttreatment environment. In other words, dietitians need to know what's going on inside and outside of their clients to foster the maintenance process.

Internal Processes

Kelman (2) described three motivational processes: compliance, identification and internalization. Self-sabotage is also an internal process, but it may be triggered by a high-risk external situation.

Compliance, a low level process, refers to participation in a program to avoid punishment or to gain rewards. Compliance examples include clients who change their eating behaviors because they fear another heart attack, derive all their reinforcement from a change in their scale weight, or dread an insulin reaction. Maintenance of change is not likely to occur if the motivational process remains at the compliance level.

A higher level of motivation, *identification*, occurs when clients do things for the counselor. Clients learn what maintaining a satisfying relationship with the counselor requires and so they alter their behaviors accordingly. They want to be liked by the counselor. Unfortunately, clients backslide once in the posttreatment phase, when the counselor becomes less available.

Internalization ranks as the highest level of the motivational processes. In this stage, the rationale for change agrees with the client's value system, and performing the behaviors becomes intrinsically rewarding. During the treatment phase, external reinforcement comes easily and often for the client. It can be a lower blood pressure or cholesterol reading, a comment from a co-worker about how great the client looks, or better blood glucose control. After treatment, when the external reinforcement wanes, the need for an internal reward system becomes apparent. The chances of maintaining behaviors will be much greater when clients internalize the motivation for change. It's easy to spot clients who internalize the motivation for change: They don't follow a diet; they've modified their lives.

Clients do not always pass through each level of motivation. Some clients you counsel may internalize right away. Other clients grow through the counseling process and pass through one or more levels. You may find that some clients may get "stuck" in the compliance or identification level. Counselors need to be prepared to gently confront clients to encourage the internalization process.

Self-sabotage can be a common problem during maintenance. It primarily involves self-talk, the messages clients give themselves. Self-sabotage can occur when clients focus on the immediate perceived benefits of an action versus the delayed benefit or negative effects. For example, faced with an urge for a high fat food, a client may think: "Oh, it would taste so good" and lose sight of how it will impact on the total fat content of the diet or the self-recrimination which may follow once the food is eaten. It must be pointed out here that high fat foods can have a place in an overall healthy diet and that eating a high fat food does not necessarily mean that self-recrimination will follow. Unfortunately, clients who have a problem with self-sabotage often develop behavioral patterns. They usually do not balance eating high fat foods with low fat foods and/or self-loathing results from behaviors which occur outside self-specified limits.

Self-sabotage also occurs when clients repeatedly deceive themselves into thinking that "one time won't hurt me." While it is absolutely true that exceptions do not derail maintenance efforts, when exceptions become the rule, self-sabotage may be at work. Rationalizing behaviors, such as eating high sodium foods because there just wasn't time to prepare an appropriate meal or dealing with stress by eating can also sabotage efforts. Finally, clients who think negatively about their abilities may deliberately set themselves up to fail, thinking, "I knew I couldn't do it."

Situational Variables

Factors outside the client also have an influence on whether or not a new behavior will be maintained. Clients must be skilled to make the appropriate food choices in many different environments, under varying conditions.

High risk situations test the abilities of client, and they differ for each client. How often have you heard, "I was doing so well until. . . ." High risk situations include social events, such as weddings, office parties, and eating out. They extend to negative life events such as divorce or changing jobs. High risk situations also include negative emotional states such as depression, anxiety, anger, and stress. Clients who deal successfully with high risk situations build confidence. Those who fail can torpedo their maintenance efforts, resulting in lapse, relapse and collapse. (3)

A *non-supportive environment* makes maintenance of any behavior difficult, especially if clients have not internalized the change process. A non-supportive environment can be a spouse who complains about the food being served or a work environment where low saturated fat food options do not exist. Dietitians must recognize that maintenance of skills requires a supportive environment. New skills are fragile at first, and need to be nurtured to grow strong. When you first work with new clients, try walking them through a typical day and explore where they get support for their new lifestyle decisions; role play how clients can ask for support or how they can deal with negative comments and lack of support. (ed. For years I have used a parable called, "Weed out the garden of your life" to help clients visualize how to deal with unpleasant things they can't keep from happening. They learn that they can control how they react and no longer allow it to be a problem. K.K.H.)

Relapse

Throughout the treatment phase and maintenance process, relapses often occur. Relapse can be better understood as a process rather than an outcome. (3) Marlatt and Gordon (4) describe the process of relapse as a specific series of cognitions and behaviors. Their relapse model integrates internal and external factors: cognitive function, self-efficacy (defined as an individual's expectation concerning his or her capacity to cope effectively with whatever it is that the present situation demands)(5), environment and situational variables. For example, the person is depressed and feeling sorry for himself (cognitive), then the person doesn't feel confident that he has the ability to handle new stresses at this time (self-efficacy), and finally, a high risk situation presents itself (environmental/situational). The person may return to old behaviors briefly and take the relapse in stride while determining other ways to handle depression or his response to it, or he may choose to believe that the return to old behaviors was out of his control or inevitable given his internal weakness or flaws.

A person is most vulnerable to relapse when he or she is angry, depressed, upset or feeling sorry for him/herself. Following are steps to take to better control the relapse event: (6)

- Stop the behavior EARLY
- Stay calm
- Renew eating vows
- Analyze what's happening
- Take charge
- Ask for help

It has often been said that the relapse itself is not the problem; it is how clients deal with the relapse that determines the ultimate outcome. Many times, people who try to change their behaviors expect perfection of themselves. When they slip, self-recrimination occurs and they view their failure to live up to their expectations as a character flaw. Called the Abstinence Violation Effect, this type of thinking sets the individual up for a downward spiral of deteriorating behaviors. (6) Danish has suggested instead that we encourage our clients to think of maintenance of change like a basketball game—no one expects 100% of the shots to make it through the hoop—a strategy for handling rebounds is part of the game plan. (7) You can help your clients understand that learning to rebound is part of what must take place for change to be maintained.

As individuals begin the journey towards lifelong maintenance, they need to expect to encounter difficulties. Individuals must be counseled to learn the strategies that work for them when faced with high risk situations that can result in a relapse. When they do relapse, they need to remove the moral overtones. (It is not the end of the world and they are not bad people; they just ate some food. That's all.) Viewing changing eating behaviors as an ongoing learning process can help, because learning involves testing boundaries, making mistakes and growing from them. As clients practice their new eating skills in different environments, they may make errors in judgement, but continued practice will build self-confidence and strength to deal with even the most challenging situations. Relapse prevention is a self-control program that combines training in coping skills, cognitive interventions, and lifestyle changes. (6)

Maintenance Skills

While most of the research on maintenance skills was completed with individuals who lost weight, each of the principles can be generalized to any dietary change. Although exercise seems more related to weight loss and maintenance than to other dietary issues, it is actually vital to every person's health as well as for recovering from illness or injury. Research supports that individuals who incorporate exercise into their lives appear to be able to maintain their weight loss better than those who do not exercise. (6) The exercise not only increases calorie expenditure, but it also seems to facilitate other positive maintenance behaviors.

Other maintenance skills that have been identified include self-monitoring, planning, setting goals, setting boundaries, and developing coping skills.

Self-monitoring refers to an awareness of eating behaviors. Clients need to be conscious of what they eat. During the treatment phase, keeping written records or oral accounts (through audiotapes) of eating behaviors help clients increase their understanding of what, where, when and how much they eat. During the maintenance phase, it becomes easy to lose track of eating as other priorities surface. Dietitians must help clients stay focussed enough to retain treatment gains.

Planning refers to meal-planning and strategy development for high risk situations. Haphazard eating can derail the best intentions and allow the environment to control the client. Skills in meal-planning and developing strategies for high-risk situations such as social occasions or negative emotional states (depression, anxiety) give clients concrete plans to use rather than entering situations blindly hoping for the best.

Setting goals, a critical life skill, was described in Chapter 7. Clients can often be so vague about what they want to achieve that they never know when they have achieved anything. Goals need to be specific, realistic and under the client's control.

Clients should *set boundaries* that have meaning for them. For example, a client concerned with weight control may set a boundary of five pounds or how a particular piece of clothing fits. Individuals trying to maintain a low cholesterol, low saturated fat eating style may set boundaries in terms of types of foods. Still other boundaries may have to do with quantities of food—protein amounts on a restricted protein diet, for example. Boundaries should be salient so they can trigger the client to take action when nudged.

A common factor in everyone's life continues to be stress. Learning how to cope with stress and with other life problems without turning to food or backsliding will be vital during the maintenance phase. Clients may need to learn to be more assertive, to deal with problems head on, or to learn how to relax. *Coping skills* will differ with each client. The counselor must actively listen to understand the client well and to help design appropriate strategies. (See FYI "What do you say when a client calls at 10PM?")

In addition to these skills, strategies such as learning how to develop a support system and continued therapist contact also encourage the maintenance of change. Family, friends and the dietitian can support the client through the maze of maintenance. Change can be stressful and difficult and the problems clients encounter are numerous and varied. Knowing the type of support needed and how to ask for it will help clients in the toughest times and provide the needed encouragement. Posttreatment contact which specifically targets maintenance skills has been found to be helpful. (9)

Our Responsibility

When beginning to counsel a new client, it is our responsibility to accurrately assess which stage of change the client is in and not present strategies for change that the client is not prepared to take (see Chapter 2). This will only discourage the client more and set him or her up for repeat failure. Far too often counselors focus on the action stage without adequately exploring clients' motivation and commitment. (6)

Developing good treatment plans for clients addresses only half of the behavior change issue. Without a formal posttreatment program, the chances for maintenance of any dietary change will be slim. In the author's opinion, dietitians have an ethical responsibility to include a specific maintenance program that may last one year or longer.

Maintenance programs should be tailored to meet each client's needs; however, general guidelines exist which can increase the effectiveness of any plan you devise. The program should include an assessment of situations the client finds most difficult (10), skills training to equip clients to cope with posttreatment challenges, strategies for helping clients develop support, and continued professional guidance through formal contact. (9)

LEARNING ACTIVITIES

1. Utilizing the FYI on page 221-222,
    a. identify external situational variables that hampered the client's efforts
    b. describe manitenance skills that were utilized in assisting the client refocus her efforts.
2. Identify one personal lifestyle issue you would like to change to enhance your own health.
    a. what motivational processes can you identify for yourself?
    b. what barriers (external forces) limit your success?
    c. what maintenance skills have/can you utilize to enhance your change process?
    d. how will you measure success?

REFERENCES

1. Danish SJ, Galambos NL, Laquatra I. Life development intervention: skill training for personal competence. In: Felner, RD, Jason, LA, Moritsugu, JN, Farber, SS, eds. *Preventive Psychology*. New York: Pergamon Press; 1983:49-61.
2. Kelman HC. Compliance, identification and internalization: three processes of opinion change. *Journal of Conflict Resolution*. 1958;2:51-60.
3. Brownell KD. Relapse and the treatment of obesity. In: Wadden TA, Van Ittallie TB, eds. *Treatment of the Seriously Obese Patient*. New York, NY: The Guilford Press; 1992:437-455.
4. Marlatt, GA, Gordon, J, eds. *Relapse prevention: maintenance strategies in the treatment of addictive behaviors*. New York, NY: The Guilford Press; 1985.
5. Bandura A. Self-efficacy: toward a unifying theory of behavioral change. *Psychosoc Rev.* 1977; 84: 191-215.
6. Shattuck, DK. Mindfulness and metaphor in relapse prevention: an interview with G. Alan Marlatt. *J Am Diet Assoc.* 1994;94:846-848.
7. Danish S. "Advanced counseling skills." Presentation at American Dietetic Association Annual Meeting, Orlando, FL, October 1994.
8. Kayman, S, Bruvold, W, Stern, JS. Maintenance and relapse after weight loss in women: behavioral aspects. *Am J Clin Nutr.* 1990;52:800-807.
9. Perri, MG. Improving maintenance of weight loss following treatment by diet and lifestyle modification. In: Wadden TA, Van Ittallie TB, eds. *Treatment of the Seriously Obese Patient*. New York, NY: The Guilford Press; 1992:456-477.
10. Schlundt, DG, Rea, MR, Kline, SS, Pichert, JW. Situational obstacles to dietary adherence for adults with diabetes. *J Am Diet Assoc.* 1994;94:874-879.

FOR YOUR INFORMATION

What Do You Say When a Client Calls at 10PM to Say She Is Eating everything in Sight?

Kathy King Helm, RD, LD

Marge, a 46-year-old divorced CPA with grown kids, has lost 30# the last seven months through increased exercise, a lower fat diet, and a lot of psychological support by the nutrition therapist. Marge and the nutrition therapist, Laura, have a close professional relationship. This is the first time Marge has ever taken Laura's offer to "call if you need me."

Marge, *"Hi, Laura, I hope I'm not calling too late."*

Laura, "No, that's just fine. How are you doing?"

Marge, *"I'm getting really depressed and I'm putting food in my mouth just to have it there. I can't still be hungry, I've eaten too much."*

Laura, "Ok. Let's talk this through. Are you feeling OK otherwise? *(yes)* Can you tell what lead you into this? What has changed?"

Marge, *"It's the craziest thing. This week I started wearing my new clothes and I was in a good mood and everyone at work started telling me how great I looked. They could finally tell how much I had lost."* (both patient and therapist laugh)

Laura, "So, the attention is new and scary for you? *(yes)* You know that it was bound to happen when you finally stopped wearing your baggy clothes. Thirty pounds is a lot to lose. What about it made you so scared?"

Marge, *"I started to feel anxious because I've lost weight before and then couldn't keep it off. I didn't want it to happen again this time."*

Laura, "You didn't want to regain your weight like before, so you started overeating to help calm your nerves? (both laugh) Would you rather gain the weight back instead of dealing with the attention?"

Marge, *"I can't gain the weight back because I'd have to go back on the blood pressure medicine and my chemistries will go back up."*

Laura, "There are other very important reasons besides your appearance to keep the weight down. So what can you do to deal with the comments?"

Marge, *"I can do something besides say, 'Oh, thank you,' become embarrassed and leave the room."*

Laura, "Your answer is fine, but is there something you could do besides becoming embarrassed and leaving?"

Marge, *"I could remember the other reasons why I needed to lose the weight. I may not tell them why. I may just say, 'I feel so much better now.'"*

Laura, "That's good. You need to remember all the other changes you have accomplished besides weight loss. Let's remember what they are. Your cholesterol. . ."

Marge, *"My cholesterol dropped from 250 to 202; my triglycerides are down from 455 to 230 and I don't have to take blood pressure medicine anymore, so I don't have all the side effects from that."*

Laura, "Great! It puts all of this in perspective better doesn't it? *(yes)* Is your anxiety the only thing you are dealing with when they compliment you? Are you proud of yourself?"

Marge, *"Yes, I feel proud, but then I feel pressure to succeed, and then I feel anger."*

At this point, Laura can tell that not all of the issues have been explored. She could either take more time at this stage to identify and work through the new issues or suggest that Marge think about her anger and write it down so they could discuss it at the next visit. Laura chooses to continue while the discussion is flowing.

Laura, "What are you angry about?"

Marge, *"Just for a moment I feel angry because people who haven't talked to me in months are now taking the time to tell me two or three times in a week how nice I look."*

Laura, "It angers you that people treat you differently because of your weight. That's understandable. Our society has an obsession about weight. Let me ask you this though. You said in the beginning that you were in a good mood this week. You bubble when you look good. I don't know if you have ever noticed it?"

Marge, *"I know I do. I know what you are getting at. It wasn't just my weight. I wore my new clothes, I felt good and looked good, so people started saying things to me."*

Laura, "Would you rather that they didn't talk to you or didn't say that you looked nice? (both laugh) You know in a little while people will be used to your appearance and won't say anything. Then will you miss it?"

Marge, *"Of course, that's how I am."*

Laura, "Are feeling better? *(yes)* Do you want to go eat now?"

Marge, *"I've eaten enough. But it doesn't interest me now at all. I wasn't eating because I was hungry; I was eating because I was stressed out and I didn't know how to cope."*

Laura, "Do you deserve to lose weight and look good? *(yes)* What are you going to say and do the next time someone tells you that you look so good?"

Marge, *"I will smile and say 'Thank you and I feel good too.' Then I'll let myself enjoy the moment."*

Laura, "Fantastic! Now I want you to call me the next few days and let me know how you are doing. Is that OK?"

Marge, *"That's fine. I feel much better."*

The next day when Marge called, she said, *"The crisis has passed and I had a great day. I ate normally and I told people some simple answer when they said I looked good."*

The following day Marge said, *"I ate well again today. I'm not hungry. I feel good about me and I walked each morning the last two days."*

PART III
Maximizing Success

14
Counseling Tactics That Work and Those That Don't

Donna Israel, PhD, RD, LD, Preferred Nutrition Therapists and President/ Founder, The Fitness Formula, Inc., Richardson, TX

After reading this chapter, the reader will be able to:
- ☐ identify personal attributes of a successful nutrition therapist
- ☐ evaluate own strengths/weaknesses as a nutrition therapist
- ☐ critique implementation of counseling strategies

The purpose of this chapter is to highlight the major points that make a nutrition therapist successful. As you will see, although the majority of our training is in the clinical aspects of nutrition, when you counsel clients many other skills and abilities contribute to success.

Are You Right For Counseling?

In counseling, as in business, the one attribute that almost all successful counselors have, and unsuccessful ones rarely have, is the ability to relate to other people in a cheerful, positive, forthright, empathic and assertive manner. (1) Successful counselors like other people and are liked in return. If you are not certain how good your "people skills" are, here are some questions to ask yourself: (1)

- Do you expect the best from people? Do you assume that others will be conscientious, trustworthy, friendly and easy to work with until they prove you wrong?
- Are you appreciative of other people's physical, mental and emotional attributes—and do you point them out frequently?
- Are you approachable? Do you make an effort to be outgoing? Do you usually wear a pleasant expression on your face?
- Do you make the effort to remember people's names?
- Are you interested in other people—all kinds of people? Do you spend far less time talking about yourself than encouraging others to talk about themselves?
- When someone is talking, do you give him or her 100 percent of your attention—without daydreaming, interrupting or planning what you are going to say next?
- Are you accepting and nonjudgmental of others' choices, decisions and behavior?
- Do you wholeheartedly rejoice in other people's good fortune as easily as you sympathize with their troubles?
- Do you refuse to become childish, temperamental, moody, inconsistent, hostile, condescending or aggressive in your dealings with other people—even if they do?
- Are you humble? Not to be confused with false modesty, being humble is the opposite of being arrogant and egotistical.
- Do you make it a rule never to resort to put-downs, sexist or ethnic jokes, sexual innuendoes or ridicule for the sake of a laugh?
- Are you reliable? If you make commitments, do you keep them—no matter what? If you are entrusted with a secret, do you keep it—no matter what?

- Are you willing to listen to opposing points of view without becoming angry, impatient or defensive?
- Are you able to hold onto the people and things in your life that cause you joy and let go of the people and things in your life that cause you sadness, anger and resentment?
- Can you handle a reasonable amount of pressure and stress without losing control or falling apart?
- If you make a mistake, are you willing to acknowledge and correct it without excuses?
- Do you like and approve of yourself most of the time?

"Yes" is the answer that shows the most likelihood of being able to successfully relate to other people.

Temper Your Advice With Common Sense

George Burns' 10 Don'ts for a Long Life:

Don't Smoke. Don't Drink. Don't Gamble. Don't Eat Salt. Don't Eat Sugar. Don't Eat Fats. Don't Overexercise. Don't Overeat. Don't Undereat. Don't Play Around. To which he added the note, "You may not live longer, but it will seem longer."

Live comedy routine

To be successful, nutrition counseling strategies must emphasize the importance of pleasing rather than punishing. People eat food to stop their hunger and fuel their bodies, but they also eat because of the pleasure it gives them. The number one reason why people choose to eat a food is taste. Dietitians must learn how to make food changes interesting, tasty and appealing—it isn't enough to make food metabolically correct! Most clients don't care about the magnesium level in their daily food intake. We must see food from the clients' perspective to be successful in counseling.

Ornstein and Sobel have gathered scientific evidence that pleasure from chocolate to charity and positive attitudes, from hot baths to afternoon naps, from happiness to optimism are not only enjoyable but also good for you in settings varying from therapeutic to preventive. (2)

Historically, dietitians have not been associated with pleasurable foods and eating, but that can and must change. Nutrition, food and health are intricately linked. The robust, octogenarian Julia Child forever will be associated in our minds with fine food. Julia feistily states, "The health fanatics and obsessed nutritionists would have us believe we're all doomed by what we eat, and if these scareheads succeed in taking over, they're going to kill gastronomy. You can lead a beautiful, healthy, fun life if you observe the old rules of variety and moderation." (3)

Three More Keys: Rapport, Helping Skills and Caring Interdependence

Once an effective relationship is established with a client, you help the client identify specific goals, develop the necessary steps to achieve the goals, and then become involved with the client in skill-training to achieve the goals. (4) The keys are:

- establishing rapport, trust and credibility with the client—through empathy, warmth, and respect or positive regard,
- using the helping skills, which facilitate the clients' movement through exploring, understanding and acting,
- fostering caring interdependence—the counselor is there to support and closely work with the client but the client learns to take responsibility and eventually act independently.

The client is provided positive choices through appropriate counseling strategies and then "respected" and "trusted," to choose and implement from the positive choices. (5) Does the client always choose and implement the positive choices? No, yet the data is far and away better for this strategy than for counseling strategies that do not deal with the whole person and all his or her feelings, and which operate on the premise of control instead of trust. (See FYI at the end of this chapter on Counseling a Client with Multiple Personalities.)

Practical Counseling "Do's" (6)

- Concentrate counseling days and times so that you take time to regenerate yourself
- Engage in "small talk" briefly and show interest in client's special people and events
- Allow freedom for client and yourself to feel and explore
- Validate the differences between client's approach and your's—it's OK
- Do give nontechnical explanations and define the terms you use
- Be specific on why you are both there
- Negotiate the process
- Summarize often: what happened, what's expected by next visit, what client expects

- Review treatment plan
- Use self-monitoring, verification of results (glucometer, biological data), questionnaires and rating scales (what helped the most?)
- Help clients see that taking the risk to change the most negative behaviors has more benefits than costs
- Teach clients how to identify what social support is needed to maintain behaviors; who is best to give support; and how to ask for help
- Adopt a "coping" model (control over time; do the best you can) instead of a "mastery" model (no variance; perfection)
- Use a problem-solving approach (collaborative and specific)
  1. define the problem
  2. identify options (long list)
  3. weigh the pros and cons of each option
  4. once client and you make a choice; teach client how to incorporate changes or skills into client's lifestyle, monitor over time, and modify as needed
- Negotiate reachable goals focused on behaviors and thoughts with lots of options instead of focused on the outcome or results
- Return phone calls promptly

Practical Counseling "Don'ts" (6)

- Don't be impolite, inattentive, or insensitive; don't take phone call unless emergency
- Don't act unorganized, scattered, or too willing to please; act mature and logical
- Don't refuse to answer or skirt questions, or give 10 minutes dialogs in order to discourage further questioning
- Don't make the patient suffer because you are under time pressures—treat the client as if he or she is the most important person in your life during the appointment time
- Don't pass judgment on the client's decisions, lifestyle, behaviors, or family
- Use sarcasm cautiously, if at all
- Do not act condesending—let the clients know that soon they will be the experts
- Do not scold—you will lose clients by treating adults as children
- Do not keep interrupting this makes you and the client feel you have all the answers
- Don't focus on results—focus on small steps to reach goals
- Don't "grill" the client with a series of close-ended questions
- Don't mistakenly believe that if clients recognize that certain behaviors are harmful—they will change them
- Don't mistakenly believe that if you give enough facts and information the client will change
- Don't tell clients what they must, should or have to do
- Don't talk too much and fail to let the client talk enough (patients forget half of what they hear in five minutes)

Other counseling strategies that don't work are provided by Landreth, PhD, counseling educator at the University of North Texas. (7) I call them "Rules of Thumb. . .To Avoid."

RULES OF THUMB. . .TO AVOID

1. Harming the clients self concept with your words
2. Being insensitive to how the world is perceived by others
3. Listening only with your ears and not your eyes
4. Doing things for others that they can do for themselves, which teaches dependency and weakness
5. Giving generic praise
6. Giving mixed messages
7. Being a thermometer with a client instead of a thermostat (think about it)
8. Ignoring the basic tenet: the important thing is not what a person knows but what he believes about himself
9. Giving direction when the client needs diversion; giving diversion when the client needs direction
10. Asking questions you already know the answers to
11. Failing to realize that the most important thing may not be making a mistake with a client, but rather, what you do after you make the mistake

12. Not understanding that the important thing is not what other people do, but what you and significant others do with the client
13. Failing to follow through
14. Focusing on the hole and not the doughnut

Three Successful Counseling Strategies

Following are the author's favorite examples of strategies that work well in counseling. They are favorites because clients rank them as the most successful.

Modeling: Clients check out for home use, or observe in the office learning room, a video tape which demonstrates the behavior change modeled by others who are successfully achieving similar goals. A video (for example, *Body Trust* [8] is designed to be used with client's who wish to address healthy weight management) will allow the client to learn the new behavior by watching others.

Thought-stopping: Clients call this the "Devil's and Angel's Lists." In one column, the Devil's, we list all the demon thoughts that chase around in the client's head, which result in devaluing the client, slowing progress, or predicting certain failure. Opposite each devil, we come up with an appropriate response that will stop the negative thought in its tracks. The positive responses are, of course, the Angel's List. Each client must practice replacing the Devil's thought many times in order to automatically think of the newer, more positive thought.

Stimulus control: Clients list all their behaviors they can remember in a "relapse to old behaviors" day. When the behavior which led to or preceded the unhealthy lifestyle behavior is identified, the problem is identified and the problem-solving behaviors and thoughts are implemented.

Checklist For Implementing Counseling Strategies

A counseling strategy is a program for implementation. A comprehensive plan is developed after goal behaviors have been set with a client (described in Chapter 7). In nutrition counseling a strategy is the plan for changing a client's existing eating behavior to one which will result in the client's achieving the stated goals. Often the majority of the client's and the counselor's time is devoted to this aspect of the counseling process. Following is a checklist adapted for the nutrition therapist for implementation. (9)

Checklist

Initial agreement
- Did the nutrition therapist provide a rationale and overview of the strategy?
- Did the counselor obtain the client's willingness to try the strategy?

Modeling goal behavior
- Did the therapist model the correct behavior for the client?
- Was the client instructed on what to look for in the demonstration?
- Did the model demonstrate the goal behaviors in a coping manner (versus perfection)?
- Did the client review or summarize the goal behaviors after the modeled demonstration?

Rehearsal of goal behaviors
- Did the client rehearse the goal behaviors until he/she felt comfortable with them?
- Is the client able to direct the practice him/herself and correct actions or statements?
- Did the counselor critique each practice and provide positive feedback?

Homework
- Was rehearsal homework assigned for the client to try at home/work?

Did the homework assignment include the following? (Check any that apply):
____ situations the client could easily initiate
____ graduated tasks: allow the client to gradually try harder elements
____ a number indicating the times to try the behavior
- Did the therapist arrange for a telephone follow-up after client's completion of some of the homework?

LEARNING ACTIVITIES

1. Divide a piece of paper into three columns. Head each column as follows: Column 1—People Skills Utilized, Column 2—People Skills Not Utilized or Utilized Infrequently, Column 3—Strategies to Increase People Skills. Review

the 17-point list of questions on pages to and evaluate your personal "people skills." For those skills used infrequently, describe personal strategies you can work on to strengthen those "people skills."

2. Observe a nutrition counseling session. What counseling "Do's" and "Don'ts" do you observe? What would you do differently given that specific counseling session?

REFERENCES

1. Scott N. Success often lies in relating to other people. In: Working Woman newspaper column. *Dallas Morning News*, April 20, 1995.
2. Ornstein R, Sobel D. *Healthy Pleasures*. Reading, MA: Addison-Wesley Publishing Co, Inc., 1990.
3. Interview, *Town and Country*. December; 1994.
4. Carkhuff RR. *The Art of Helping VII*. Amherst, MA: Human Resource Development Press, Inc; 1993.
5. Steinhardt M. Pleasure Principle. *Shape* Magazine. 1992.
6. Snetslaar L, Danish S, Raczynski J, Laquatra I. *Advanced Counseling Skills*. Presentation at American Dietetic Association Annual Meeting, Orlando, FL, October, 1995.
7. Landreth G. Denton, TX: University of North Texas; Class handout.
8. Hayes, D. *Body Trust*. Billings, MT, 1993. Video.
9. Cormier WII, Cormier LS. *Interviewing Strategies for Helpers*, 2nd ed. Pacific Grove, CA: Brooks/Cole Pub; 1985.

FOR YOUR INFORMATION

Counseling a Client with Multiple Personalities Disorder (MPD)

Kathy King Helm, RD, LD

Last year a woman called for information on my services to help her lose weight. "Shirley" was 47-years-old, a consultant and teacher, working on her PhD in language skills. She told me she had irritable bowel syndrome (IBS) and esophageal reflux that caused occasional problems. Then she said, "I also have multiple personalities. Thirty-two different ones at last count." I was honest with her and said, "I've never worked with anyone who admitted that before, but I'm certainly willing to work with you if you have a therapist I can talk to about what you need." We agreed to a date and time and she gave me her psychologist's name and phone number. As I worked with her over the next year, I adapted the lessons taught in this book: collaboration, continued learning, helping skills, patient-paced learning, nonjudgmental acceptance of the client and so forth, to this new counseling challenge.

I made three phone calls to get prepared for my appointment with Shirley. Her psychologist said she was very delightful, not dangerous, and probably would not arrive as different people on my doorstep. When I asked if the personalities were a defense mechanism that she developed as a child to cope with something awful in her reality, he just said, "yes."

Then I called two dietitians with extensive counseling experience. Theresa Wright, MS, RD, CDE, Germantown, PA, had a patient with multiple personalities who changed one time into a child as the appointment ended and said, "I'll wait for my mommy to come and pick me up." Theresa put her in the lobby and then called the client's psychotherapist who said, "She'll be fine. She waits until her adult personality returns in a little while and then drives home." Another time the woman arrived with her male biker personality "out." Theresa told the "biker" that it wasn't fair for him to hear the information since Joan was going to pay for the visit and she wanted Joan to come out. In a few minutes the dominant personality returned and the session went on as usual.

Bridget Klawitter, co-author, Racine, WI, had a dietitian on staff who worked with a woman with MPD. It was difficult to work with her on weight loss because one personality had anorexia and one was a compulsive overeater. There was a constant battle in which one personality or the other prevailed and the woman's eating habits went from one extreme to the other.

Shirley arrived at my door anxious, but ready to talk. She weighed over 280 pounds, but didn't want to weigh on the scale. She brought her food record from the past week. It was full of malts, Big Macs, fried foods, and sweets. We laughed together as I read some of the meals. She said, "In anticipation of coming here, I ate everything I knew you wouldn't want me to have after I start." I answered, "Actually, that's not true. There's no food that you can't have. You just can't have them as often if you want to weigh less than you do now." We went over her blood chemistries, GI problems, allergies, physical limitations due to back problems, and family situation.

She explained that she was diagnosed with MPD just three years before and had denied it at first and went into severe depression just thinking about it. She was hospitalized twice, but now lives at home with her husband and teenage son. Two daughters are grown and on their own. When she told her family the diagnosis they said, "We've known mom had many personalities all our lives." One daughter insists on driving because Shirley misses turnoffs too easily, but otherwise everyone is accepting and loving. Some of Shirley's women friends pulled away from her when they found out about her diagnosis, but she is cultivating new acquaintances and working hard on her studies.

I asked Shirley to explain how MPD affects her life, and she said, "Right now I'm being distracted by something happening in that corner over there. Part of me wants to go see what it is and part of me wants to stay here and concentrate on our discussion. I've read that a person's vision can be different, depending upon which personality is 'out.' Like right now, my glasses are off, and Shirley wears glasses, so I don't know who is 'out.' Sometimes I'm co-conscious and know what's happening. Other times my dominate personality, Shirley, sort of blacks out, and then comes back to find out that lots of things have happened without her. I have a great wardrobe: professional suits mixed with colorful, ruffled gypsy skirts. Shirley doesn't drink alcohol because of my medicines, but someone has been drinking margaritas recently! Sometimes one personality will sabotage what I've decided to do and get me lost driving or hide my homework. I've been signaling to make an exit off the highway and I'll wake up 45 minutes later on my way to Austin, Texas."

Our next discussion centered upon what she was willing and able to do. We discussed what she could eat on the run, in between jobs and classes, and what kinds of foods to eat more often. She cooked very little and seldom wanted to go to the grocery store to purchase interesting produce or other items, so meal planning had to be simple and fast. A revisit was scheduled for one week later.

At the second visit Shirley arrived 25 minutes late. She had turned at my corner on time but then got "lost." The same thing happened for several days with her food records—they kept disappearing. Overall, her eating had greatly improved with only two high fat meals in the whole week. We talked about her work on her PhD and her present career path. She indicated that walking was difficult but she loved to swim and had a place to go that she enjoyed. She said she could only control her eating when she is really active and that when school is out in May there could really be problems.

During the third and fourth visits Shirley disclosed that she developed her multiple personalities in response to her mother's violent behavior that began when she started menopause. Shirley was a change-of-life baby, 18 years younger than her younger half sister. Her mother would "snap" and threaten to kill Shirley while she held a butcher knife over her. Many times Shirley's dad would save her life by grabbing the knife handle. At the time we were meeting, Shirley's mom lived in Missouri close to Shirley's older sisters. Her mom was in her eighties and totally denied that she ever committed such atrocities.

Over the next weeks, Shirley was erratic in keeping her appointments, food records, and exercising. She started feeling depressed and went to her physician who diagnosed that Shirley was starting into menopause. In some ways it was a relief, but in other ways, Shirley was afraid she might react the same way as her mother, and it scared her. Besides talking about her food intake, which varied greatly, we discussed ways Shirley could enjoy herself besides through eating: she taught quilting classes on weekends, she wanted to spend more time with her husband, she wanted to fix up their house, and she wanted to have a massage more often.

In the fourth month of working together Shirley called one morning early and said she needed to cancel that week's appointment because her mother had just died and she would be gone a week or two. I asked if she was OK, and she said, "I haven't cried until now." I said, "You know this will be a big change for you. This wasn't just a normal mother-daughter relationship. Take Larry's (her psychologist) and my number with you in case you feel the need to talk."

When Shirley called in three weeks for an appointment, she was in a better mood than I had ever heard before. At our meeting she was laughing and joking more than usual. She was looking forward to May when she finally had some time for herself, which was a change in attitude from when she first began coming to see me. Her food intake was better than when she started, but still erratic at times. She reported that her other personalities didn't come out often.

Over the summer, she seldom made appointments. In August when I called to see how she was doing, she reported that she was working through some issues.

By the end of September, Shirley was back into school and her work routines. She was being asked to speak regionally at conventions in her field. However, her knees were more painful due to her weight and her blood lipids had gone up over the summer. Her physician suggested that she go on a strict fat gram counting diet, which she had started on her own. At our first visit in many months, we discussed what short term goals she would work for the next month, including regular swimming 2-4 times per week. She seemed confident, relaxed, and more motivated than ever before (probably due to the pain) to make consistent food and lifestyle changes. Her weight is dropping slowly.

My plan for the future is to be here for Shirley when she needs me. This has been a wonderful year of growth and change for her. As she becomes more confident and stronger, her other personalities seldom appear. She is merging into one dominant personality, Shirley.

15
Seizing Opportunities in Future Markets

Bridget Klawitter, MS, RD, FADA and Kathy King Helm, RD, LD

After reading this chapter, the reader will be able to:
- ☐ **identify current trends in the changing healthcare arena**
- ☐ **describe the implications of managed care on dietetic practice**
- ☐ **describe the role of dietetic practitioners in home healthcare and private practice**
- ☐ **identify growing dietetic counseling opportunities**
- ☐ **identify business skills that will be more crucial for dietitians to know in the future**
- ☐ **describe the importance of outcome data to dietetic practice**

As research shows the profoundly significant role nutrition plays in people's health and quality of life, dietitians will have to struggle to maintain our prominence in the field that was once ours by default. The answer is not to entrench ourselves and protect our present turf, now is the time to blossom! The following suggestions for the profession and for individual practitioners will help:

- assess the market trends (health care, medical care, payment systems, client preferences, nomenclature, other professionals' scope of practice, and so on);
- identify new emerging areas of opportunity in traditional and nontraditional dietetic acute and chronic care, food, fitness, wellness and health markets;
- determine the skills and abilities that will be needed to succeed in those markets;
- upgrade skills, abilities and knowledge, as a profession and individually, in the specific areas we want to practice, *but do not expect each person to be qualified in each area;*
- look for collaborators and colleagues in fields outside of dietetics in order to expand your sphere of influence;
- consider title changes to match the new, more specialized areas of clinical practice: "Nutrition Therapist" (for psychotherapy-based counseling, especially in outpatient counseling), "Medical Nutrition Therapist" (for clinical nutrition care in acute care setting and home health IV service); (1)
- collect the outcome data to show your effectiveness;
- communicate your messages to your target markets;
- market and promote your services and products for the world to know.

THE IMPACT OF HEALTH CARE REFORM
Edward H. O'Neil, PhD, MPA, and Serena D. Seifer, MD, Pew Health Professions Commission,
U of Calif. S.F., San Francisco, CA (Used with permission.)

Since the early part of 1994, the nation has been engaged in a great debate regarding the future of its health care system. The debate has progressed from discussing whether health care reform is feasible to addressing questions of when and to what extent the current arrangements for health care will be altered. Gone is the reaction that there is nothing fundamentally wrong with the system of care in America. Also gone is the chorus denying that one-seventh of the nation's resources is too much to pay for health care. There seems to be an emerging consensus that reform of a significant nature is necessary.

Presented here is a discussion of the broad forces currently driving health care reform, the competencies needed to compete in the new health care delivery system created by the forces, and some suggestions as to what you need to do to meet these challenges.

Dynamic Tensions of Health Care

The transformation of health care is emerging at many levels, i.e. federal, state and local. Daily employers move their employees to capitated systems of care and hospitals, insurance companies, and professional practice groups buy out one another in an effort to create new health care organizations and systems.

As chaotic as all of this may seem, these developments are actually driven by underlying principles. For the past four years, the Pew Health Professions Commission has been working from these principles. The first Commission report Healthy America: Practitioners for 2005 (2) assessed the forces that would likely impact the health care system and all of its providers by the year 2005. These forces are characterized as a set of tensions between what currently exists as the dominant paradigm in the health care system and what will emerge over the next 15 years (see Table 15-1).

Table 15-1 Dynamic Tensions of Health Care

Current Paradigm	Emerging Paradigm
Specialized care	Primary care
Technologically-driven	Humanely balanced
Cost unaware	Cost aware
Institutionally-based	Community-based
Governed professionally	Governed managerially
Acute treatment	Chronic management
Individual patient focused	Population perspective
Curative care	Prevention orientation
Individual provider	Team provider
Competition	Cooperation

(Source: Pew Health Professions Commission. Used with permission.)

The trends are deliberately presented as tensions that will seek a balance point between the left and right sides indicated in Table 15-1. These tensions pervade health care delivery and financing, the provider-client relationship, the provider-payer relationship, and the atmosphere within health professions educational institutions. These tensions also provide the framework for examining and redefining the higher education mission of professional schools. A shift in orientation or balance of these tensions seems inevitable and it is important for individual practitioners to understand and make the necessary strategic accommodations. Some professions, institutions and practitioners will remain close in orientation to the current paradigm. The nation's health system will need some to do that, but it is important to realize how difficult and increasingly competitive it will become to have such an orientation.

Dynamic Tensions Drive Reform

Closer examination is needed to fully understand how these dynamic tensions are driving reform:

Specialized Care vs. Primary Care. The nation has experienced a 43-year period in which health care disciplines have grown more specialized with the expansion of highly reductionistic knowledge. Although this trend has served the public's needs, it is recognized as a major contributor to the rapid escalation of costs, isolation of patients, and lack of coordination of treatment. In the future the nation will recapture a better balance between the generalist and the specialist, with the system turning more to the generalist for direction and integration of care. (3) Dietitians will need to show how they can serve the primary health care needs of the public by following patients for longer periods to make sure of recovery and by helping contain cost through prevention and health promotion.

Technology-Driven vs. Humanely Balanced. Americans will continue to demand advanced technologies but they also increasingly recognize and value the balancing of technology with more hands-on approaches such as health promotion and disease prevention. This demand for "high tech/high touch" will present a major opportunity to those professionals and delivery systems that can successfully demonstrate effectiveness, efficiency, and cost savings of using particular technologies to payers and purchasers of care. Dietitians should be willing and able to manage and use large volumes of scientific, technological, and patient information.

Cost Unawareness vs. Cost Awareness. As the population ages and utilizes more health care, even greater pressure will be placed on health care costs. The single most important reality for all of health care over the next 20 years will be finding ways to deliver more care of higher quality for fewer dollars.

Institutionally-Based Care vs. Community-Based Care. The growth in size of the hospital system and its related expenses have made health care unnecessarily expensive. With cost containment incentives such as diagnosis-related groups (DRGs), improved technology and consumer preferences, hospital stays have shortened and a greater percentage of inpatients are sicker. The most successful players in the future health care system will be those who are accessible to the public, responsive to consumer demand, and able to accommodate the patterns of contemporary lifestyles. More jobs and opportunities will be available for dietitians in the outpatient clinic, managed care, wellness, private practice, and home health care arenas.

Professional Governance vs. Managerial Governance. The only way to succeed under a new management environment is to fully understand those elements of the managerial paradigm and begin the process of incorporating them into the basic professional values and patterns of practice. All health professionals will need to develop the skills and capacities to utilize outcomes data, develop practice guidelines, and incorporate cost-effective strategies that do not compromise quality. Professionals and institutions that do this will be in a position to control more of their own destiny and still be responsive to the changing demands of the public.

Acute Treatment vs. Chronic Treatment. The challenge of the future is to move to an approach that focuses on the prevention of disease and the management of chronic disease in a fashion that enhances the quality of life. This development has important implications for dietitians. More opportunities in health education in wellness, prenatal, lactation, adolescent and adult obesity, geriatric/longevity, disease prevention and so on are available right now for appropriately trained and experienced dietitians (see Appendix 15-A and B on counseling on lactation and becoming a Certified Lactation Consultant). More practice settings will change (see side bar on page 237 about WIC counseling in Dade County Medicaid HMO). A growing phenomenon in many metropolitan areas is Medicare HMOs for people over 65 years.

Individual Patient Focus vs. Population Perspective. The US health care system will continue to be concerned about the treatment of individuals, but the reality of the demands of the future calls for a balancing of this demand with one that both prevents disease and disability in populations and does a better job of managing the needs of individuals better given the available resources.

Curative Care vs. Preventive Orientation. The future will demand more generalists having more knowledge in a broader spectrum, rather than specialized knowledge. However, the management of patients and clients will grow increasingly complex as the population ages. Successful professionals will broaden their identities as team members and providers. Those professionals most valued by clients and systems of care will be those that have the capacity and skills to lead multidisciplined teams. Dietitians should think about getting more education and training/experience in management.

Competition vs. Cooperation. Finally, the tension, legal and economic forces that have kept professionals and professional groups from cooperating will play out and a better system of care will evolve. Since health care resources will be scarce, it must be understood that downsizing will eliminate over two million health care jobs over the next five years. (4) Dietitians need to forge strategic partnerships with the public, insurers, and managed care providers. There is a question about whether physicians will be the gatekeeper or a case manager; whichever it is in your area of practice, you need to work with the gatekeepers and let them know what you do whether you work in an institutional setting or outpatient.

The most pervasive factor affecting allied health workers over the next decade will be cross-training or multi-skilled training across several disciplines. The reality is that these accommodations are occurring in the care delivery system independent of the accreditation and licensure regulations that have served to limit such developments. If these individuals prove to give more comprehensive care at a lower cost they will be in demand inside the health system and out. For example, if a dietitian can teach stress management, take vital signs, take fitness and anthropometric measurements, manage a clinic or wellness center, or follow women as they go through their pregnancy and try to breastfeed, he or she will have more to offer. At the same time, if every pharmacist, nurse and physician is taught how to interpret nutrition science, educate clients and do nutrition assessments, dietitians who only do those things will feel strong competition. It saves administrators money to employ someone who can not only take vital signs or dispense drugs but also can assess a person's nutritional needs and drug/diet interactions. Consider learning new skills yourself and become certified if necessary in order to improve your positioning in the market.

WHAT IS MANAGED HEALTHCARE?

From 1970 to 1990, healthcare expenditures have increased at an annual rate of approximately 12%, nearly 3% faster than the gross national product. (5) Healthcare expenditures in the United States are the highest in the world and continue to grow faster than any other country (6).

A growing number of Americans, including healthcare professionals themselves, are being ushered into a new world of healthcare. It is a world in which we are not readily admitted to a hospital or automatically placed in the care of a therapist. Medical care is no longer "delivered," it is "managed." Managed care organizations are paid a set amount by employers, state or federal governments, or private individuals to cover the health care needs of subscribers. The managed care organization may hire its own staff of care providers (Health Maintenance Organization—HMO) or it may contract with physicians and other health providers who will see clients at their private offices for a reduced fee (Preferred Provider Organization –PPO). Every day there are new combinations and strategies for doing the basic services in a more effective manner. Managed care operates on the premise that actual medical practice and resultant outcomes are monitored and information regarding the costs and quality are compared to an expected standard. Expensive therapies or ones with little or no medical benefit are closely scrutinized and often eliminated.

Changes in the provision of healthcare have been facilitated by businesses striving to control costly medical expenses for their employees, services many businesses believed in the past were dispensed too liberally and, perhaps, inappropriately. This has raised many concerns by healthcare professionals, including dietitians, that clients receive care based on affordability and not on true needs.

Although managed care is expanding, it is not at the same pace in all parts of the United States. Adjusting to healthcare being managed has been difficult for many individuals accustomed to free access of services and a blessing to others, especially those on Medicare who often get more coordinated care without the piles of paperwork (generated when they see several different physicians and carry a supplemental policy too). Some companies are controlling costs by setting limits on the number of outpatient visits or hospital days an individual can use each year. This may be an easy way for employers to cut costs by cutting services.

Opportunities in Managed Care

For hospital dietitians, it is important to seize the opportunity to establish a billing system for nutrition so that nutrition services are considered in the negotiation of managed care contracts. Although it varies somewhat, the basic mechanism for hospital billing and collection practices should be important for dietetic practitioners to explore and pursue.

Before billing for outpatient services, dietitians should contact third party payers for information regarding policies for reimbursement of nutrition counseling. This information can then be used as a guide in evaluating potential contract negotiation points. To be recognized as a provider, it helps to work with a referring physician or institution that already gets coverage. The issue of cost containment may be addressed with a variety of cost control measures for the utilization of outpatient nutrition counseling. One may be a client copayment that is identical to the amount required for any other outpatient medical visit. Another strategy may be the establishment of an annual benefit cap that would limit the number of sessions with the dietitian to a certain number per calendar year per plan participant. Additional visits usually require approval from the plan administrators or the person pays for the services him or herself. Defining the boundary in terms of visits is not a problem except for weight control, diabetes and other more long-term therapies, and it avoids annual readjustments as the fee schedule changes. Psychologists, like nutrition therapists, are also feeling the pressure to help clients make changes faster or pay for the visits themselves. An actual dollar amount per client is preferred by other practitioners. It is also feasible to provide phone follow-ups as a professional service after the annual benefit cap has been used in order to provide continuity of care and enhance outpatient compliance.

As the trend continues towards prospective payment, stressing that nutrition intervention can decrease complications and promote faster recovery will be important in the promotion of nutrition services. The team approach may become important to dietetic practitioners as the solo practice of nutrition like medical practice may not carry the clout to negotiate larger contracts.

CONTINUUM OF CARE INTO OUTPATIENT SETTINGS

Although the need for nutrition counseling is recognized in the inpatient setting, shortened lengths of stay limit the opportunities to provide the services. Ambulatory care services are one of the fastest growing segments in the healthcare arena (7) yet the increased need for dietitians to be involved in these settings has been more slow to evolve.

A standard health benefits package of comprehensive health services should include outpatient therapeutic nutrition services, delivered by registered staff, to ensure the highest quality and most cost-effective care. Preventive nutrition services for vulnerable populations is important across the lifespan, from prenatal care to old age. No period in life is more important to good health than the months before birth.

Early nutrition intervention can substantially change the course of events to improve pregnancy outcomes. Parents of children with special needs need to have access to professional advice on diet and feeding methods. This may include children with physical or developmental disabilities or those with chronic medical conditions caused by or associated with genetic/metabolic disorders, birth defects, prematurity, trauma, infection, or perinatal exposure to drugs.

Common nutrition problems among children, i.e. obesity, failure-to-thrive, diabetes, undernutrition, iron deficiency, constipation with encoparesis, and dental caries, can have significant short and long-term consequences. The establishment of healthy eating practices at an early age is particularly important. Nutrition problems among adolescents include obesity, chronic dieting, eating disorders, hyperlipedemia, and dental caries. The potential cost of these diseases could be prevented or significantly reduced with nutrition counseling for youth in primary care and other preventive healthcare settings.

Disease prevention is more than just keeping people well. It includes keeping people healthy in their communities, reducing the incidence and severity of preventable diseases, improving health and quality of life, and reducing total medical costs, particularly costs for medication, hospitalization, and extended care. It is much simpler and more cost-effective to lower a client's cholesterol level through diet changes and exercise than to perform open heart surgery. (See sidebar on counseling at the worksite.)

Clinical nutrition treatment, previously provided to inpatients who need to follow special diets after discharge, may need follow-up reinforcement as an outpatient. For example, for people with diabetes released from the hospital, maintenance of a diet plan can be critical to the stabilization of health and the prevention of rehospitalization. In an early study, it was reported that expanding nutritional counseling for diabetics decreased hospital costs for ketoacidosis and lower extremity amputations by over $3 million from 1971 to 1978. (8) Appropriate clinical nutrition counseling is a cost-effective use of dietetic professionals to keep patients healthy by providing individualized training on the incorporation of therapeutic diets into a healthy lifestyle.

HOME HEALTH CARE

The 1980's brought an increase in the number of individuals discharged from the acute care setting to home health care agencies. Due to decreased length of inpatient stays, many patients now go home sicker and requiring further care. (9) In many instances, home health care agencies may provide this continued care. Unfortunately, not many home health care agencies employ dietitians in any capacity, except perhaps on infusion teams, despite the fact that a substantial number of clients require therapeutic diets for nutrition-related diagnoses. (9,10) Part of the difficulty arises from the fact that many third-party payers, including Medicare, private insurance and preferred providers, do not automatically cover nutrition services provided by a registered dietitian. Some dietitians report however, that they have been hired as consultants to home health agencies because the agencies' lawyers felt it reduced their medical liability and showed more comprehensiveness of services. If an agency values the services of a dietitian, it will find a way to pay for his or her services.

Jessup (11) states that dietitians in the state of Texas are having success obtaining reimbursement for medical nutrition therapy by proactively contacting insurance companies and case managers to discuss the cost-effectiveness of services. Other state associations have documented similar findings. (12,13,14)

Why should home healthcare agencies utilize the services of registered dietitians? Jessup suggests the following: (11)

- medical nutrition therapy can assist in improving patient outcomes;
- dietetic services can prevent or decrease hospital readmissions and consequently loss of revenue for the agency;
- the development and implementation of a nutrition screening protocol can identify clients at nutritional risk earlier and facilitate early intervention;
- the provision of in-service education to homecare staff regarding the benefits of medical nutrition therapy and early interventions;

Taking WIC Counseling Into The Private Sector

Denise West, MPH, RD, Public Health Nutrition Program Director, Dade County, State of Florida

In 1984 the Dade County WIC and Nutrition Program initiated a paradigm shift in the delivery of health care to Medicaid recipients in Florida. Two Florida Medicaid Prepaid Health Plans (HMO's) began enrollment of Medicaid participants. Ten years later, 15 Medicaid HMO's operate in Dade County serving 89,000 Medicaid recipients; statewide 371,000 are served by HMO plans.

The private sector is rapidly replacing the public sector as the source of medical care for Medicaid recipients in Florida. As Medicaid recipients shift away from traditional locations of medical care, WIC and Nutrition Services have relocated to follow the client in order to continue fulfilling WIC's mission.

Working with the private sector results in advantages for all parties, especially the client. The HMO's receive:

- Cost savings because WIC funds and paid staff help cover and take care of qualified clients
- Documented cost-effective health benefits for its pregnant clients
- Nutrition assessment, nutrition counseling, breast feeding promotion and support for its WIC eligible clients
- On site access to WIC services for their clients

The WIC Program benefits by:

- Locating with a medical facility serving its target population, often in unserved or underserved geographic locations
- Reduced overhead because the HMO's provide free or reduced cost office space, utilities, security, lab and anthropometric data
- Caseload expansion into Medicaid and low income medically insured population
- Better patient care coordination.

The client benefits by having:

- One stop Medical/ WIC services
- Care coordination
- Supplemental nutritious food, and comprehensive nutrition counseling
- More locations from which to receive WIC benefits.

As medical care delivery changes, nutrition programs must be flexible and proactive to ensure that nutrition services remain an integral part of patient care.

Nutrition Counseling at the Worksite

Denice Ferko-Adams, RD, President, Wellness Resources & Services

What could be a better way to reach people in a timely, cost-effective and efficient manner than by providing counseling services at the worksite?

The average employee spends over half of their daytime hours at the work place. With the current shift in extending the workday instead of hiring new employees, people do not have time to attend evening nutrition programs or counseling sessions. Company executives are becoming more aware of how nutrition counseling can help reduce their health care costs directly by reducing the need for medications or other more expensive means of intervention.

One of my corporate contracts included providing nutrition counseling services for top executives at a Fortune 200 company who have poor annual physical examinations. The medical department, consisting of a physician and several nurses, supported nutrition intervention. The clinical indicators for referrals often included elevated cholesterol, obesity, and high blood pressure. Spouses were encouraged and invited to attend the hour long sessions. Counseling sessions included a nutritional assessment, food history, and a computerized analysis of food records when necessary. Weight loss clients required the most follow-up sessions and were most often men with sever obesity. Patient materials were customized for this corporate client and presented in professional folders. The executives were given the option of having the counseling session in their own office or in the medical department. I billed the company directly, so there was no expense to the executive.

Growth follows Success

The subsequent ripple effect of these executive counseling sessions was a welcome growth in a variety of wellness services. Soon, I was providing individual counseling for non executives with similar medical problems. Within the year, my services extended to working with the corporate chef on a more healthful year-round menu for the executive cafeteria. I also provided other group sessions of for employees, such as weight loss contest, cholesterol education, and brown bag lunch seminars.

There is strong business potential for the corporate-minded dietitian who is able to educate medical directors and human resource managers on the benefits of nutrition counseling for a wide spectrum of health care services. From diabetes education to cholesterol and weight control counseling, medical nutrition therapy provided by a registered dietitian is one of the primary interventions in controlling these costly medical conditions. With the increased use of health risk appraisals, specific preventive counseling services can even be tailored to best meet the needs of the company's high risk employees.

Nutrition services can be provided to the employee at the worksite and the company can be billed directly. A second option is to incorporate medical nutrition therapy into the corporate health care benefits plan. A third option is to offer corporate services that reach many people, such as weight loss and walking programs. Seize the opportunity to diversify services and educate the local companies on how nutrition services can make an important difference in their medical costs and in their employees' health!

- provides a channel of communication regarding medical nutrition therapy that can coordinate both acute and chronic nutrition interventions and provide for "seamless" continuity of care for the client;
- can assist the agency in developing and implementing critical pathways that include the role of nutrition in determining patient outcomes.

Home care services themselves are going through an evolutionary process. While referrals and case loads increase, staffing levels do not necessarily keep pace. Home care staff must focus more on increasing client responsibility and self-care. Health promotion literature emphasizes the need to create an environment in which clients' can grow in their ability to take control over their health decisions. A published overview of the challenges incurred by Vancouver Canada's Home Care program (15) closely correlates trends in the United States home care industry as well:

- absorbing increasing numbers of medically fragile and technologically dependent clients with multiple diagnoses
- identification of community needs as a whole
- supporting families overwhelmed by increased demands such as caregivers for aging family members and/or single parent and working households
- examining needs for group and community level interventions as related to public policy

OPPORTUNITIES IN PRIVATE PRACTICE AND CONSULTING

As mentioned many times in this book, the market is wide open for entrepreneurial dietitians who want to pursue the public's interest in receiving nutrition therapy on a variety of nutrition-related problems, plus health promotion/disease prevention, sports/fitness nutrition and weight control. The author encourage you to consider adding healthy food and food preparation to the variety of products or services you offer. Although the medical model has become very dependent upon third-party funding sources, it should never be overlooked that if the public wants something bad enough it will pay for it! The challenge is to assess what people are buying, use good judgment to determine future trends, create the services and products that will sell, package them with flair, and promote them. This of course must be supported with good business decisions, adequate funding and a willingness to take risks.

FUTURE DIRECTIONS

Dietetic practitioners must be prepared to work with markets of the future. The development of skills in counseling, group process, adult learning, physical activity (movement), and such business aspects as proposal writing, negotiation and marketing can serve to strengthen your position. Knowledge on the gathering of outcome data, understanding managed and home health care and how to work with them, and gaining the confidence and respect of referral sources will broaden the populations you serve. Evaluation of state-of-the-art information systems and looking for opportunities as changes evolve will further your professional progress. Flexibility, innovation and creativity in designing your service and product line will clearly define your role in markets of the future. Always remember, you will be considered good at counseling when your clients are successful.

LEARNING ACTIVITIES

1. Visit with a dietetic practitioner in two of the following settings.
   - acute care
   - longterm care
   - home care

- public health
- business and industry/ corporate wellness
- private practice

a. How has their practice changed in the last five years? 10 years?

b. How has healthcare reform specifically impacted their practice?

c. What have these practitioners done to personally help them adapt to the changes (i.e. new affiliations, education, etc.)?

d. What implications does this activity have on your vision of your future as a Nutrition Therapist or Medical Nutrition Therapist or as a dietetic practitioner?

REFERENCES

1. Dan Reiff, MPH, RD. Personal interview on April 21, 1995.
2. Shugars DA, O'Neil EH, Bader JD, eds. *Healthy America: Practitioners for 2005, An Agenda for Action for U.S. Health Professional Schools.* Report of the PEW Health Professions Commission. Durham, NC: The Pew Health Professions Commission, 1991.
3. Starfield B. *Primary Care: Concept, Evaluation and Policy.* New York: Oxford University Press; 1992.
4. *Future Search Conference,* The American Dietetic Association, Itasca, IL, June 12-14, 1994.
5. Jencks SF, Schieber GJ. *Containing US health care costs: what bullet to bite?* Washington DC: US Government Printing Office; 1992. HCFA publication 03322.
6. Kosterlitz J. A sick system: diagnosing the ailments. *National Journal.*1992; 2:3763-88.
7. DeMuth JS. Patient teaching in the ambulatory care setting. *Nursing Clinics of North America.* 1989; 24:645-654.
8. Davidson JK, Delcher HK, Englund A. Spinoff cost/benefits of expanded nutritional care. *J Am Diet Assoc.* 1979; 75:250-257.
9. Sandall MJ, Massey LK. The impact of diagnosis related groups/prospective payment system on nutritional needs in home health and extended care facilities. *J Am Diet Assoc.* 1989; 89:1441-1447.
10. Posner BM, Krachenfels MM. Nutrition services in the continuum of healthcare. *Clinics in Geriatric Medicine.* 1987; 3:261-274.
11. Jessup K. Finding new partners under healthcare reform: home healthcare agencies. *TDA Today.* 1994; 62:1,6-7.
12. Nuhlicek DR, Braun J. eds . *Nutrition services: health effective, cost effective evidence from Wisconsin.* 1994; Madison: Wisconsin Dietetic Association.
13. Folkman JW, Johnson EQ, Lynch M, Rowan ML, Tiller S, eds. *Nutrition services improve health and save money: evidence from Massachusetts.* 1993; Newton: Massachusetts Dietetic Association.
14. Road RS, Griffith M. The Ohio NSPS statewide survey on third party reimbursement policies for nutrition services. *J Am Diet Assoc.* 1993;93:181-182.
15. Wearing J. The new emphasis on homecare. *The Canadian Nurse.* 1994; 22-26.

HERMAN

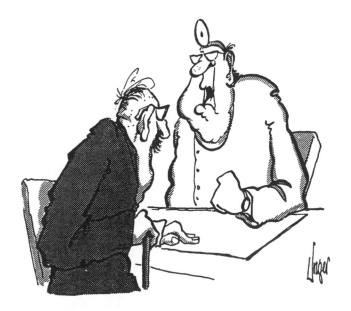

"I'm well aware you're only 28 years old. That's why I'm telling you to take better care of yourself."

Appendix 15-A

Nutrition Counseling for the Lactating Woman

Miriam Erick, MSRD, CDE, Senior Dietitian/Manager (Obstetrics). Brigham and Women's Hospital. Department of Nutrition Services. Boston, MA

One goal of the Surgeon General of the United States in the Healthy People Report for the year 2000 is to increase the number of women who choose to breastfeed their infants. There is ample evidence of the immunological qualities ascribed to lactation, some financial savings and certainly a benefit to the ecosystem as the amount of waste packaging is reduced. One secondary benefit conferred to lactation is maternal weight loss. (1) However, there appears to be some controversy in the professional literature, as to whether women lose weight during lactation or not. (2) As dietitians we should be concerned about the quality of nutrition provided throughout the life-cycle, we can facilitate this occurring by supporting women better who want to breastfeed their infants.

When counseling overweight women, they will often point to their pregnancies as the start of their weight problems stemming from an inability to return to their prenatal weight. This may be caused by tiredness from lack of sleep and too many demands, disruption of personal routines leading to lack of regular exercise, or changes in their eating habits brought on by erratic eating or overeating during their pregnancy and when breastfeeding.

Calories Used For Lactation

The standard recommendation for energy prescription for lactation is established by the Recommended Dietary Allowances at 500 kcals/day (1), which is predicated on an average milk output of 750 ml/day for the first six months and 600 ml/day for the second six months. The RDA (1) acknowledges that "fat stores accumulated in pregnancy can theoretically provide about 100-150 kcals/day during the first six month period." Some studies, however, do not support the hypothesis that fat deposited during pregnancy is necessarily mobilized later during lactation. (3) The energy utilization of producing one cc.(ml) of breast milk is about .8 calories (1); so that producing 100 cc of breast milk requires approximately 80 calories. In the first week or two of lactation, the usual breast milk output of a neophyte lactating woman, is generally less than 750 cc's; hence real need may not parallel recommendation. It is easy for a lactating mother to overconsume calories. However to evaluate the appropriateness of the current allowance for an individual, one needs to start with a prepregnancy weight assessment and track pregnancy weight gain. (2,4)

The National Academy of Sciences (1) suggests that the underweight woman (85% IBW) gain 35 pounds, the reference woman gain 28-35 pounds while the overweight woman (125% IBW) should aim for 15 to 20 pounds. In actual fact, there are many deviations from these recommendations in clinical practice due to: severe nausea and vomiting of pregnancy, subacute nausea which is abated slightly by constant eating, cravings that are difficult to control, smell aversions can reduce appetite, and deliberate attempts to control changing body size and image. Each of these clinical realities may be undetermined and uncalculated if dietary counseling has not been part of prenatal care.

Fluid Weight Gain

Eventually the "big day" arrives, the day of delivery! Unless the woman is in a special birthing unit or has requested differently, protocols in most major hospitals suggest that intravenous (IV) fluid be started on the laboring woman. Intravenous fluids replete expected fluid losses through perspiration, increased breathing and blood loss. An IV also provides a readily available access to administer anesthetic agents in case of an emergency.

On postpartum units, dietitians may counsel a new mother who has done her math-weight homework and expects to see a substantial weight loss. The mother undoubtedly knows her total weight gain in pregnancy and has subtracted the birth weight of her child. Armed with this information, she expects to get on the postpartum scale and see a weight loss if she's gained the recommended 28-35 pounds. Depending upon how long she has been on IV, she may face an enormous (and depressing) surprise. She even may find herself weighing more than before delivery due to administration and retention of IV fluids. Although this weight gain is temporary, it is often misinterpreted.

Nursing women have frequently been told to drink plenty of fluids and not to lose weight too quickly or it might have an adverse impact on breastfeeding the infant. The first few days there is a "postpartum" diuresis as the extra intrapartum fluid weight is shed. New mothers understandably want to do "the right thing" and may react by eating more food and higher calorie fluids than they actually need in order to maintain their weight.

The reality of weight loss from fluid is often confused with the party line of "don't lose more than 1/2 pound a week while you are breastfeeding." Because the amount of breast milk is not seen nor easily accounted for unless the mother uses a breast pump, a woman has very little idea of how much breast milk is being produced.

Education Tool

To illustrate breast milk output to the new mother collect four 10-ounce paper cups, marking a line at the eight ounce point on three of them and a point half way up on the fourth cup. The total amount shown on the four cups is approximately 750 ml, or the amount of breast milk upon which the 500 calories per day allowance for breastfeeding was established. This amount of output assumes that the other calories comes from adipose stores, and hence the lactating mother loses weight.

The new mother needs to be aware that if her calorie intake equals her breast milk output, no real weight loss will ensue, however the postpartum diuresis may create the illusion that milk output is significant as there is a negative or downward trend on the scale. Once the diuresis is over, the true picture appears.

Postpartum Counseling

The nutrition therapist who engages in consultation with the postpartum client needs to be able to assess prepregnancy weight, weight gain or lack thereof in pregnancy, number of births, previous lactation experience (successes and failures), and create calorie guidelines on a case by case basis, *which may differ from the standing recommendations*.

At this point, women may have difficulty finding time to seek a daytime appointment with a dietitian as issues of child care, fatigue, return to work, and the juggling act of a new combined role of mother/provider surface. New frustrations and loss of control over one's own schedule may result in a slow and chronic state of overeating or oversnacking. Women often report voracious appetites while lactating which is difficult to curb. The constant presence of food in the home, which is vastly different from the lack of visible food during the day in most work environments and an ever-present reminder to "eat because of the baby" threatens any control they may try to establish.

Because few clinical dietitians are available for in-depth individual nutrition assessment on maternity units in many hospitals, printed generic information often given to lactating women reiterates the "500 calories extra per day"; for a single birth. Books written by dietitians acknowledge that recommendations for lactation calories may be excessive (6) or an increased weight loss in the first few weeks postpartum are due to a high fluid gain, but mothers seldom hear these message. (3,7)

Group Classes

Getting the postpartum woman into weekly weight classes has been attempted (8) with some success, but drop-out rates can be considerable. Clifford-Murphy, RD gives these statistics about her series of classes: 10 women will call for information, five women will register, three women will show up and be very loyal to the group. (9) This particular program is a flexible series of five meetings, which meets in the evenings at a time convenient to the attendees. The series has been tried two different ways: over five consecutive weeks and five times over the course of three months. She found that once a woman enrolls, weight control is a serious matter to her, especially after the second and third child. Behavior modification within the new role of mother is a focus for many, as well as changing their beliefs about how much to eat. Another variation is to have one or two on-site group meetings and build in three or four once a week phone check-ups where the client reviews her food intake with the dietitian and reports her lactation progress.

Summary

With an annual birth rate of approximately 3.5 million babies there is a tremendous need for pre- and postpartum nutrition counseling. We must actively market our services before a disappointed new mother either quits breastfeeding or fails to lose weight and starts the never-ending cycle of dieting and regaining weight. (To become a Certified Lactation Consultant read the following appendix.)

REFERENCES

1. Food and Nutrition Board. Recommended Dietary Allowances. 10th edition. National Academy of Sciences. Washington, D.C. 1989.
2. Worthington-Roberts B, Williams SR. *Nutrition in Pregnancy and Lactation.* (5th ed.). St. Louis, MO: Times-Mirror, Mosby; 1993.
3. Institute of Medicine. *Nutrition During Pregnancy: Weight Gain. Nutrient Supplementation.* Food and Nutrition Board, National Academy of Sciences. Washington, D.C. 1990.
4. Erick M. Nutritional Management of Gestational Diabetes. In: *Dietitians in General Clinical Practice Newsletter.* Vol. IX, No. 2: 35, 1991.
5. Bullard AM. Personal Communication. November 1994.
6. Sweeney, B. *Eating Expectantly.* Colorado Springs, CO: Fall River Press; 1993.
7. Somer, E. *Nutrition for Women: the complete guide.* New York: Henry Holt and Co; 1993.
8. Department of Media Relations. *Losing baby fat.* BWH Magazine. Brigham and Women's Hospital, Summer 1994.
9. Clifford-Murphy J. Personal Communication. November 1994 .

SUGGESTED READING/ VIEWING

Video: Erick, M., Weiss, E. *Morning Sickness: All Day and All Night*. Woburn, MA: LemonAid Films, Inc; 1994.

Erick, M. Hyperolfaction as a Factor in Hyperemesis Gravidarum: Considerations for Nutritional Management. Perspectives in Applied Nutrition. Vol. 2: 2: 39. Oct/Dec. 1994.

Erick, M. *No More Morning Sickness: a survival guide for pregnant women*. New York: Plume/Penguin; 1993.

Appendix 15-B

How to Become a Certified Lactation Consultant

Robin Blocker, MA, RD, IBCLC

Dietitians should consider becoming a certified lactation consultant if you are currently involved in, or are interested in, lactation counseling. Through the process of studying for certification, you will concentrate on the entire subject of lactation including anatomy, physiology, and the vast number of circumstances that complicate breastfeeding success. Many well-paying jobs are available in public health and health education for Certified Lactation Consultants.

Certification validates special knowledge and skills. The International Board of Lactation Consultant Examiners, Inc. (IBLCE) administers the certification exam and will send you a brochure containing detailed information on how to apply. A fee is required to take the exam. All Registered Dietitians with experience counseling breastfeeding mothers can qualify to take the exam, which consists of two components, a didactic section (of about 150 multiple choice questions) and a clinical component with 35-50 multiple choice questions on clinical problem identification photographs. In order to pass the test, it helps to have experience working with many different breastfeeding problems.

Once the exam is passed, the lactation consultant is certified for five years and must maintain certification through continuing education. At the end of five years, there are two options: submit 75 Continuing Education Recognition Points (CERPS), or successfully complete the IBLCE certification exam. The person must retake of the exam at least once every ten years to maintain certification status. The IBLCE will provide a list of suggested resources to read to stay current or to study for the exam. Many certified lactation consultants become members of International Lactation Consultant Association (ILCA) and receive the Journal of Human Lactation (a quarterly publication).

New mothers who want to breastfeed their children are anxious for information. With the growing body of research in breastfeeding and its known benefits for health of the infant, this area of practice will continue to be a growing career option.

Write to:
The International Board of
Lactation Consultant Examiners
P.O. Box 2348
Falls Church, VA. 22042

REFERENCE
The International Board of Lactation Consultant Examiners. Falls Church, VA: IBLCE; 1994. (brochure)

Appendix 15-C

Dietitian as Team Leader In Caring For a Child With a Feeding Disability

Harriet H. Cloud, MS, RD

Increasing numbers of children are referred to dietitians for feeding disabilities. Often the child may be classified as "failure to thrive" (FTT), which is a syndrome of growth failure due to inadequate intake, retention or utilization of nutrients to allow normal growth for age. (1) Feeding disabilities often result in FTT or growth failure. Traditionally the causes have been classified as organic, stemming from a medical condition, or nonorganic implying a social, emotional or behavioral factor.(2) In actuality, the cause of FTT or growth failure may include a combination of organic or nonorganic factors.(3)

Identification of the cause of the feeding disability is essential when counseling the child's family in a counselling mode. It requires careful assessment of the clinical history of the child and is best served when that assessment is provided in a team setting.(4) The team often includes an occupational therapist, physical therapist, social worker, nurse, psychologist and dietitian/nutritionist. Team makeup can vary and also may include a speech therapist, special educator, dentist and physician. Understanding the role or contribution of each discipline is important for good team interaction. Training in working with children and adults with developmental disabilities and interdisciplinary teams may be required for dietitians wishing to provide counseling and nutrition intervention. Training programs exist in University Affiliated Programs in almost every state.

Following is an overview of the principles involved in caring for a child in this setting.

ASSESSMENT

The team assessment should include a review of medical records, socioeconomic status, nutrition assessment to determine height, weight, head circumference, fat fold measures, usual food intake, an oral motor assessment, positioning, and developmental evaluation. Watching the child eat or be fed by a parent or caregiver is necessary for adequate determination of any problems that exist.(4)

INTERVENTION

Once a list of problems and family strengths is generated, the team in concen with the parent, will prioritize the various problems to solve. Including the parent in problem selection and intervention also reflects the legislative language for children with disabilities which recommends that "all services be comprehensive, family centered, culturally appropriate and community based." (5)

If the child is enrolled in a state funded "early intervention" or school program, the strategies selected for intervention should be included in the child's Individualized Education Program (IEP).This increases the possibility of intervention occurring both in the home and in the school. The following case study is an example of the principles just outlined.

Case Study

Sarah is a two-year-old girl with a diagnosis of spastic quadriplegia (Cerebral Palsy), hydrocephalus and esotropia (eyes don't focus). She receives ongoing health care from the Children's Rehabilitation Service. Her problems include developmental delays, inability to walk, shunting for hydrocephalus secondary to intraventricular hemorrhage, visual problems for which glasses were prescribed, and since birth inadequate nutritional intake leading to growth failure.

History

Sarah had a birthweight of four pounds and a gestational age of 30 weeks. As an infant feeding was difficult due to her weak suck, and poor tolerance of milk-based formula. The mother is a single parent with three other children. Sarah is receiving S.S.I. benefits, and the mother receives Aid to Dependent Children and Food Stamps, but Sarah was not on the WIC program.

Nutrition Information

On Sarah's first visit to the nutritionist, anthropometric measurements were taken: length was 29 1/8", weight 14 1/2 lbs, both below the 5%tile. Her mother reported an intake of 12 small jars of baby food mixed with six ounces of infant formula, given in a 24-hour period (mostly at night from the "infa-feeder," which totalled approximately 540 calories/day). Vomiting was reported if milk was given in a cup or bottle. She never slept through the night, but took naps throughout the day. Following her first visit, the dietitian referred Sarah to the feeding clinic where occupational and physical therapy, and social work services were provided through Children's Rehabilitation Services, a state agency. The dietitian served as the team coordinator for Sarah's care.

Feeding Evaluations

During these evaluations it was determined that Sarah was attending a program for children with disabilities, but no feeding intervention had occurred since birth. Positioning while feeding was identified as a problem since she was held in her mother's lap for feeding or was fed lying down in bed. At school Sarah was fed sitting in a wheel chair. Her oral motor problems were multiple: immature sucking from the "infa-feeder", difficulty swallowing liquids, and resistance in the form of crying when a therapist tried to evaluate her oral-motor skills. She appeared to have resistance to tactile stimulation inside her mouth, but less resistance around her mouth. Although she could move her tongue laterally, spoon feeding caused her great distress. All of this resulted in inadequate energy, nutrient and fluid intake. Sarah was video taped while she ate in order to be evaluated at a parent/ team meeting which would enable collaboration in problem identification and selection.

Recommendations

1. Gradually discontinue the use of the infa-feeder.
2. Feed in her wheel chair at all feeding times.
3. Thicken fruit juice and lactose-free milk to increase calories and enhance swallowing.
4. Feed blended table foods, gradually added to baby foods.
5. Introduce a high calorie, lactose-free commercial beverage to replace the food given in the infa-feeder as the transition to spoon feeding is made.
6. Regular follow-up visits through school, Children's Rehabilitation Services, and the feeding clinic.

Follow-up

All of the recommendations were acceptable to the mother; however she elected starting with feeding in the wheel chair as her first priority. She was willing to thicken beverages and utilize the high calorie, lactose-free beverage. The Department of Human Resources provided a homemaker to give support in the home and the school reinforced all of the feeding recommendations. The nutritionist also accessed WIC to cover the cost of the supplemental beverage. The health department monitored Sarah's growth and she returned for feeding clinic evaluations every 4-6 weeks. At the end of a year, her weight gain had improved, she was fed in her wheel chair, and she was eating by spoon.

For this example of nutrition therapy, the nutritionist/dietitian was the coordinator of the team assessment and follow-up. The multifactoral nature of Sarah's problems made the need for a team approach imperative. This represents the type of counseling and intervention frequently required for successful management of children with feeding disabilities.

REFERENCES

1. Ramsay M, Gisel EG, Boultry M. Nonorganic failure to thrive,; growth failure secondary to feeding skills disorder. *Develop Med & Child Neurol.* 1993; 35:285-297.
2. Bithoney WG, Dubowitz H, Egan H. Failure to thrive/Growth deficiency. *Pediatr in Rev.* 1992; 13:453-459.
3. Bithoney WG, Dubowitz H. Organic concomitants of nonorganic failure to thrive: Implications for research. In: Drotar D, ed. *New Directions in Failure to Thrive.* New York, NY: Plenum Press; 1985: 47-68.
4. Lane SJ, Cloud HH. Feeding problems and intervention: an interdisciplinary approach. *Topics Cl Nutr.* 1988; 3:23-32.
5. Lichtnwalter l,Freeman R, Lee M, Cialone J. Providing nutrition services to children with special needs in a community setting. *Top Clin Nutr.* 1993; 4:75-78.

INDEX